CANCER ETIOLOGY, DIAGNOSIS AND TREATMENTS

# LIVER CANCER: CAUSES, DIAGNOSIS AND TREATMENT

# CANCER ETIOLOGY, DIAGNOSIS AND TREATMENTS

Additional books in this series can be found on Nova's website under the Series tab.

Additional E-books in this series can be found on Nova's website under the E-books tab.

# HEPATOLOGY RESEARCH AND CLINICAL DEVELOPMENTS

Additional books in this series can be found on Nova's website under the Series tab.

Additional E-books in this series can be found on Nova's website under the E-books tab.

CANCER ETIOLOGY, DIAGNOSIS AND TREATMENTS

# LIVER CANCER: CAUSES, DIAGNOSIS AND TREATMENT

## BENJAMIN J. VALVERDE
### EDITOR

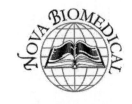

Nova Science Publishers, Inc.
*New York*

Copyright © 2011 by Nova Science Publishers, Inc.

**All rights reserved.** No part of this book may be reproduced, stored in a retrieval system or transmitted in any form or by any means: electronic, electrostatic, magnetic, tape, mechanical photocopying, recording or otherwise without the written permission of the Publisher.

For permission to use material from this book please contact us:
Telephone 631-231-7269; Fax 631-231-8175
Web Site: http://www.novapublishers.com

## NOTICE TO THE READER

The Publisher has taken reasonable care in the preparation of this book, but makes no expressed or implied warranty of any kind and assumes no responsibility for any errors or omissions. No liability is assumed for incidental or consequential damages in connection with or arising out of information contained in this book. The Publisher shall not be liable for any special, consequential, or exemplary damages resulting, in whole or in part, from the readers' use of, or reliance upon, this material. Any parts of this book based on government reports are so indicated and copyright is claimed for those parts to the extent applicable to compilations of such works.

Independent verification should be sought for any data, advice or recommendations contained in this book. In addition, no responsibility is assumed by the publisher for any injury and/or damage to persons or property arising from any methods, products, instructions, ideas or otherwise contained in this publication.

This publication is designed to provide accurate and authoritative information with regard to the subject matter covered herein. It is sold with the clear understanding that the Publisher is not engaged in rendering legal or any other professional services. If legal or any other expert assistance is required, the services of a competent person should be sought. FROM A DECLARATION OF PARTICIPANTS JOINTLY ADOPTED BY A COMMITTEE OF THE AMERICAN BAR ASSOCIATION AND A COMMITTEE OF PUBLISHERS.

Additional color graphics may be available in the e-book version of this book.

**Library of Congress Cataloging-in-Publication Data**

Liver cancer : causes, diagnosis, and treatment / editor, Benjamin J.
Valverde.
    p. ; cm. -- (Cancer etiology, diagnosis, and treatments)
  Includes bibliographical references and index.
  ISBN 978-1-61209-115-0 (hardcover : alk. paper)
  1. Liver--Cancer. I. Valverde, Benjamin J. II. Series: Cancer etiology,
diagnosis, and treatments.
  [DNLM: 1.  Liver Neoplasms--diagnosis. 2.  Liver Neoplasms--etiology. 3.
Liver Neoplasms--therapy.  WI 735]
  RC280.L5L5763 2011
  616.99'436--dc22
                                    2010047017
  ISBN 978-1-61209-115-0

*Published by Nova Science Publishers, Inc.* † *New York*

# Contents

| | | |
|---|---|---|
| **Preface** | | **vii** |
| **Chapter I** | Plant Polyphenols for Prevention and Therapy of Liver Cancer<br>*Brahma N. Singh, Braj R. Singh, Shi W. Jiang,*<br>*and Harikesh B. Singh* | **1** |
| **Chapter II** | Mechanisms of Hepatocarcinogenesis: A Dialogue<br>Between Exogenous Factors and the Endogenous Response<br>*Jordan C. Woodrick and Rabindra Roy* | **53** |
| **Chapter III** | Liver Cancer Prevention and Treatment with Resveratrol<br>*Anupam Bishayee* | **103** |
| **Chapter IV** | Signaling Pathways in Hepatocellular Carcinoma<br>*Edith Y. T. Tse and Judy W. P. Yam* | **137** |
| **Chapter V** | Health-related Quality of Life in Patients with Liver Cancer<br>*Sheng-Yu Fan* | **161** |
| **Chapter VI** | Diagnosing Liver Cancer: A Multi-Modal Approach<br>*Marco L. H. Gruwel, Eilean McKenzie-Matwiy and Erika Lattová* | **173** |
| **Chapter VII** | Cost Effectiveness Analysis of Liver Transplantation<br>*Haruhisa Fukuda and Hirohisa Imai* | **195** |
| **Chapter VIII** | Imaging Hepatocellular Carcinoma Using Positron Emission<br>Tomography<br>*Zhenghong Lee, Nicolas Salem, Yu Kuang, Haibin Tian and Pablo*<br>*Ros* | **223** |
| **Index** | | **239** |

# Preface

Primary liver cancer, mainly hepatocellular carcinoma (HCC), is the third leading cause of cancer-related deaths worldwide. The incidence is increasing worldwide and the overall survival of patients with HCC is grim because most patients are diagnosed late, when curative treatment is not possible. This book presents topical research in the study of liver cancer, including plant polyphenols for the prevention of HCC and therapy of liver cancer; cytotoxic effects of reservatrol against liver cancer; the molecular mechanisms of HCC and the identification of prognostic markers and health-related quality of life for patients with liver cancer.

Chapter I – Primary liver cancer, mainly hepatocellular carcinoma (HCC), is the third leading cause of cancer-related deaths worldwide. The incidence of HCC is increasing worldwide; the overall survival of patients with HCC is grim because most patients are diagnosed late, when curative treatment is not possible and is the direct cause of about 1 million deaths annually. Chronic infection with hepatitis B viruses, toxic industrial chemicals, food additives (N-nitrosodiethylamine; NDEA), fungal toxins (aflatoxins), air, water pollutants and chronic heavy alcohol use leading to cirrhosis of the liver remain the most important causes. The great challenge in cancer prevention and control is how to manage those who have already been exposed to carcinogens, such as individuals who are HBsAg carriers and have long-term aflatoxin and NDEA exposure. The development of tumor markers that can detect HCC at even earlier stages is essential. In recent years, clinically useful tumor markers for HCC diagnosis have included $\alpha$-fetoprotein (AFP), a fucosylated variant of the AFP glycoprotein which has a high affinity to the sugar chain of lens culinaris (AFPL3), des-$\gamma$-carboxy prothrombin (DCP), carcinoembryonic antigen (CEA) glypican-3 (GPC3) golgi protein 73 (GP73), growth factors or cytokines, insulin-like growth factor (IGF), interleukin (IL)-6 and IL-10, $\gamma$-glutamyl transferase (GGT) and $\alpha$-L -fucosidase (AFU) etc. Chemoprevention has been proposed as the good tool to target these high-risk populations. Among various identified chemopreventive agents, plant polyphenols have been shown to be safe and high effective in inhibition of carcinogen-induced mutagenesis and tumorigenesis in bioassays and animal models for different target organ sites. The compounds derived from the plants are of considerable interest among oncologists. Many plant-derived, plant polyphenols have been studied for their chemopreventive and chemotherapeutic properties against human HCC, including green tea polyphenols, genistein (found in soy), apigenin (celery, parsley), luteolin (broccoli), quercetin (onions), kaempferol (broccoli, grapefruits), curcumin (turmeric), etc. The more authors will discuss their involved molecular mechanisms and cellular targets, the better they could utilize these "natural gifts" for the prevention and treatment of HCC. Furthermore, better understanding of their structure-activity relationships will guide synthesis of analog compounds with improved bio-availability, stability, potency and specificity. In this article, for the sake of better understanding, the effective plant polyphenols against HCC will also be discussed, with more emphases on the basic conceptions of phenolics with strong antioxidant activity.

Chapter II - The World Health Organization (WHO) estimated in 2004 that primary liver cancer, claiming the lives of 610,000 people worldwide, is one of the top five cancers that contribute to the 7.4 million deaths due to cancer globally each year. In the United States, primary liver and bile duct cancers are the 6th and 9th leading causes of cancer death in men and women, respectively. In 2009 there were 22,620 newly diagnosed cases and 18,160 deaths of primary liver cancer, and the Surveillance, Epidemiology, and End Results (SEER) Program reported a dismal overall 5-year survival rate of primary liver cancers at 13.8% between 1999 and 2006. As is the case with many other diseases, understanding the underlying causes of liver cancers provides potentially useful information regarding prevention as well as diagnosis and treatment. This chapter will elucidate what is currently known concerning the causes of various types of hepatic malignancies. The major etiologic agents discussed here include infectious agents, such as hepatitis B and C viruses, Helicobacter, and liver flukes, as well as toxic agents, such as alcohol, metal accumulation, and Aflatoxin B. This chapter will also explore the role and known molecular mechanisms of inflammation in primary liver cancers, as it is one of the most influential risk factors for these diseases and plays a role in the carcinogenic effects of many of the etiologic agents. Liver cancers are heterogeneous in nature, so the multifactorial genetic and epigenetic alterations that drive hepatocarcinogenesis will be discussed. Finally, this chapter will also review current knowledge on the potential role of hepatic stem cells in the development of liver cancer.

Chapter III- Primary liver cancer, the majority of which represents hepatocellular carcinoma (HCC), is one of the most lethal cancers in the world with an annual incidence of over 700,000 cases. HCC most commonly develops in patients with chronic liver disease, the etiology of which includes viral infections (hepatitis B and C), alcoholic liver damage and ingestion of dietary carcinogens, such as aflatoxins and nitrosamines. Although, surgical resection and liver transplantation are currently available treatment options, only 10% of HCC patients qualify for these modalities. In view of the limited therapeutic alternatives and poor prognosis of liver cancer, chemoprevention and novel therapeutic approaches could be extremely valuable in lowering the present prevalence of the disease. Oxidative stress and inflammation are intimately connected to each other in the multistage hepatocarcinogenesis and these have been proposed as potential targets for the prevention and therapy of inflammation-associated HCC. A variety of bioactive food components, obtained from various fruits, vegetables, nuts and spices, have been shown to modify molecular targets involved with oxidative stress and chronic inflammation with resultant attenuation of carcinogenesis. Resveratrol, a naturally occurring antioxidant and antiinflammatory agent found in grapes and red wine, has emerged as a promising molecule that inhibits carcinogenesis with a pleiotropic mode of action. Although anticancer activities of resveratrol have been studied extensively in various cancer models, the preventive and therapeutic potential of resveratrol in liver cancer is only beginning to be unraveled. This chapter reviews the current cutting-edge discoveries on the potent cytotoxic effects of resveratrol against various liver cancer cells *in vitro* as well as the chemopreventive and therapeutic potential of this dietary agent *in vivo*. Available toxicity and pharmacokinetic data are also presented for clinical relevance. The current limitations, potential challenges, innovative approaches as well as the future directions of resveratrol research to explore its full potential in the prevention and therapy of liver cancer are also critically examined.

Chapter IV - Hepatocellular carcinoma (HCC) is a prevalent malignancy worldwide. It is often diagnosed at the advanced stage and the overall prognosis is unsatisfactory due to high rates of postoperative recurrence and metastasis. High incidence and severe casualty have led to the attention of the public health problem caused by HCC. HCC is developed from a multistep process which emerged through chronic hepatitis/cirrhosis and dysplastic nodules from normal liver. The genomic alterations and dysregulations of multiple intracellular signaling pathways reveal the heterogeneity and complexity of HCC. Profound evidence has demonstrated that cross-talks between different signaling pathways have made the pathogenesis of HCC even more intriguing. In this review, the authors provide a comprehensive overview on the salient signaling pathways in HCC, including growth factors regulated pathways and Rho-ROCK signaling cascad, zero in on the molecules along these pathways which are the key players in the initiation and progression of HCC. A better understanding of the molecular mechanisms of HCC would facilitate and advance the identification of prognostic markers, the improvement of therapeutic management and the development of novel therapies.

Chapter V - Liver cancer is one of most common cancers in the world and is associated with considerable impact on not only physical but also psychosocial functioning. Health-related quality of life (HRQOL) is increasingly seen to be an important endpoint in health care. The aims of this chapter are to consider issues in the definition and measurement of HRQOL, as applied specifically to patients with liver cancer. HRQOL in patients with liver cancer can be considered both from a generic viewpoint in comparison with the general population, and in terms of disease-specific issues. In this regard, pain, fatigue, nausea, jaundice, weight loss, and body image need to be considered. Current research suggests that patients with liver cancer have substantially compromised HRQOL compared with the healthy population, both in physical and psychological dimensions. Suggestions are made for improving assessment of HRQOL in this population, and the timing and evaluation of programs to improve HRQOL over the course of treatment.

Chapter VI - Liver cancer is the $3^{rd}$. leading cause of death world wide for which the WHO estimates at least 550,000 fatalities per year. In many cases chronic Hepatitis B infection results in the development of hepatocellular carcinoma. As Hepatitis B infection is endemic in China and other parts of Asia, a large part of the world population has the potential to develop liver cancer. The high morbidity rate of liver cancer is related to the late diagnosis when treatment is no longer effective. Diagnosis is usually performed using standard imaging modalities including ultrasonography (US), magnetic resonance imaging (MRI), computed tomography (CT) and positron emission tomography (PET), used for the detection of focal liver lesions. Diagnosis by imaging is usually limited by the skill of the operator (US), the detection limit of the lesion size (MRI, CT) or the cost factor (PET). People at risk, those chronically infected with Hepatitis B (and C), are often screened for liver cancer using the serum $\alpha$-1 fetoprotein level as a liver cancer biomarker. Unfortunately, the current diagnostic use of the alpha-fetoprotein serum level is limited due to numerous complications. Liver cancer patients, or patients at risk, will thus benefit from a better, accurate diagnosis which allows for effective, timely treatment and provides a higher survival rate. Mass spectrometry (MS) has the potential to become a major clinical test for liver cancer biomarkers providing a rapid, accurate and the most sensitive screening procedure. When increases in biomarkers occur,MR imaging and spectroscopy can be used to screen the liver of patients for lesions to localize the tumor and initiate treatment planning. Post-translational modifications in proteins have been shown to associate with cancer diseases and MS analysis of human and animal sera revealed alterations in N-glycans between healthy individuals and those with hepatocellular carcinoma. MALDI-MS, in combination with MS/MS, helped to identify N-glycan structures in a woodchuck model of hepatocellular carcinoma of which some showed elevated levelsin animals with liver cancer. $^{31}$P MR spectroscopy showed elevated levels of phosphomonoesters, particularly phosphocholine, in selectively imaged voxels within the tumor.

Chapter VII - For patients with end-stage liver disease (ESLD), liver transplantation is an established therapy. The efficacy of deceased donor liver transplantation (DDLT) has been verified in various studies, and the procedure is a socially acceptable medical technique. On the other hand, one current challenge is the increase in the number of DDLT cases, causing longer waiting periods for available organs, a situation that has been recognized as a social issue. Living donor liver transplantation (LDLT) is performed as an alternative.

Chapter VIII - Hepatocellular carcinoma (HCC) is the fifth most common tumor and the third most common cause of cancer death worldwide with a dismal survival rate < 3 month. Positron emission tomography (PET) played a minor role in HCC imaging so far largely due to the fact that the commonly used radiotracer, 2-$[^{18}$F]-2-deoxy-D-glucose (FDG) has little uptake in a number of HCC cases leading to a high false positive rate. In addition, the cost associated with a PET scan prevented it from becoming surveillance or screening tool. Several existing small molecule PET tracers, which were initially developed for other studies, have shown uptake in HCC. These include $[^{11}$C]-acetate, $[^{11}$C]-methionine, $[^{11}$C]-choline as well as $[^{18}$F]-labeled fluorinated choline analogs. For each of these tracers, the uptake mechanisms were studied extensively with an animal model of hepatitis viral infection induced HCC for correlation with preliminary clinical PET scans of HCC using the same tracer if performed. However, the full clinical utility of each tracer needs to be further investigated through patient studies to determine if any of them is useful for early detection, staging, and/or treatment evaluation. The promising PET tracers such as 3'-deoxy-3'-fluorothymidine (FLT) or 2'-$[^{18}$F]fluoro-5-methyl-1-β-D-arabinofuranosyluracil (FMAU), both thymidine analogs designed for imaging tumor proliferation, may not be suitable for imaging HCC due to their degradation in the liver. Currently, an imaging biomarker for tumor proliferation in HCC is actively sought after. The combined PET/CT scanner offers advantage than the stand-alone PET by providing anatomical reference for localizing tumor uptake as well as CT-based attenuation correction for PET tracer uptake quantification.

In: Liver Cancer: Causes, Diagnosis and Treatment
Editor: Benjamin J. Valverde

ISBN: 978-1-61209-115-0
© 2011 Nova Science Publishers, Inc.

*Chapter I*

# Plant Polyphenols for Prevention and Therapy of Liver Cancer

*Brahma N. Singh,[1] Braj R. Singh,[2] Shi W. Jiang,[3] and Harikesh B. Singh[1\*]*

[1]Department of Mycology and Plant Pathology, Institute of Agricultural Sciences, Banaras Hindu University, Varanasi, Uttar Pradesh, India
[2]DNA Research Chair, College of Science, King Saud University, Riyadh, Saudi Arabia
[3]Department of Biomedical Science, Mercer University School of Medicine at Savannah, Savannah, Georgia, USA

## Abstract

Primary liver cancer, mainly hepatocellular carcinoma (HCC), is the third leading cause of cancer-related deaths worldwide. The incidence of HCC is increasing worldwide; the overall survival of patients with HCC is grim because most patients are diagnosed late, when curative treatment is not possible and is the direct cause of about 1 million deaths annually. Chronic infection with hepatitis B viruses, toxic industrial chemicals, food additives (N-nitrosodiethylamine; NDEA), fungal toxins (aflatoxins), air, water pollutants and chronic heavy alcohol use leading to cirrhosis of the liver remain the most important causes. The great challenge in cancer prevention and control is how to manage those who have already been exposed to carcinogens, such as individuals who are HBsAg carriers and have long-term aflatoxin and NDEA exposure. The development of tumor markers that can detect HCC at even earlier stages is essential. In recent years, clinically useful tumor markers for HCC diagnosis have included $\alpha$-fetoprotein (AFP), a fucosylated variant of the AFP glycoprotein which has a high affinity to the sugar chain of lens culinaris (AFPL3), des- $\gamma$-carboxy prothrombin (DCP), carcinoembryonic antigen (CEA) glypican-3 (GPC3) golgi protein 73 (GP73), growth factors or cytokines, insulin-like growth factor (IGF), interleukin (IL)-6 and IL-10, $\gamma$-glutamyl transferase (GGT) and $\alpha$-L -fucosidase (AFU) etc. Chemoprevention has been proposed as the good tool to

---

\* Corresponding author:* hbs1@rediffmail.com.

target these high-risk populations. Among various identified chemopreventive agents, plant polyphenols have been shown to be safe and high effective in inhibition of carcinogen-induced mutagenesis and tumorigenesis in bioassays and animal models for different target organ sites. The compounds derived from the plants are of considerable interest among oncologists. Many plant-derived, plant polyphenols have been studied for their chemopreventive and chemotherapeutic properties against human HCC, including green tea polyphenols, genistein (found in soy), apigenin (celery, parsley), luteolin (broccoli), quercetin (onions), kaempferol (broccoli, grapefruits), curcumin (turmeric), etc. The more we will discuss their involved molecular mechanisms and cellular targets, the better we could utilize these "natural gifts" for the prevention and treatment of HCC. Furthermore, better understanding of their structure-activity relationships will guide synthesis of analog compounds with improved bio-availability, stability, potency and specificity. In this article, for the sake of better understanding, the effective plant polyphenols against HCC will also be discussed, with more emphases on the basic conceptions of phenolics with strong antioxidant activity.

# 1. Introduction

Primary liver cancer, mainly hepatocellular carcinoma (HCC), remains one of the most common malignancies in the world and the most common in men in many developing countries [1]. HCC is the third leading cause of cancer-related deaths worldwide with poor diagnosis and accounts for approximately 549,000 deaths each year [2]. It is also the first human cancer largely amenable to prevention using hepatitis B virus (HBV) vaccines and screening of blood and blood products for the hepatitis C virus (HCV). It has been estimated that worldwide some 564,000 new cases (398,000 in men and 166,000 in women) occurred in 2000 [3,4]. PLC (primary liver cancer) accounts for 5.6% of all human cancers (7.5% among men and 3.5% among women). In Europe, for the 1985-1989 period and in North America, for 1983-1988, the 5-year relative survival rate (mortality from LC adjusted for mortality from competing causes) was 5% and 6%, respectively. In developing countries LC is inevitably fatal [5]. The geographic areas at highest risk are located in Eastern Asia, Middle Africa and some countries of Western Africa. Low-risk areas include Northern Europe, Australia, New Zealand, and the Caucasian populations in North and Latin America. In high-risk countries, incidence rates are typically 2 to 3-fold higher than those in developed countries. An excess of LC incidence among men compared to women has been well documented (range of the sex ratios in the AAIRs is 1.4 to 3.3). In high risk countries, sex ratios tend to be higher, and the male excess is more pronounced around 40-50 years of age. In populations with low incidence, the highest sex ratios occur later, around 60-70 years of age [6].

Time trends analyses have reported significant increasing rates for the Black, White and Hispanic populations in the US. The interpretation made by the authors suggest that HCV exposure in the relevant generations in the period 1960-70 may explain most of the cases observed [6]. In Japan, increasing LC incidence and mortality trends since the early 1970s have been largely attributed to increasing consumption of alcohol, to massive exposure of the population to HCV through blood transfusion or contaminated needles in vaccination campaigns against tuberculosis after World War II and to illegal intravenous drug abuse. Other registries that have suggested increasing trends in LC incidence among men included

Australia, India, Israel, Canada, Italy, Spain and Finland. Decreasing incidence trends are observed in several registries in Scandinavia, parts of China, and among Japanese populations in the USA [5].

Several chemicals are known to possess chemopreventive properties against a broad spectrum of cancers. Chemoprevention serves as an attractive alternative to control malignancy [7]. Several herbal drugs have been evaluated for their potential as liver protectant against different carcinogens-induced hepatotoxicity [8,9]. Recently, identification of bioactive ingredients from medicinal plants to inhibit tumorigenesis in a variety of animal models of carcinogenesis, involving organ sites, such as the skin, lungs, oral cavity, esophagus, stomach, liver, pancreas, small intestine, colon, and prostate is gaining considerable attention [10]. A number of non-nutrients including polyphenolic compounds have chemopreventive role in cancer through the induction of enzymes affecting carcinogen metabolism and inhibiting various activities of tumor promoters which are involved in the process of carcinogenesis [10,11]. Moreover, numerous medicinal plants and their formulations are also used for liver disorders in ethnomedical practices as well as traditional system of medicine (Ayurveda) in India.

In addition to many essential nutritional components, plants contain phenolic substances, a large and heterogeneous group of biologically active non-nutrients. Flavonoids are divided into many categories, including flavonols, flavones, catechins, proanthocyanidins, anthocyanidins and isoflavonoids. Phenolic acids present in plants are hydroxylated derivatives of benzoic and cinnamic acids [12]. Flavonoids and phenolic acids have many functions in plants. They act as cell wall support materials and as colourful attractants for birds and insects helping seed dispersal and pollination. Phenolic compounds are also important in the defence mechanisms of plants under different environmental stress conditions such as wounding, infection, and excessive light or UV irradiation [13].

The biological potency of secondary plant phenolics was found empirically already by our ancestors; phenolics are not only unsavoury or poisonous, but also of possible pharmacological value [14]. Flavonoids have long been recognised to possess anticancer, anti-inflammatory, antiviral and antiproliferative activities [15]. Flavonoids and phenolic acids also have antioxidative and anticarcinogenic effects. Inverse relationships between the intake of flavonoids (flavonols and flavones) and the risk of liver and stomach cancer have been shown in epidemiological studies [2]. Phenolics and flavonoids normally scavenge the free radicals and play an essential role in prevention and therapy of cancer [10], cardiovascular diseases [16] neurodegenerative diseases and inflammation [17] by inducing antioxidant defense system, drug metabolizing enzymes [9], modulating diverse events in cellular signaling, inhibiting inflammation, hyperplasia, proliferation and oxidative DNA damage [2,18,19,20]. Polyphenolic compounds including quercetin [21,22], protocatechuic acid [23,24], ellagic acid [21], gallic acid [25], and caffeic acid [26] are natural antioxidants, which decrease oxidation of biomolecules essential for life. They are also having anti-carcinogenic and anti-tumorigenic activities against several chemically-induced hepatocarcinogenesis.

Many so-called secondary products can act as potent bio-antimutagens. Anticancer action of polyphenols has been studied, for which many compounds seems to be most responsible [22]. Therefore, there is currently a strong interest in the study of natural compounds with free radical scavenger capacity and their role in human health and nutrition [27]. Dietary polyphenols may contribute to the decrease of cancer disease by reduction of free radical formation as well as oxidative stress in general, by protection of low density lipoprotein (LDL) oxidation and platelet aggregation and by inhibiting synthesis of proinflamatory cytokines [2]. In this article, for the sake of better understanding, the effective plant polyphenols against liver cancer will also be discussed, with more emphases on the basic conceptions of phenolics with strong antioxidant activity.

# 2. Risk Factors of HCC

## 2.1. N-Nitrosodiethylamine

*N*-Nitrosodiethylamine (NDEA) is a potent hepatocarcinogenic dialkylnitrosoamine present in tobacco smoke, water, cheddar cheese, cured and fried meals and in a number of alcoholic beverages [28]. NDEA is known to cause perturbations in the nuclear enzymes involved in DNA repair/replication and producing reproducible HCC after repeated administration in experimental animals [8]. Investigations have provided evidence that NDEA causes a wide range of tumors in all animal species and such compounds are hazardous to human health [29]. The formation of reactive oxygen species (ROS) is apparent during the metabolic biotransformation of NDEA resulting in oxidative stress. Oxidative stress leads to carcinogenesis by several mechanisms including DNA, lipid and protein damage, change in intracellular signaling pathways and even changes in gene expression. Together, these oxidative modifications promote abnormal cell growth and carcinogenesis [30]. DNA damage includes the formation of 8-hydroxydeoxyguanosine (8-OHdG), which is the most studied DNA oxygen adduct implicated in carcinogenesis [31]. Lipid peroxidation (LPO) may result in several sequelae, including structural and functional membrane modifications, protein oxidation and generation of oxidation products such as acrolein, crotonaldehyde, malondialdehyde (MDA) and 4-hydroxy-2-nonenal (HNE), which are considered strong carcinogens [2].

## 2.2. Viral Hepatitis B (HBV) and/or C (HCV)

However, the importance of these different factors varies in different geographic areas. Major factors affecting progression to HCC are older age at infection, older age at diagnosis of cirrhosis, male sex and stage of compensated cirrhosis at presentation [32]. HBV is more predominant in Chinese, Southeast Asian and African patients with HCC, whereas HCV is common in HCC patients in developed countries (Japan, France, Italy and others). The prevalence of hepatitis B surface antigen (HBsAg) and antibody to HCV (anti-HCV) in HCC patients were reported to be 63.2% and 11.2% respectively in China [33] which was similar to that reported in the past. In China, HBV and HCV (mainly HBV) contamination of drinking water (such as microcystin, a promoter of hepatocarcinogenesis) remain as major risk factors of HCC. The 5-year cumulative risk for HCC in patients with cirrhosis is 16% in Europe and the United States and 32% in Japan. Prospective studies showed that there is an additive effect of HCV and HBV infection on HCC development [34,35,36]. Cirrhotic patients infected with HCV type 1b carry a significantly higher risk of developing HCC than patients infected by other HCV types [37]. An association was found between high serum alanine aminotransferase levels and more rapid development and high incidence rate of HCC in patients with HCV-associated cirrhosis [38]. In a transgenic mouse, it was found that the core protein of HCV induces HCC [39]. Additional prognostic factors are HBV coinfection (2-6-fold increased risk) and heavy alcohol intake (2-4- fold increased risk). There is growing evidence that occult HBV coinfection and HIV coinfection as well as liver steatosis may increase the HCC risk. No conclusions can be drawn on the role of HCV genotype in HCC risk.

## 2.3. Aflatoxins

Aflatoxins are a group of approximately 20 related fungal metabolites. The four major aflatoxins are known as $B_1$, $B_2$, $G_1$, and $G_2$. Aflatoxins $B_2$ and $G_2$ are the dihydro-derivatives of the parent compounds $B_1$ and $G_1$ [40]. Aflatoxin $B_1$ (AFB1) is the most potent (in some species) naturally occurring chemical liver carcinogen known. Naturally occurring mixes of aflatoxins have been classified as a Group 1 human carcinogen by the International Agency for Research on Cancer (IARC) and has demonstrated carcinogenicity in many animal species, including some rodents, nonhuman primates, and fish [International Programme on Chemical Safety (IPCS)/WHO 1998)]. Specific P450 enzymes in the liver metabolize aflatoxin into a reactive oxygen species (aflatoxin-8,9-epoxide), which may then bind to proteins and cause acute toxicity (aflatoxicosis) or to DNA to cause lesions that over time increase the risk of HCC [41].

HCC as a result of chronic aflatoxin exposure has been well documented, presenting most often in persons with chronic HBV infection [42]. The risk of liver cancer in individuals exposed to chronic HBV infection and aflatoxin is up to 30 times greater than the risk in individuals exposed to aflatoxin only [41]. These two HCC risk factors—aflatoxin and HBV—are prevalent in poor nations worldwide. Within these nations, there is often a significant urban–rural difference in aflatoxin exposure and HBV prevalence, with both these risk factors typically affecting rural populations more strongly [43].

Aflatoxin also appears to have a synergistic effect on HCV-induced liver cancer [44], although the quantitative relationship is not as well established as that for aflatoxin and HBV in inducing HCC. Other important causative factors in the development of HCC, in addition to HBV or HCV infection and aflatoxin exposure, are the genetic characteristics of the virus, alcohol consumption, and the age and sex of the infected person [45].

## 2.4. Alcohol

The magnitude of risk of HCC in cirrhosis caused by diseases other than viral hepatitis is not known accurately. Most of the studies of the incidence of HCC in alcoholic cirrhosis date from before the identification of HCV. Given that hepatitis C is relatively frequent in alcoholics, the reported incidence rates must be too high for pure alcoholic cirrhosis. Nonetheless, that alcoholic cirrhosis is a risk factor for HCC is clear. Excessive, long-term use of alcohol can cause liver damage caused cirrhosis, a condition marked by scarring of the liver. Several studies have documented that the presence of alcoholic liver disease correlates with the development of HCC [46,47]. In the United States, the approximate hospitalization rate for HCC related to alcoholic cirrhosis is 8 to 9 per 100,000 per year compared with ~7 per 100,000 per year for hepatitis C [48]. This study did not determine the incidence of HCC in alcoholic liver disease, but it confirmed that alcoholic cirrhosis is a significant risk factor for HCC, probably sufficient to warrant screening for HCC.

## 2.5. Others

With the new recognition of steatohepatitis as a cause of cirrhosis has come the suspicion that this too is a risk factor for HCC. No study to date has followed a sufficiently large group of such patients long enough to describe an incidence rate for HCC. In one cohort study of patients with HCC, () diabetes was found in 20% as the only risk factor for HCC. Whether or not these patients were cirrhotic was not noted. Nonalcoholic fatty liver disease (NAFLD) has been described in cohorts of patients with HCC [49]. Because the incidence of HCC in cirrhosis related to NAFLD is unknown, it is not possible to assess whether screening might be effective or cost efficient.

In Japan, alcohol consumption and cigarette smoking were also risk factors of HCC, and synergism between them was observed [50,51]. In Italy, for attributable risk (AR) of HCC, heavy alcohol intake ranked first (45%), HCV second (36%) and HBV third (22%) [52]. The risk of dietary iron overload was 4.1 for HCC in black Africans, which is similar to that of haemochromatosis in Caucasians. A role of family history independent from and interacting with known risk factors for HCC was also reported, the odds ratio was reported to be 2.4 [53].

Patients with genetic hemochromatosis (GH) who have established cirrhosis have an increased risk of HCC [54,55]. The relative risk of HCC is ~20 [56]. The standardized incidence ratio for HCC in cirrhotic GH is 92.9 (95% confidence interval [CI], 25 to 237.9) [54]. Another study suggested that the relative risk of HCC in GH was only 1.1 [55]. Nonetheless, the incidence of HCC in cirrhosis related to GH is probably sufficiently high (~3 to 4%/year) that these patients should be included in screening programs. Whether this will reduce mortality from the disease is not known. The incidence of HCC in primary biliary cirrhosis is about the same as in cirrhosis related to hepatitis C [57]. For cirrhosis related to $\alpha_1$-antitrypsin deficiency [58,59].

# 3. Tumour Markers of HCC

In accordance with the unified medical language system and according to the dictionary of the National Cancer Institute (NCI) a tumor marker is a substance found in the blood, urine, or body tissues that can be elevated in cancer, among other tissue types. There are many different tumor markers, each indicative of a particular disease process, and they are used in oncology to help detect the presence of cancer. An elevated level of a tumor marker can indicate cancer; however, there can also be other causes of the elevation. These markers are commonly used in diagnosis, staging and prognosis of cancer, and can be useful to localise the tumour burden, as well as to monitor therapeutic effectiveness, detect recurrence or localisation of the tumour, and screen the general population or groups at risk. Tumour markers, also called biomarkers, have been classified as follows: enzymes, isoenzymes, hormones, oncofoetal antigens, carbohydrate epitopes, oncogene products and genetic alterations. Unfortunately, to date, none of the known biomarkers fit the ideal specificity profile. The most important characteristics for a biomarker are measurement by easy techniques, reliability, reproducibility, minimal invasiveness and low cost.

In recent years, clinically useful tumor markers for HCC diagnosis have included α-fetoprotein (AFP), a fucosylated variant of the AFP glycoprotein which has a high affinity to the sugar chain of Lens culinaris (AFPL3), carcinoembryonic antigen (CEA) and des-γ-carboxy prothrombin (DCP). Among them, AFP and AFP-L3 tests were approved by the Food and Drug Administration (FDA) and the DCP test is currently under review. These markers will definitely be helpful in evaluating and managing patients with HCC or those at risk for HCC in medical practice.

## 3.1. α-Fetoprotein (AFP)

The most widely used tumor marker for diagnosis of HCC is AFP, which is a unique immunomodulatory glycoprotein (65 kDa) normally made by the immature liver cells in the fetus [60]. AFP, discovered in 1963 by Abelev et al. [61], is an oncofetal glycoprotein that is normally produced by the fetal liver. AFP levels decline gradually after birth, reaching low levels in normal adults. However, because AFP levels are usually increased in patients developing HCC, it is widely accepted as a candidate tumor marker in the detection of HCC. Its detection during monitoring of HCC treatment is well accepted in patients with increased AFP levels prior to therapy, and is recommended by the European Association for the Study of the Liver (EASL). Since its FDA approval in the early 1980s, AFP has been studied extensively as a tumor marker of HCC. Previous studies have demonstrated that the sensitivity and specificity of AFP for HCC diagnosis are 41–65 and 80–94%, respectively, with a cutoff value of 20 ng/ml [62]. This variability in the sensitivity in different studies is thought be due to several factors including study design (retrospective vs. prospective study), insufficient sample size, etiologic factors of HCC, race and the different cutoff values used for AFP. In addition, given that serum AFP levels can be increased in benign conditions such as liver cirrhosis, chronic hepatitis or acute hepatitis, it is difficult to determine the appropriate value at which sensitivity and specificity are maximized. Nevertheless, AFP remains the most commonly used marker in screening and surveillance programs of HCC to date. Because early detection of HCC significantly affects patient survival and prognosis, a surveillance program using serum and liver ultrasonography every 3 or 6 months has been recommended in different countries of the world. However, it is still debatable whether this surveillance program provides any survival benefit for HCC patients, and therefore further large-scale prospective studies are required in the future.

AFP is quite specific, but sensitivity is poor, thus a more effective tumor marker than AFP has been required. Recently, the AFP-L3 test has gained FDA approval as a risk marker for primary liver cancer. Since the introduction of AFP-L3 by Taketa et al. [63], subsequent studies of AFP-L3 have shown sensitivities and specificities ranging from 30.9 to 75 and 63 to 99.5%, respectively, in the detection of HCC ( Table 1 ) [64,65,66,67,68]. The AFP-L3 test has higher specificity than total AFP in the detection of HCC, but similar sensitivity.

However, clinical utility of AFP-L3 for HCC screening is still limited because the test is very troublesome and difficult to standardize.

**Table 1. Sensitivity and specificity of AFP-L3 in the diagnosis of HCC**

| References | Study design | Cases (n) | Cutoff value, % | Sensitivity, % | Specificity, % |
|---|---|---|---|---|---|
| Sato et al. [66] | Prospective | LC (361) | 15 | 55 | 68 |
| Wang et al. [68] | Prospective | LC (1,500) | 35 | 75 | 83 |
| Oka et al. [65] | Prospective | HCC (388) | 10 | 36.1 | 93.4 |
|  |  | CLD (212) | 15 | 30.9 | 99.5 |
| Sterling et al. [67] | Prospective | HCC (40) | 10 | 36.5 | 91.6 |
|  |  | CLD (212) |  |  |  |
| Leerapun et al. [64] | prospective | HCC (160) | 10 | 71 | 63 |
|  |  | CLD (106) |  |  |  |

CLD = Chronic liver disease; LC = liver cirrhosis.

## 3.2. Carcinoembryonic Antigen (CEA)

CEA, a member of the immunoglobulin supergene family, is a 180–200 kDa heavily glycosylated protein was originally described by Gold and Freedman in 1965 [69]. Frequently it is detected in a high concentration in the serum of individuals with malignancies in the digestive system, particularly the colon. In contrast, the occurrence of high serum levels of CEA is most unusual in HCC. Maeda and their group [70] had a patient with HCC and a marked elevation of the serum CEA level, which was demonstrated immunohistologically in the cytoplasm of the tumor cells. It functions as an adhesion molecule that can form both homotypic and heterotypic aggregates between cells. CEA is cleared from the circulation by the liver with significant traces taken up by the spleen and lungs.

## 3.3. Des-$\gamma$-Carboxy Prothrombin (DCP)

DCP has been used widely in Japan for HCC diagnosis and surveillance [71]. DCP is an abnormal prothrombin molecule that is generated as a result of an acquired defect in the posttranslational carboxylation of the prothrombin precursor in malignant cells; this prothrombin defect in malignant cells is similar to the deficit in vitamin K deficiency and has been called *prothrombin inducedby vitamin K absence* [72]. Since Liebman et al. [72] firstly reported DCP as a candidate marker for the diagnosis or prognosis of HCC, its diagnostic accuracy has been investigated in several studies. In initial studies, the sensitivity of DCP for HCC was poor, ranging from 23 to 41% [73], but recent studies document higher sensitivities and specificities ranging from 44.3 to 92% and 93 to 97%, respectively (Table 2 ) [74,75,76]. In particular, compared with total AFP and AFPL3, DCP showed the highest sensitivity in the early detection of small HCC [76]. Due to these promising results, DCP is under review as a candidate marker for HCC by the FDA.

## Table 2. Sensitivity and specificity of DCP in the diagnosis of HCC

| Study design | Cases (n) | Cutoff value mAU/ml | Sensitivity, % | Specificity, % | References |
|---|---|---|---|---|---|
| case-control | HCC (55) | 125 | 89 | 95 | Marrero et al. [74] |
| | CLD (104) | | | | |
| case-control | HCC (1,377) | 40 | 58 | 97 | Nakamura et al. [75] |
| | CLD (355) | | | | |
| case-control | HCC (84) | 150 | 86 | 93 | Volk et al. [76] |
| | LC (169) | | | | |

AU = Arbitrary unit; CLD = chronic liver disease; LC = liver cirrhosis

## 3.4. Glypican-3 (GPC3)

GPC3 is an oncofoetal protein, being a member of the glypican family of heparin sulfate proteoglycan that is anchored to the plasma membrane via glycosyl phosphatidylinositol [77]. GPC3 has been reported to play an important role in the development and regulation of cellular proliferation and apoptosis [78]. GPC3 has been reported to be down-regulated in breast cancer, ovarian cancer and lung adenocarcinoma but upregulated in HCC [79,80,81,82]. Recent studies suggest GPC3 as a candidate marker for HCC based on previous results showing that GPC3 is overexpressed or increased in the tissue or serum of patients with HCC [83]. In HCC, GPC3 has been shown to stimulate growth forming complexes with Wingless-type MMTV (Wnt) interaction site family [84]. In patients with advanced liver cirrhosis, early detection of HCC based solely on imaging is very limited. Therefore, the development of new markers to be able to differentiate early HCC from dysplastic or regenerating nodules of liver cirrhosis is imperative in clinical practice. Interestingly, GPC3 was found to be specifically overexpressed in tumor tissue of most HCC patients. In this regard, Di Tommaso et al. [84] showed that immunostaining for GPC3 was very helpful in distinguishing early and grade-1 HCC from dysplastic nodules arising in cirrhosis, suggesting GPC3 as a tissue marker for the early detection of HCC. To date, few studies have been reported concerning the diagnostic value of serum GPC3 for HCC [83]. In a study by Capurro et al. [83], GPC3 was significantly increased (53%) in the sera of HCC patients compared with healthy controls or patients with hepatitis. In a subsequent study by Hippo et al. [85], the sensitivity and specificity of serum GPC3 were reported to be 51 and 90%, respectively. No systematic data are available concerning its sensitivity and specificity, furthermore the use of this marker mainly in histological procedures hampers its use in surveillance programs and in the clinical setting.

## 3.5. Golgi Protein 73 (GP73)

GP73, is a resident Golgi protein localized in the membrane of the Golgi complex, is significantly upregulated in hepatitis virus-related HCC patients [86]. Sensitivity of 69% and a specificity of 75% in HCC versus cirrhotic patients, using 10 relative units as cut-off, calculated by densitometric scanning of immunoblotting [87]. Based on these interesting findings, few studies have attempted to investigate the diagnostic value of GP73 in HCC. In an initial study, the level of GP73 was significantly increased compared to normal controls or colorectal cancer in immunoblot analysis. This result highlighted the potential of GP73 as a reliable HCC biomarker [88]. Further study conducted by Marrero et al. [89] demonstrated that GP73 had a sensitivity of 69% and a specificity of 75% at the optimal cutoff point of 10 relative units for HCC diagnosis. Also, regarding the early detection of HCC in liver cirrhosis, GP73 showed significantly higher sensitivity than AFP in diagnosing early HCC (62 vs. 25%, respectively), suggesting that it may be a more precise marker than AFP in the detection of early HCC. However, it is very unlikely that this marker could be used in clinical practise because the technique used to quantify it does not make the molecule suitable as a routine biomarker, since it does not fit the ideal technical criteria defining a reliable clinical marker for large-scale use in diagnosis. Thus, the development of a simple quantitative serum assay such as ELISA is urgently needed.

## 3.6. Growth Factors or Cytokines

Transforming Growth Factor- β1 (TGF- β1) TGF-β1, a member of the gene superfamily involved in the regulation of cell growth and differentiation, plays a complex and multifaceted role in the regulation of tumorigenesis. It has been reported to be strongly expressed in tumorous tissue and elevated in the sera of human HCC [90]. A recent study by Song et al. [91] demonstrated that at a cutoff value of 800 pg/ml in plasma the sensitivity and specificity of TGF-β1 for the detection of small HCC were 68 and over 95%, respectively, suggesting TGF-β1 to be a useful serologic marker in detecting early HCCs. Interestingly, TGF-β1 was also evaluated as a urinary tumor marker for HCC by Tsai et al. [36]. At the optimal cutoff value of 32 mg/g creatinine, sensitivity and specificity of urinary TGF-β1 were 67.4 and 91.0%, respectively. Tumor markers in the urine are superior to blood testing in terms of invasiveness. Therefore, further large-scale studies are needed to confirm their diagnostic value in discriminating HCC from liver cirrhosis.

## 3.7. Insulin-Like Growth Factor (IGF)

IGF-II, a polypeptide involved in cellular proliferation and differentiation, was reported to be overexpressed in both mRNA and at protein level in tumorous tissue of HCC [92]. In an earlier study on the diagnostic value of IGF-II as a tumor marker for HCC, the sensitivity, specificity and diagnostic accuracy of IGF-II for HCC at the optimal cutoff value of 4.9 mg/g prealbumin were demonstrated to be 31, 100 and 65.5%, respectively [93]. According to these results, IGF-II seems to have no diagnostic advantage compared to AFP in the detection of HCC. In addition, IGF-II levels, which depend on the prealbumin concentration in the serum, are affected by the nutritional status of the patients. To develop IGF-II as a candidate marker for HCC, more convincing evidence is required.

## 3.8 Interleukin (IL)-6 and IL-10

IL-6 and IL-10, multifunctional cytokines produced by various cells, play an important role in host defense mechanisms and the modulation of immune response [94]. A previous study showed that plasma IL-6 and IL-10 levels were frequently elevated in HCC patients [95]. Hsia et al. [96] compared the accuracy of IL-6 and IL-10 as candidate markers for HCC. The sensitivity of IL-6, IL-10, hepatocyte growth factor (>1,000 pg/ml) and AFP (>20 ng/ml) was 46, 50, 58 and 62%, respectively, and the specificity was 95, 96, 53 and 88%, respectively, suggesting that IL-6 and IL-10 may be candidate markers for HCC [96]. However, further large-scale studies confirming the role of IL-6 and IL-10 as tumor markers for HCC are required.

## 3.9. γ-Glutamyl Transferase (GGT)

Total GGT secreted from hepatic Kupffer cells and endothelial cells of the bile duct can be divided into 13 isoenzymes. Among them, the diagnostic value of hepatoma-specific GGTII was evaluated as an HCC marker complementary to AFP [97]. The overall accuracy, sensitivity and specificity of GGTII for the detection of HCC were 77.6, 74.2 and 82.2%, respectively. Subsequent analysis for small HCC revealed a sensitivity of 43.8% and a specificity of 82.2% [97]. Consequently, serum GGTII may be a useful tumor marker complementary to AFP in the diagnosis of HCC.

## 3.10. α-L -Fucosidase (AFU)

AFU is a lysosomal enzyme responsible for hydrolyzing fucose glycosidic linkages of glycoproteins and glycolipids. Since increased AFU activity was reported in HCC [98], few studies have attempted to validate the diagnostic value of AFU in HCC [99]. However, although serum AFU may be useful in the early detection of HCC, its activity is also increased in other diseases such as diabetes, pancreatitis and hypothyroidism [100]. Therefore, further studies assessing the accuracy of AFU as a tumor marker for HCC diagnosis are warranted.

## 3.11. Others

Human Cervical Cancer Oncogene (HCCR) known to be a negative regulator of the p53 gene was overexpressed in tumorous compared with non-tumorous cirrhotic tissue of HCC [101]. Serological studies revealed 78.2% sensitivity for HCCR (cutoff value, 15 µg/ml), being significantly higher than the 64.6% of AFP, and 95.7% specificity for HCC. The positive rate of 69.2% in HCC patients with tumor sizes <2 cm was higher than that of AFP. Furthermore, sensitivity and specificity were 88.1 and 79.0%, respectively, at a cutoff value of 8 µg/ml, suggesting that the HCCR assay may have an advantage over the AFP assay in the detection of HCC [101]. This EDRN phase II study needs further validation.

Although autoantibodies are almost exclusively detected in autoimmune diseases, they are also found in some malignant diseases. With respect to HCC, some autoantibodies were reported to be increased during malignant transformation from non-malignant chronic liver diseases to HCC [102]. In a recent study, on average 3.6 antibody specificities of five candidate tumor-derived autoantibody (TAA) were found in HCC [103]. In addition, TAA can be a potential target for immunotherapy against cancer. Thus, more extensive studies are needed to document the clinical utility of TAA for diagnosis or as therapeutic targets of HCC.

## 4. Polyphenols Are Miracle Agents

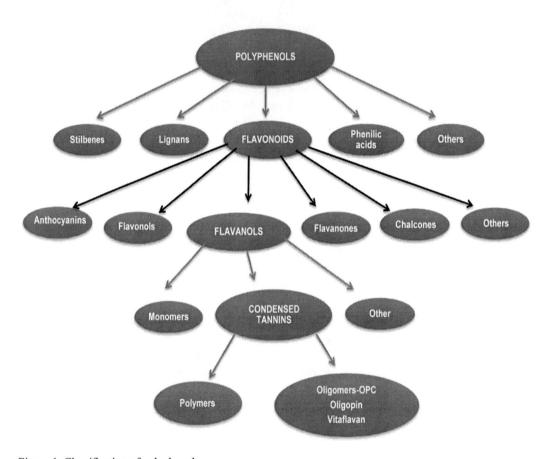

Figure 1. Classification of polyphenols.

The term polyphenols or phenolics refer precisely to those chemical compounds, which have an aromatic ring with hydroxyl substituent(s), including their derivatives like esters, methyl ethers and glycosides [104]. On the basis of chemical structure, they can be classified into phenolic acids, flavonoids, stilbenes and lignans. Polyphenolic compounds are ubiquitous in plants, in which they function in various protective roles [104-106]. A 'recommended' human diet contains significant quantities of polyphenolics, as they have long been assumed to be 'antioxidants' that scavenge excessive, damaging, free radicals arising from normal metabolic processes. There is recent evidence that polyphenolics also have 'indirect' antioxidant effects through induction of endogenous protective enzymes [104]. There is also increasing evidence for many potential benefits through polyphenolic mediated regulation of cellular processes such as inflammation and cancer. Inductive or signalling effects may occur at concentrations much lower than required for effective radical scavenging. Flavonoids and phenolic acids also have antioxidative and anticarcinogenic effects [2,20,105,106]. Inverse relationships between the intake of flavonoids (flavonols and flavones) and the risk of coronary heart disease and stomach cancer have been shown in epidemiological studies. Many so-called secondary products can act as potent bio-antimutagens. Antimutagen action of green tea extract has been studied, for which epigallocatecin gallate seems to be most responsible. Therefore, there is currently a strong interest in the study of natural compounds with free radical scavenger capacity and their role in human health and nutrition. Dietary antioxidants may contribute to the decrease of cardiovascular disease by reduction of free radical formation as well as oxidative stress in general, by protection of LDL oxidation and platelet aggregation and by inhibiting synthesis of proinflamatory cytokines [27].

**Table 3. The major classes of phenolics in plants**

| No. of C atoms | Basic skeleton | Class | Example |
|---|---|---|---|
| 6 | C6 | Simple phenols – benzoquinones | Catechol, hydroquinone2, 6-dimethoxybenzoquinone |
| 7 | C6-C1 | Phenolics acids | p-hydroxybenzoic, salicylic,Gallic acid, Syringic acid |
| 8 | C6-C2 | Acetophenones phenyiacetic acid | 3-Acetyi-6-methoxybenzaldehyde, p-Hydroxyphenylacetic |
| 9 | C6-C3 | Hydroxycinnamic acids coumarin, isocoumarin, chromones | Caffieic, ferulic myristicin, eugenol umbelliferone, aesculetin, bergenin, eugenin, |
| 10 | C6-C4 | Napthoquinone, | Juglone, plumbagin |
| 13 | C6-C1-C6 | Xanthones | Mangiferin |
| 14 | C6-C2-C6 | Stilbenes, anthraquinone | Lunularic acid, emodin |
| 15 | C6-C3-C6 | Flavonoids, isoflavonoids | Quercitin, cyaniding, genistein |
| 18 | $(C6-C3)_2$ | Lignans, neolignans | Pinoresinol eusiderin |
| 30 | $(C6-C-3-C6)_2$ | Biflavonoids | Amentoflavone |
| N | $(C6-3)n(C6)_6(C6-C3-C6)$ n | Lignins, catechol, melanins, flavolans (condensed tannins) | |

Some classes of polyphenol, such as the condensed tannins, have many catechol and phloroglucinol groups in their struture. A purely chemical definition of a plant phenol, however is not entirely satisfactory, since it would mean including some compounds such as the phenolic carotinoid or the phenolic female sex hormone orstrone, which are principally terpinoid in origin. For this reason a biogenetic definition is preferable. The natural plant phenol arises biogenetically from 2 main pathways. The Shikimate pathway which directly provide phenylpropanoids such as hydrxoxycinnamic and coumarins and the polyketide pathway (acetate) which can produce simple phenols and also many quinines. Major classes of phenolics have been described in Table 3 [13].

They are the most abundantly occurring polyphenols in plants, of which flavonoids and phenolic acids accounts for about 60% and 30% of total dietary phenols respectively [109,110]. Antioxidant activity and biological properties of polyphenols from berries, red wine, ginkgo, onions, apples, grapes, chamomile, citrus, dandelion, green tea, hawthorn, licorice, rosemary, thyme, fruits, vegetables and beverages have been studied. They are rich sources of phenols that can enhance the efficacy of vitamin C, reduce the risk of cancer, act against allergies, ulcers, tumors, platelet aggregation and are also effective in controlling hypertension [111].

## 4.1. Classification of Polyphenols

### (a) Hydroxy-Benzoic Acid

Hydroxybenzoic acids have a general structure of C6-C1 derived directly from benzoic acid (Fig 2). Variations in the structures of individual hydroxybenzoic acids lie in the hydroxylations and methylations of the aromatic ring. Four acids occur commonly: p-hydroxybenzoic, vanillic, syringic, and protocatechuic acid [112].

### (b) Hydroxy - Cinnamic Acids

The four most widely distributed hydroxycinnamic acids in fruits are *p*-coumaric, caffeic, ferulic and sinapic acids (Figure 3) [112].

### (c) Flavonoids

Flavonoids are formed in plants from the aromatic amino acids phenylalanine and tyrosine, and malonate. The structural basis of all flavonoids is flavone nucleus (2 phenyl-benzo-Ɣ-pyrone) (Figure 4) but, depending on the classification method, the flavonoids group can be divided into several categories on the basis of hydroxylation of flavonoids nucleus and linked sugar [113].

Flavonoids and their relatives are derived biosynthetically from the Shikimate pathway. They share a three-ring structure of two aromatic centers, ring A and B and a central oxygenated heterocycle moiety, ring C (Figure 4). They have a flavone nucleus (2 phenyl-benzo-γ-pyrone) and on the basis of variation in the heterocyclic C ring may be classified into flavones, flavonols, flavanones, flavanols, isoflavones, anthocyanidins and proanthocyanidins. Chalcones such as butein, isoquirtigenin (Figure 5) are considered to be members of the flavonoids, despite of lacking heterocycle ring C [111]. Flavones and flavonols have a double bond between C-2 and C-3 (Figs. 6 & 7). Flavonols have a hydroxy group at the C-3 position that is lacking in flavones. Flavanones and flavanols are characterized by the presence of a saturated three-carbon chain. Flavanols differ from flavanones by having a hydroxyl group at C-3 position (Figs. 8 & 9). Isoflavones (Figure 10) are derived by cyclization of chalcones in such a way that the B ring is located at C-3 position. Anthocyanins (Figure 11) are composed of aglycon called anthocynidins and sugar moiety(ies). Proanthocyanidins are condensed tannins or polymeric flavonols, which are generally formed as a result of coupling between electrophilic and nucleophilic flavanyl units [110,114].

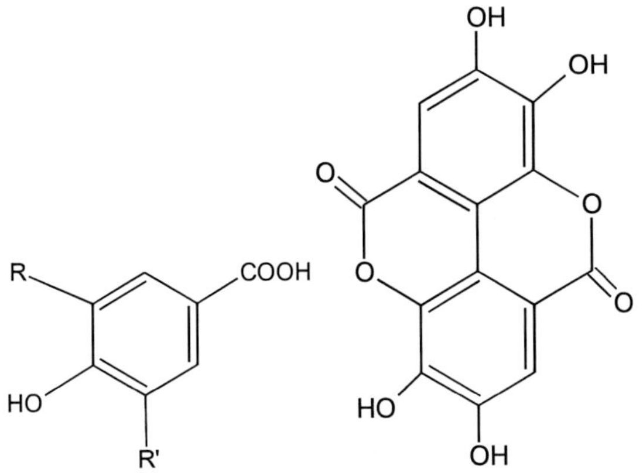

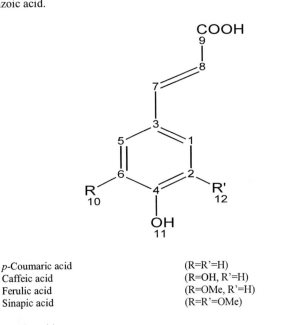

(a)

Protocatechuic acid

Gallic acid
Syringic acid

p-Hydroxybenzoic acid

Vanillic acid

(b)

(R= OH, R'=H)

(R=R'=OH)

(R=R'=OMe)
(R=R'=H)

(R=OMe, R'=H)

Figure 2. Hydroxy-benzoic acid.

p-Coumaric acid
Caffeic acid
Ferulic acid
Sinapic acid

(R=R'=H)
(R=OH, R'=H)
(R=OMe, R'=H)
(R=R'=OMe)

Figure 3. Hydroxy- cinnamic acids.

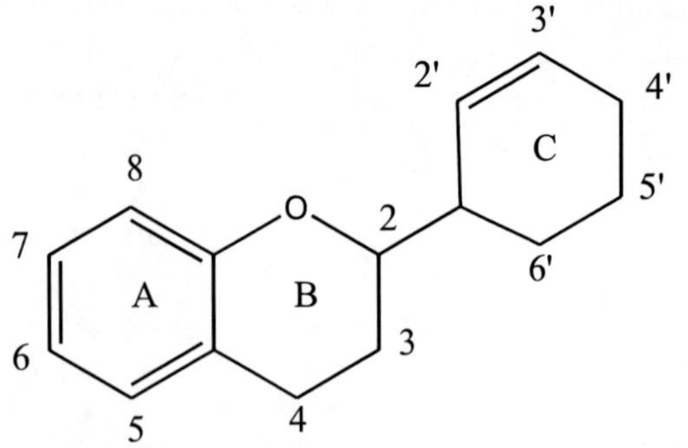

Figure 4. Flavone nucleus (2 phenyl-benzo-Υ-pyrone).

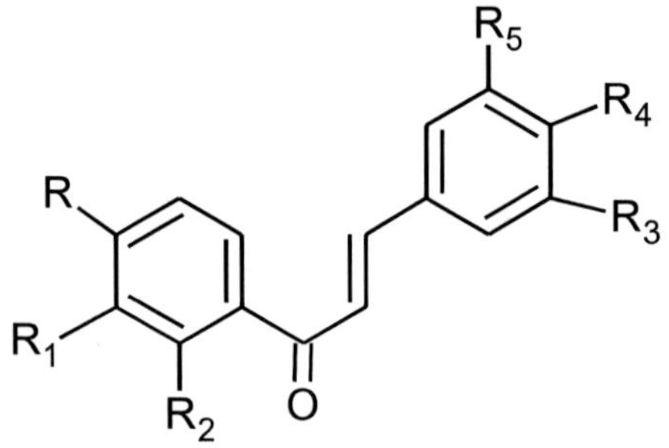

|  | R | $C_2$-$C_3$ |
|---|---|---|
| Flavone | H | Double bond |
| Flavonol | OH | Double bond |
| Flavanone | H | Single bond |
| Flavanol | OH | Single bond |

|  | R | $R_1$ | $R_2$ | $R_3$ | $R_4$ | $R_5$ |
|---|---|---|---|---|---|---|
| Butein | OH | H | OH | H | OH | OH |
| Isoquirtigenin | OH | H | OH | H | OH | H |

Figure 5. Chalcones.

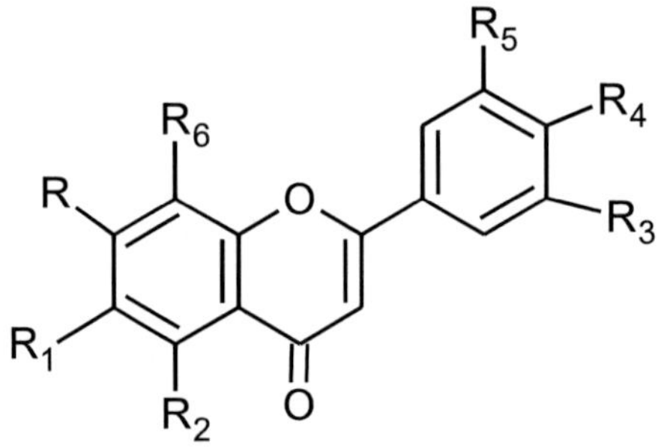

|  | R | $R_1$ | $R_2$ | $R_3$ | $R_4$ | $R_5$ | $R_6$ |
|---|---|---|---|---|---|---|---|
| Apigenin | OH | H | OH | H | OH | H | H |
| Vitexin | OH | H | OH | H | OH | H | O-Glucose |
| Isovitexin | OH | O-Glucose | OH | H | OH | H | H |
| Luteolin | OH | H | OH | H | OH | OH | H |

Figure 6. Flavones.

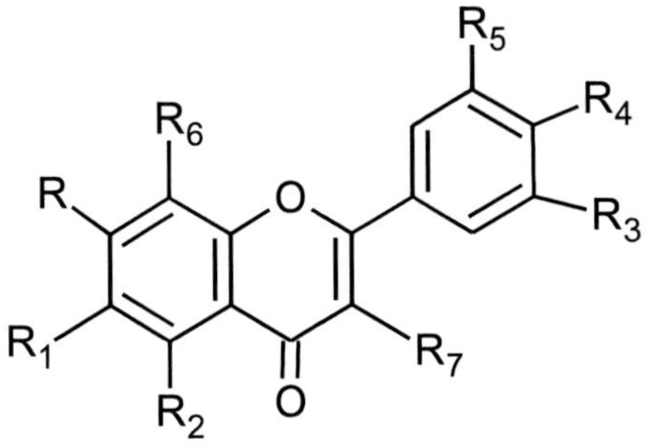

|           | R  | $R_1$ | $R_2$ | $R_3$ | $R_4$ | $R_5$ | $R_6$ | $R_7$     |
|-----------|----|-------|-------|-------|-------|-------|-------|-----------|
| Kaempferol| OH | H     | OH    | H     | OH    | H     | H     | OH        |
| Quercetin | OH | H     | OH    | H     | OH    | OH    | H     | OH        |
| Quercetrin| OH | H     | OH    | H     | OH    | OH    | H     | O-Glucose |
| Rutin     | OH | H     | OH    | H     | OH    | OH    | H     | O-Rutinose|
| Myricitin | OH | H     | OH    | OH    | OH    | OH    | H     | OH        |

Figure 7. Flavonol.

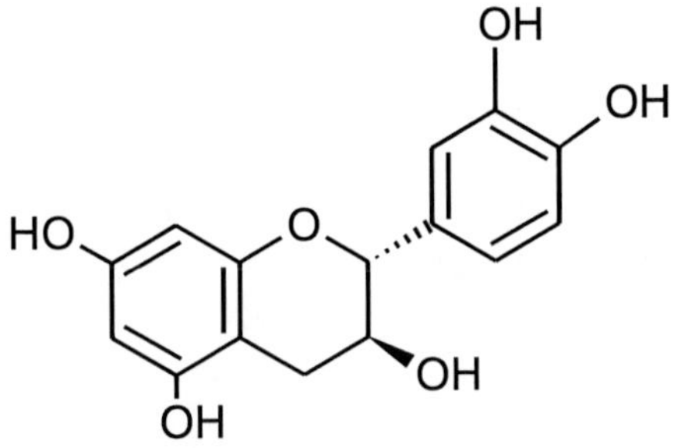

Catechin

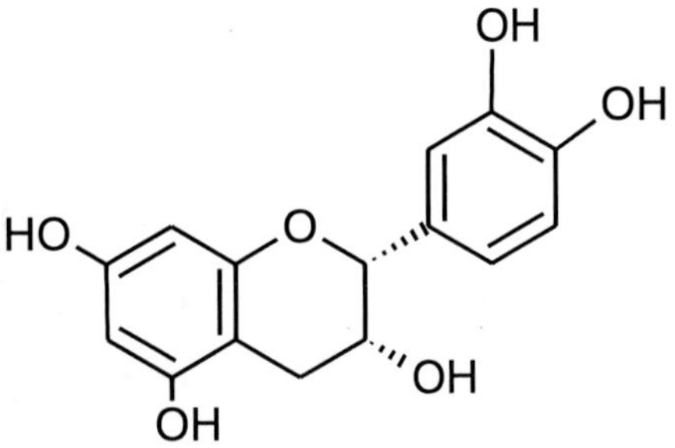

Epicatechin

Figure 8 (Continued).

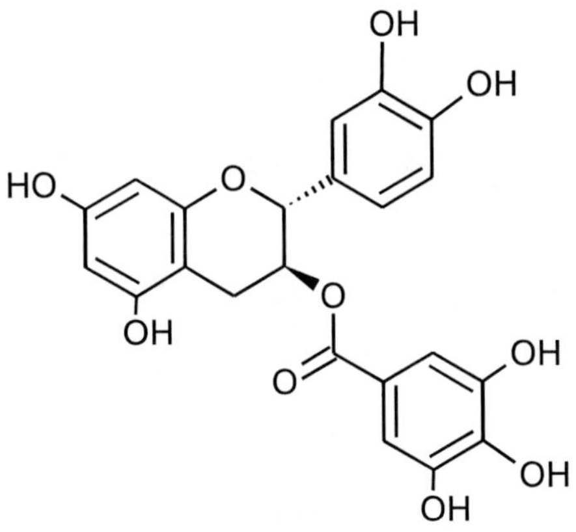

Catechin gallate

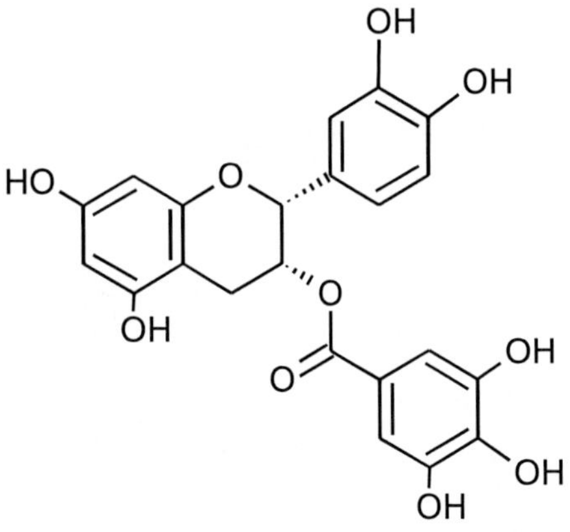

Epicatechin-3-gallate (EGCG)

Figure 8. Flavanol (Flavan-3-ols).

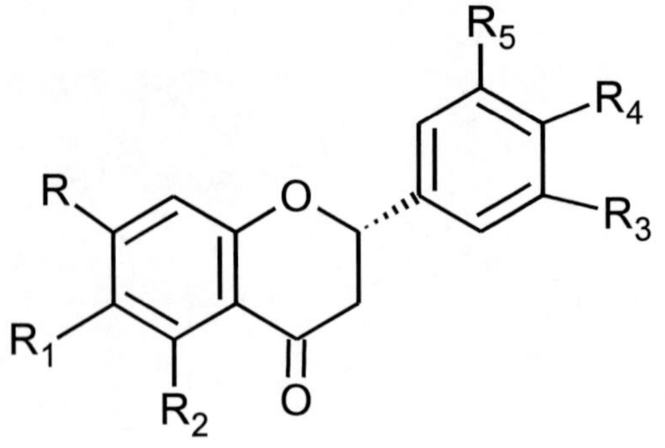

| | R | $R_1$ | $R_2$ | $R_3$ | $R_4$ | $R_5$ |
|---|---|---|---|---|---|---|
| Naringenin | OH | H | OH | H | OH | H |
| Hesperitin | OH | H | OH | H | OCH3 | H |

Figure 9. Flavanone.

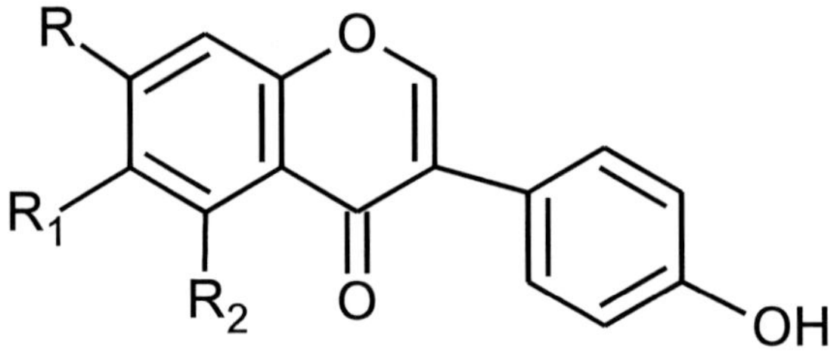

| | R | $R_1$ | $R_2$ |
|---|---|---|---|
| Daidzein | OH | H | OH |
| Genistein | OH | H | H |

Figure 10: Isoflavones.

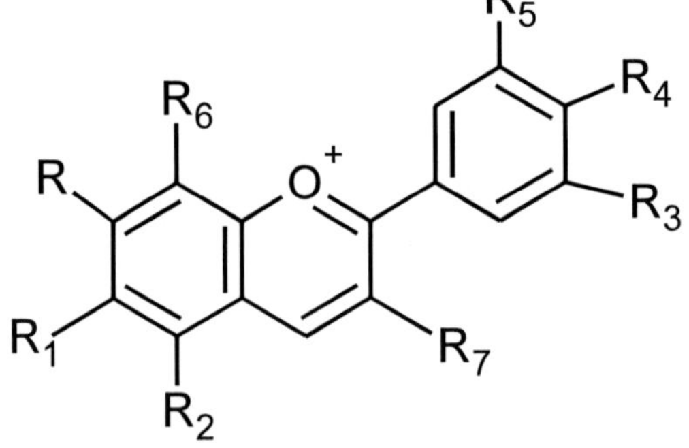

| | R | $R_1$ | $R_2$ | $R_3$ | $R_4$ | $R_5$ | $R_6$ |
|---|---|---|---|---|---|---|---|
| Pelargonidin | OH | H | OH | H | OH | H | H |
| Cyanidin | OH | H | OH | H | OH | OH | H |
| Delphinidin | OH | H | OH | OH | OH | OH | H |

Figure 11. Anthocyanin.

Flavonoids possess ideal structure for free radicals scavenging activity and have been found to be more effective cancer preventive agents *in vitro* than tocopherols and ascorbates. They are efficient reducing agents that can stabilize the polyphenols derived radicals and delocalise the unpaired electrons. It has been reported that flavonoids with strong antioxidant activity are excellent hydrogen donors and have a 3', 4'-dihydroxy configuration. Interestingly the hydroxyl groups on the chromane ring do not appear to participate directly in the redox chemistry. Instead it is the hydroxyl group of catechol moiety present in the B ring that donates or accepts hydrogen. However, while the flavonoids nucleus does not undergo direct redox modification, it does affect redox behaviour of substituents on B ring. Therefore, flavonoids containing catechol structure can exert a powerful radical scavenging activity. The position and number of hydroxyl groups also plays an important role in antioxidant activity. For example in apigenin (Figure 6), the three-hydroxyl groups at position 5, 7, 4' were associated with a small but definite antioxidant effect, while kaempferol (Figure 7) with an additional hydroxyl at position 3 was more potent than apigenin. Quercetin with additional hydroxyl group at 3' and myrcetin at 3', 5' positions (Figure 7) were still more effective [111,114,115]. Flavonoids can also generate $H_2O_2$ by donating a hydrogen atom from their pyrogallol or catechol structure to oxygen, through a superoxide anion radical. The pyrogallol-type compounds generate more $H_2O_2$ than that of catechol. $H_2O_2$ has been reported to raise levels of intracellular $Ca^{2+}$, activate transcription factors, repress expression of certain genes, promote or inhibit cell proliferation, be cytotoxic, activate or suppress certain signal transduction pathways, promote or suppress apoptosis [116,117].

More than 4000 flavonoids have been identified in plants, which are responsible for the color of vegetables, fruits, grains, seeds, leaves, flowers, bark and products derived from them [109,114]. Luteolin, kaempferol, quercetin, quercitrin, rutin, myricetin and vitamin C are powerful antioxidants that inhibit the oxidation of LDL, a major factor in the promotion of atherosclerosis, which is the plaque build up in arteries that can lead to heart attack or stroke. In general, the aglycones were found with greater antioxidant potential than their glycosides [109,115]. Use of comet assay to assess DNA damage during oxidative stress showed that quercetin was more potent antioxidant as compared to rutin and vitamin C. Isoflavones like genestein and daidzein found abundantly in legumes such as lentils, chickpeas and soybeans, have nutraceutical properties against tumor growth and cancer and they form one of the main classes of oestrogenic substances in plants (Figure 10). Anthocyanins, another major group of flavonoids play a significant role in collagen protein synthesis and sport medicines (Figure 11). Athletes who exercise a lot produce free radicals that can be tackled by anthocyanidins [118,119].

# 5. Polyphenols and their Targets for Prevention and Therapy of Liver Cancer

Fruits, vegetables, and spices have drawn a great deal of attention from both the scientific community and the general public owing to their demonstrated ability to suppress cancers. The questions that remain to be answered are which component of these dietary agents is responsible for the anti-cancer effects and what is the mechanism by which they suppress cancer? Dietary agents consist of a wide variety of biologically active compounds that are ubiquitous in plants, many of which have been used in traditional medicines for thousands of years. As early as 2500 years ago, Hippocrates recognized and professed the importance of various foods both natural and those derived from human skill in the primary constitution of the person.

Fruits and vegetables are excellent sources of polyphenols, but they also contain components like fiber, vitamins, and minerals, terpenes, and alkaloids that may provide substantial health benefits beyond basic nutrition. Research over the last decade has shown that several micronutrients in fruits and vegetables reduce cancer [10; Table 4). The active components of dietary phytochemicals that most often appear to be protective against cancer are curcumin, genistein, resveratrol, ellagic acid, quercetin, rutin, morin, diallyl sulfide, S-allyl, lycopene, ellagic acid, epicatechin gallate, gallic acid, silymarin, catechins, isothiocyanates, isoflavones, Vitamin C, lutein, Vitamin E, and flavonoids. These dietary polyphenols are believed to suppress the inflammatory processes that lead to transformation, hyperproliferation, and initiation of carcinogenesis. Their inhibitory influences may ultimately suppress the final steps of carcinogenesis as well, namely angiogenesis and metastasis (Figure 12).

**Table 4. Molecular targets of polyphenols for prevention and therapy of cancer**

| Polyphenols | Plant name | Molecular target |
|---|---|---|
| Resveratrol | Grapes (*Vitis vinifera*) | ↓COX-2, ↓iNOS, ↓JNK, ↓MEK, ↓AP-1, ↓NF-κB, ↑P21 Cip1/WAF1, ↑p53, ↑Bax, ↑caspases, ↑TNF, ↓survivin, ↓cyclin D1, ↓cyclin E, ↓Bcl-2, ↓Bcl-xL, ↓CIAP, ↓Egr-1, ↓PKC, ↓PKD, ↓casein kinase II, ↓5-LOX, ↓VEGF, ↓IL-1, ↓IL-6, ↓IL-8, ↓AR, ↓PSA, ↓CYP1A1, ↓TypeII-Ptdlns-4kinase, ↓Cdc2-tyr15[a], ↑HO-1, ↑Nrf2, ↓endothelin-1 |
| Caffeoylquinic acids | Quince (*Cydonia oblonga*) | ↓IFN-γ, ↓IL-2, ↓ERK1/2, ↓AKT, ↓NF-κB, ↓NO, ↓iNOS |
| Ellagic acid | Pomegranate (*Punica granatum*) | ↓NF-κB, ↓COX-2, ↓cyclin D1, ↓MMP-9, ↓PDGF, ↓VEGF, ↑GST, ↑p21/WAF1, ↑p53 |
| Genistein | Soyabean (*Glycine max*) | ↓NF-κB, ↑caspase-12, ↑p21/WAF1, ↑glutathione peroxidase |
| Flavonoids, catechins | Tea (*Camellia sinensis*) | ↓NF-κB, ↓AP-1, ↓JNK, ↓COX-2, ↓cyclin D1, ↓MMP-9, ↑HO-1, ↓IL-6, ↓VEGF, ↓IGF, ↑p53, ↓Bcl-2, ↑p21/WAF1 |
| Quercetin | Citrus fruits, apple (*Citrus* sp.) | NF-κB, ↑Bax, ↓ Bcl-2, ↓cyclin D1, ↑caspase, ↑PARP, ↑Gadd 45 |
| Silymarin | *Silybum marianum* | ↓NF-kB, ↓AP-1, ↓JNK, ↓COX-2, ↓cyclin D1, ↓MMP-9 |

AR, androgen receptor; NF-κB, nuclear factor kappa B; NO, nitric oxide; PGE, prostaglandin; iNOS, inducible nitric oxide synthase; COX-2, cyclooxygenase-2; IL, interleukin; MAP, mitogen-activated protein; TNF, tumor necrosis factor; CYP7A1, cholesterol 7alpha-hydroxylase; CYP, cytochrome p450; HO, heme oxygenase; IAP, inhibitor-of-apoptosis protein; PKC, protein kinase C; PKD, protein kinase D; LOX, lipoxygenase; VEGF, vascular endothelial growth factor; PSA, prostate-specific antigen; molecules; GST, glutathione *S*-transferase; MMP, matrix metalloprotease.

Tumorigenesis is a multistep process that can be activated by any of various environmental carcinogens (such as cigarette smoke, industrial emissions, gasoline vapors), inflammatory agents (such as tumor necrosis factor (TNF) and H2O2), and tumor promoters (such as phorbol esters and okadaic acid). These carcinogens are known to modulate the transcription factors (e.g., NF-kB, AP-1, STAT3), anti-apoptotic proteins (e.g., Akt, Bcl-2, Bcl-XL), proapoptotic proteins (e.g., caspases, PARP), protein kinases (e.g., IKK, EGFR, HER2, JNK, MAPK), cell cycle proteins (e.g., cyclins, cyclin-dependent kinases), cell adhesion molecules, COX-2, and growth factor signaling pathways. In the recent years, many studies have been showed that molecular targets of polyphenols for not only prevention but also for therapy of cancers (Figure 13). NF-κB is a family of closely related protein dimers that bind to a common sequence motif in DNA called the κB site [120]. The identification of the p50 subunit of NF-κB as a member of the reticuloendotheliosis (REL) family of viruses provided the first evidence that NF-κB is linked to cancer. Under resting condition, the NF-κB dimers reside in the cytoplasm. NF-κB is activated by free radicals, inflammatory stimuli, cytokines, carcinogens, tumor promoters, endotoxins, γ-radiation, ultraviolet (UV) light, and X-rays. Upon activation, it is translocated to the nucleus, where it induces the expression of more than 200 genes that have been shown to suppress apoptosis and induce cellular transformation, proliferation, invasion, metastasis, chemo-resistance, radio-resistance, and inflammation. Many of the target genes that are activated are critical to the establishment of the early and late stages of aggressive cancers, including expression of cyclin D1, apoptosis suppressor proteins such as Bcl-2 and Bcl-XL and those required for metastasis and angiogenesis, such as matrix metalloproteases (MMP) and vascular endothelial growth factor (VEGF).

Several dietary agents like curcumin [121], resveratrol [122], ellagic acid [123], green tea catechins are natural chemopreventive agents that have been found to be potent inhibitors of NF-κB (Table 4). How these agents suppress NF-κB activation is becoming increasingly apparent. These inhibitors may block any one or more steps in the NF-κB signaling pathway such as the signals that activate the NF-κB signaling cascade, translocation of NF-κB into the nucleus, DNA binding of the dimers, or interactions with the basal transcriptional machinery. To investigate the inhibitory and apoptosis-inducing effects of flavonoids from oil-removed seeds of Hippophae rhamnoides (FSH) on liver cancer cell line BEL-7402. FSH has potent inhibitive effect on BEL-7402 cell line in a concentration-dependent manner. BEL-7402 cells exhibit typical morphological alteration of apoptosis when sub-Gl peak can be seen. FSH exerts its inhibitive effect on BEL-7402 cells by inducing apoptosis [124].

AP-1 was originally identified by its binding to a DNA sequence in the SV40 enhancer [125]. Many stimuli, most notably serum, growth factors, and oncoproteins, are potent inducers of AP-1 activity; it is also induced by TNF and Interleukin 1 (IL-1), as well as by a variety of environmental stresses, such as UV radiation [126]. AP-1 has been implicated in regulation of genes involved in apoptosis and proliferation and may promote cell proliferation by activating the *cyclin D1* gene, and repressing tumor-suppressor genes, such as p53, p21cip1/waf1 and p16.

Several polyphenols such as green tea catechins [127], quercetin [128], and resveratrol [122], have been shown to suppress the AP-1 activation process. Epicatechin-3-gallate (EGCG) and theaflavins inhibit TPA- and epidermal growth factor-induced transformation of JB6 mouse epidermal cells [127]. This finding correlates with the inhibition of AP-1 DNA binding and transcriptional activity.

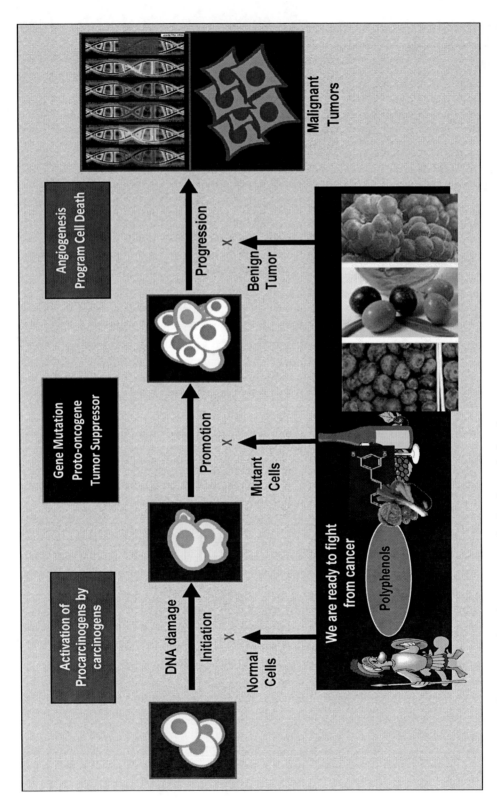

Figure 12. Diagrammatic representation of cancer prevention by plant polyphenols.

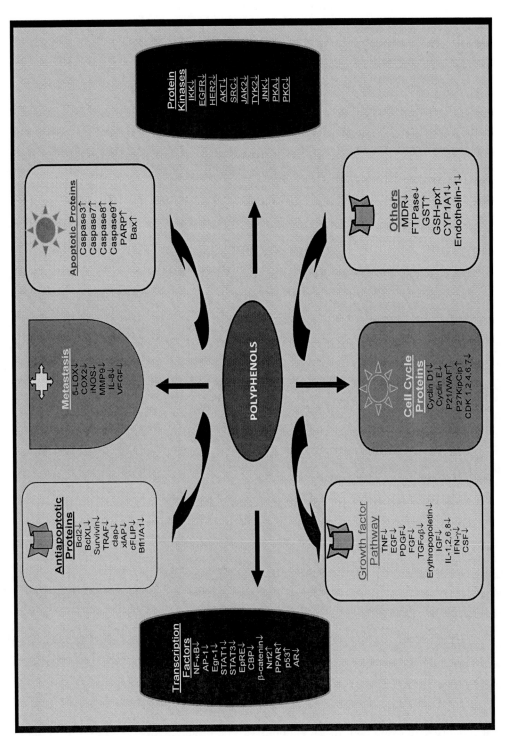

Figure 13. Molecular targets of plant polyphenols for prevention and therapy of liver cancer.

The inhibition of AP-1 activity by EGCG was associated with inhibition of JNK activation but not ERK activation. Interestingly, in another study where EGCG blocked the UVB-induced c-Fos activation in a human keratinocyte cell line HaCaT [129], inhibition of p38 activation was suggested as the major mechanism underlying the effects of EGCG. The role of MAPK pathways in the regulation of AP-1 activity by EGCG has been further investigated [130].

Treatment of Ha-ras-transformed human bronchial cells with EGCG has been shown to inhibit c-Jun and ERK1/2 phosphorylation as well as the phosphorylation of ELK1 and MEK1/2 [131]. In contrast to these reports, EGCG has been shown to markedly increase AP-1 factor-associated responses through a MAPK signaling mechanism in normal human keratinocytes, suggesting that the signaling mechanism of EGCG action could be markedly different in different cell types [132]. Lagarrigue et al. showed that the flavonoid quercetin could inhibit the transformation of the rat liver epithelial cell line overexpressing c-Fos, suggesting that regulation of c-Fos/AP-1 complexes might be involved in the antitransforming mechanism of quercetin [133]. Pretreatment of RAW 264.7 macrophages with quercetin blocked LPS-induced TNF transcription. This effect of quercetin was mediated by inhibiting the phosphorylation and activation of JNK/stress-activated protein kinase, by suppressing AP-1 DNA binding, and by down-regulating TNF transcription [133]. Resveratrol has been shown to inhibit the activity of AP-1 as demonstrated by several studies. We have found that resveratrol inhibits TNF-dependent AP-1 activation in U-937 cells, and that pretreatment with resveratrol strongly attenuates TNF-activated JNK and MEK kinases [122]. Cyclin D1, a component subunit of cyclin-dependent kinase (Cdk)-4 and Cdk6, is a rate-limiting factor in progression of cells through the first gap (G1) phase of the cell cycle [134]. Dysregulation of the cell cycle check points and overexpression of growth-promoting cell cycle factors such as cyclin D1 and cyclin-dependent kinases (CDK) are associated with tumorigenesis [135]. Several dietary agents including resveratrol [136], genistein [137], apigenin [138], and silibinin [139] have been shown to block the deregulated cell cycle in cancers. the green tea component EGCG causes cell cycle arrest and promotes apoptosis via a dose- and time-dependent up-regulation of p21/Cip1/Waf1, p27Kip1, and p16/INK4A, and down-regulation of proteins such as cyclin D1, cyclin E, Cdk2, and Cdk4 [140].

In liver cancer cells (HepG2), EGCG has been shown to induce apoptosis and block cell cycle progression at G1 [141]. These effects were accompanied by increased expression of p53 and p21/WAF1 proteins and proapoptotic Fas and Bax proteins. The serine/threonine protein kinase Akt/PKB is the cellular homologue of the viral oncogene v-Akt and is activated by various growth and survival factors. Activated Akt promotes cell survival by activating the NF-κB signaling pathway [142] by inhibiting apoptosis through inactivation of several proapoptotic factors including Bad, Forkhead transcription factors, and caspase-9 [143]. Several phytochemicals including genistein [144], and EGCG [145] are known to suppress the activation of Akt.

p53 is a tumor-suppressor and transcription factor. It is a critical regulator in many cellular processes including cell signal transduction, cellular response to DNA-damage, genomic stability, cell cycle control, and apoptosis. The protein activates the transcription of downstream genes such as p21WAF1 and Bax to induce the apoptotic process, inhibiting the growth of cells with damaged DNA or cancer cells [146]. Some of the polyphenols that are known to modulate p53 activity are resveratrol [147], EGCG [140], and silibinin [148]. Apoptosis and the expression of the non-steroidal anti-inflammatory drug-activated gene-1

(NAG-1), a member of the TGFβ superfamily that has been associated with proapoptotic and antitumorigenic activities, is induced by resveratrol-induced NAG-1 expression through an increase in the expression of p53 [149]. In a human liver cancer cell line, EGCG also significantly increased the expression of p53 and p21WAF1 protein, and this contributed to cell cycle arrest [150]. Several studies examined the potential effects of I3C and DIM on the proliferation and induction of apoptosis in human prostate cancer cell lines with different p53 status. They found that induction of apoptosis by I3C was p53-independent [151], and induction of p21WAF1 expression by DIM was independent of estrogen-receptor signaling and p53 [152].

Growth factors are proteins such as epidermal growth factor (EGF), platelet-derived growth factor (PDGF), fibroblast growth factors (FGFs), transforming growth factors (TGF)-α and -β, erythropoietin (Epo), insulin-like growth factor (IGF), interleukin (IL)-1, 2, 6, 8, tumor necrosis factor (TNF), interferon-γ (INF-γ) and colony-stimulating factors (CSFs) that bind to receptors on the cell surface, with the primary result of activating cellular proliferation and/or differentiation. Several chemopreventive phytochemicals including genistein, resveratrol, and catechins have been shown to be potent inhibitors of several growth factor signaling pathways.

TNF, initially discovered as a result of its antitumor activity, has now been shown to mediate tumor initiation, promotion, and metastasis [153]. In agreement with these observations, mice deficient in TNF have been shown to be resistant to skin carcinogenesis [154]. The induction of proinflammatory genes by TNF has been linked to most diseases. Phytochemicals such as green tea polyphenols [155], resveratrol, kaempferol and apigenin [156] have been shown to suppress TNF production. Green tea polyphenols are potent antioxidants that demonstrate both anti-cancer and anti-inflammatory effects. EGCG, the major green tea polyphenol, have been shown to down-regulate LPS-induced TNF production in a dose-dependent fashion [155]. Flavonoids have been reported to bring benefits in lowering inflammation and oxidative stress and exert positive effects in cancer and cardiovascular and chronic inflammatory diseases. Apigenin, kaempferol, and resveratrol, which are present in fruits, vegetables, and grains, exert inhibitory effects on the expression of TNF [156].

Cyclooxygenases are prostaglandin H synthase, which convert arachidonic acid released by membrane phospholipids into prostaglandins. Two isoforms of prostaglandin H synthase, COX-1 and COX-2, have been identified. COX-1 is constitutively expressed in many tissues, but the expression of COX-2 is regulated by mitogens, tumor promoters, cytokines, and growth factors. COX-2 is overexpressed in practically every premalignant and malignant condition involving the colon, liver, pancreas, breast, lung, bladder, skin, stomach, head and neck, and esophagus [158]. Several dietary components including galangin, luteolin [159], apigenin [160], 6-hydroxykaempferol, quercetagenin [161], genistein [162], wogonin [163], green tea catechins [164], and resveratrol [165] have been shown to suppress COX-2. LOXs are the enzymes responsible for generating leukotrienes (LT) from arachidonic acid. There are three types of LOX isozymes depending upon the different cells and tissues they affect. 15-LOX synthesizes anti-inflammatory 15-HETE; 12-LOX is involved in provoking inflammatory/allergic disorders; and 5-LOX produces 5-HETE and LTs, which are potent chemoattractants and lead to the development of asthma. Aberrant arachidonic acid metabolism is involved in the inflammatory and carcinogenic processes. Several dietary agents known to suppress LOX are green and black tea polyphenols [166], resveratrol [167], and flavonols [168]. Flavonols, including kaempferol, quercetin, morin, and myricetin, were found to be potent inhibitors of 5-LOX [168].

# 6. Polyphenols and HCC

## 6.1. Apigenin

Plant flavonoids may be beneficial in preventing this disease. Initial studies on plant flavonoids have shown that structural analogs designated the flavonoid 7-hydroxyl group are potent inhibitors of the human P-form phenolsulfotransferase, which is of major importance in the metabolism of many drugs, resulting in either inactivation and rapid renal elimination of the highly ionized sulfuric acid ester conjugates formed or, in some instances, formation of conjugates with increased pharmacological activity [169]. Apigenin is a well-known inhibitor of protein-tyrosine kinases and has been shown to block peroxisome proliferation regulated kinase. (ERK), a mitogen activated protein kinase (MAPK) in isolated hepatocytes [170]. Yee *et al.* [171] investigated the inhibitory effects of luteolin and apigenin on human hepatocellular carcinoma HepG2 cells. The results indicate that both flavonoids exhibited cell growth inhibitory effects which were due to cell cycle arrest and down-regulation of the expression of cyclin dependent kinase 4 (CDK4) with induction of p53 and p21, respectively. In addition, Jeyabal *et al.* [172] have shown the *in vivo* protective effects of apigenin on *N*-nitrosodiethylamine-induced and phenobarbitol promoted hepatocarcinogenesis in Wistar albino rats. Apigenin treatment at 25 mg/kg body weight for two weeks to these rats provided protection against the oxidative stress and DNA damage caused by the carcinogen.

## 6.2. Quercetin

The enhanced production of ROS to the initial oxidative stress prior to the apoptotic process, although quercetin might not require enhanced ROS production for the apoptosis induction, as reviously described for TGF-b1 in fetal rat hepatocytes [173] or IL-3 in murine myeloid cells [174]. That inhibition of Akt and ERK phosphorylation, induced by high quercetin concentrations, was coupled with a significant increase of caspase-3 and -9 levels and activities, higher expression of proapoptotic Bcl-2 family members (Bcl-xS and Bax), and lower levels of antiapoptotic Bcl-xL that contributed directly to the apoptotic process. Interestingly, the highest quercetin concentrations (75 and 100 mmol/l) reduced the expression of proapoptotic (caspase-3, -9, and Bax) and prosurvival signals (Akt and ERK) compared with lower concentrations of quercetin (50 mmol/l). Thus, the caspases implicated in the mitochondrial apoptosis pathway that showed the highest activity after 18 h of treatment with 50 mmol/l quercetin provoked the greatest activation of their Bcl-2 family substrates, whereas the apoptotic effect might have been enhanced by the inhibition of Akt and ERK. Higher concentrations further decreased cell viability due to the activation of executor apoptotic signal and the more pronounced inhibition of prosurvival pathways (Akt). Quercetin concentrations that significantly decrease HepG2 cell viability have similar effects on other cancer cell cultures, such as leukemia [175], and lung [176]. Although special attention must be given to flavonoid concentrations, quercetin may be a potential chemopreventive or therapeutic agent in HCC, and further efforts to investigate these possibilities are needed. Moreover, intravenous administration of pterostilbene and quercetin in a mouse melanoma animal model resulted in a 73% reduced metastasis of B16M-F10 cells in the liver, involving the inhibition of VCAM-1 (vascular adhesion molecule-1) by the hepatic sinusoidal endothelium [177]. In addition, flavonoids could control cell metastasis by regulating the expression of integrin partners. Resveratrol treatment of the erythroleukemia K562 cell line increased expression of tensin, a cell-matrix adhesion protein capable of binding integrins and cytoskeletal actin filaments. This resulted in increased cell adhesion to fibronectin, cell spreading, and actin polymerization. It is interesting that resveratrol induced similar cytoskeletal changes in the tensindeficient MCF7 human breast cancer cell line and abrogated estrogen-induced MCF7 cancer cell invasion [178].

## 6.3. Tea Ployphenols

The concept of cancer prevention using naturally occurring substances that could be included in the diet has gained increased attention. After water, tea is the most popular beverage worldwide and is grown in about 30 countries. All types of tea, including black, green and red (oolong), contain polyphenols with antioxidant properties [179]. Green tea is the least processed and most of the polyphenols in green tea are flavanols, commonly known as catechins. The main catechins in green tea are epicatechin, epicatechin-3-gallate, epigallocatechin, and EGCG. During fermentation of green tea, the polyphenols are oxidized to theaflavins and thearubigins, which are the main polyphenols of black tea [180]. Several epidemiological and experimental studies have shown the preventive effects of tea consumption against various diseases including atherosclerosis [181], cardiovascular diseases, and neurological diseases [182-184]. There are also abundant data, from several laboratories and epidemiological studies performed during the past 10 years, that provide strong evidences that polyphenolic antioxidants present in tea reduce the risk of cancer in many animal-tumor bioassay system esophagus, liver [181,185] cancers induced by chemical carcinogens. Green and black teas have shown cancer chemopreventive activity against ultraviolet light irradiation, as well as in chemically induced and genetic models of cancer, such as cancer of the skin, lung, prostate, bladder, liver, colon, oral cavity, esophagus, stomach, small intestine, and pancreas [186]. The antidotal capability of rats' livers can be significantly improved after long-term consumption of tea polyphenols. There are differences in changes of drug-metabolizing enzymes between the sexes induced by tea polyphenols and normal condition [187]. EGCG and theaflavins are responsible for most cancer chemopreventive properties of tea [179,188]. A significant reduction in the number of proliferating cells [185] and an increased number of apoptotic cells was found after treatment with the aflavins and EGCG in benzo(a) pyrene (B(a)P)-exposed mice [188]. A study on animals and human cell lines demonstrated tea polyphenols ability to modulate signaling pathways, [189] which have an important role in the prevention of cancer. Studies in rat liver have shown that tea polyphenols inhibit the production of mitochondrial ROS induced by chemical carcinogens, thereby preventing oxidative damage in the liver [186]. As bioactivation of the precarcinogens and detoxification of carcinogens are mainly performed by hepatic metabolizing enzymes, and previous studies investigated modulation of enzyme activities after tea consumption in animal models [190]. It was shown that tea consumption provides protection by modulating the expression of both phase I and phase II hepatic drug metabolizing enzymes in Wistar rats [191]. Cytochrome P450 (CYPs) are mainly expressed in the liver, except CYP1A1 and CYP1B1, which are extrahepatic isoenzymes in humans. Polyphenols' beneficial effects have been also attributed to their competitive inhibition of enzymes such as CYPs. Indeed, black tea polyphenols have been reported to inhibit the benzo(a)pyrene-induced activity and levels of cytochrome P4501A1 and 1A2 in mouse liver and lungs [192].

A cross-sectional study in Japanese men showed that increased consumption of green tea may also protect against liver disorders by reducing concentrations of hepatological markers in the serum [193]. Tea catechins, black tea extract and oolong tea extract (0.05% or 0.1%) significantly decreased the number and area of preneoplastic glutathione-S-transferase placental form (GST-P)-positive foci in the hepatocarcinogenesis model induced by NDEA in the male F344 rat liver (Matsumoto et al., 1996). Srivastava et al. [194] demonstrated the protective role of tea polyphenols on the development of DEN-induced altered hepatic foci (AHF) in a rat medium-term bioassay, indicating that polyphenols may prevent cancer at an early stage of rat liver carcinogenesis. These results also indicate that GTP is more effective than BTP in modulation of NDEA+2-acetyl aminofluorene (2-AAF)-induced AHF at the tested doses. Dietary administration of black tea polyphenols effectively suppressed $p$-dimethylaminoazobenzene (DAB)-induced hepatocarcinogenesis, as evidenced by reduced preneoplastic and neoplastic lesions, modulation of xenobiotic-metabolizing enzymes and amelioration of oxidative stress [195]. Thus, it can be concluded that black tea polyphenols acts as an effective chemopreventive agent by modulating xenobiotic-metabolizing enzymes and mitigating oxidative stress in an *in vivo* model of hepatocarcinogenesis.

## 6.4. Trans-Resveratrol

Few studies have evaluated the chemopreventive effects of resveratrol against liver cancer. Carbo *et al.* [196] demonstrated that resveratrol administration to rats inoculated with a fast growing tumour (the Yoshida AH-130 ascites hepatoma) caused a very significant decrease (25%) in the tumor cell content. This effect was found to be associated with an increase in the number of cells in the G2/M phase of the cell cycle. Interestingly, flow cytometric analysis of the tumor cell population revealed the existence of an aneuploid peak (representing 28% of total), which suggested that resveratrol causes apoptosis in the tumor cell population resulting in a decreased cell number. Sun *et al* demonstrated that resveratrol inhibited the growth of hepatoma cells line H22 in a dose- and time-dependent manner via the induction of apoptosis [197]. Some studied have shown that *trans*-resveratrol decreased hepatocyte growth factor-induced cell scattering and invasion [198]. However, *trans*-resveratrol did not: (i), decrease the level of the hepatocyte growth factor receptor c-met; (ii), impede the hepatocyte growth factorinducedincrease in c-met precursor synthesis; (iii), decrease hepatocyte growth factor-induced c-met autophosphorylation, or Akt-1 or extracellular-regulated kinases-1 and -2 activation; (iv), decrease urokinase expression; and (v), block the catalytic activity of urokinase. It was also demonstrated that *trans*resveratrol decreases hepatocyte growth factor-induced HepG2 cell invasion by an as yet unidentified post-receptor mechanism [198]. Resveratrol suppressed the invasion of the hepatoma cells even at low concentrations. Sera from rats orally given resveratrol restrained only the invasion of AH109A cells. Resveratrol and resveratrol-loaded rat serum suppressed reactive oxygen species-mediated invasive capacity. The antiinvasive activity of resveratrol was found to be independent of the anti-proliferative activity [199]. Further, resveratrol was found to strongly inhibit cell proliferation at the micromolar range in a time- and dose-dependent manner in rat hepatoma Fao and human hepatoblastoma HepG2 cell lines. It was suggested that resveratrol prevents or to delays the entry to mitosis. Ciolino and Yeh [200] examined the effect of resveratrol on the function of the aryl hydrocarbon receptor (AHR) and the transcription of CYP1A1 in human HepG2 hepatoma cells. Resveratrol was found to inhibit the increase in CYP1A1 mRNA caused by the AHR ligand 2,3,7,8-tetrachlorodibenzo-p-dioxin (TCDD) in a concentration-dependent fashion. The induction of transcription of an aryl hydrocarbon-responsive reporter vector containing the CYP1A1 promoter by TCDD was also inhibited by resveratrol [201]. Resveratrol was also found to inhibit the constitutive level of CYP1A1 mRNA and reporter vector transcription in HepG2 cells. The increase in CYP1A1 enzyme activity induced by TCDD was inhibited by resveratrol. Further, resveratrol was found to prevent TCDD-induced transformation of the cytosolic AHR to its nuclear DNAbinding form [201]. These data demonstrated that resveratrol inhibits CYP1A1 expression *in vitro*, by preventing the binding of the AHR to promoter sequences that regulate CYP1A1 transcription [201]. This activity was suggested to be important for the chemopreventive activity of resveratrol. Ciolino *et al.* [202] also investigated the effect of resveratrol, on the carcinogen activation pathway regulated by the aryl hydrocarbon receptor. Resveratrol inhibited the metabolism of the environmental aryl hydrocarbon benzo[a]pyrene (B[a]P) catalyzed by microsomes isolated from B[a]P-treated human hepatoma HepG2 cells. Resveratrol was found to inhibit, in a concentration-dependent manner, the activity of CYP1A1/CYP1A2 in microsomes and intact HepG2 cells [203]. Resveratrol inhibited the B[a]P-induced expression of the CYP1A1 gene, as measured at the mRNA and transcriptional levels. Resveratrol also abolished the binding of B[a]P-activated nuclear aryl hydrocarbon receptor to the xenobiotic-responsive element of the CYP1A1 promoter but did not bind to the receptor [203]. These data demonstrated that resveratrol inhibits aryl hydrocarbon-induced CYP1A activity *in vitro* by directly inhibiting CYP1A1/CYP1A2 enzyme activity and by inhibiting the signal transduction pathway that up-regulates the expression of carcinogen activating enzymes [203].

*trans*-Resveratrol decreased the secretion of MMP-2 by cultured human liver myofibroblasts [204] and delphinidin inhibited the activity of MMP-2 and MMP-9 in human fibrosarcoma HT-1080 cells, an effect that may be responsible for its ability to inhibit tumor cell invasiveness [205]. Luteolin and quercetin suppressed EGF-induced secretion of MMP-2 and MMP-9 in A431 [206] and MiaPaCa-2 cells [207]. Proanthocyanidins from grape seeds inhibit the expression of matrix metalloproteinases in human prostate carcinoma DU145 cells [208]. Moreover, resveratrol was found to inhibit aryl hydrocarbon-induced CYP1A1 enzyme activity and expression in HepG2 cells. In addition, *trans*-resveratrol inhibited CYP1B1 activity and expression in MCF7 cells [209] while resveratrol has been reported as inhibitor of CYP3A4 and CYP2E1 in liver cells [210]. Finally, epsilonviniferin, a dimer of resveratrol, displaced a strong inhibitory effect for CYP1A1, CYP1B1, and CYP2B6, and to a lesser extent for CYP1A2, CYP2A6, CYP2E1, CYP3A4, and CYP4A [210]. The findings of Li et al. [211] indicated that resveratrol inhibited proliferation, induced apoptosis, and influenced cell cycle of Bel-7402 cells at a dose-and time-dependent manner in vitro. Furthermore, resveratrol could exert a dose-related down-regulatory effect on IL-8 in Bel-7402 bearing mice. It suggestes resveratrol might have chemotherapeutic potential and immunomodulation action to Bel-7402 to cellular carcinoma both *in vitro* and *in vivo*.

## 6.5. Gallic Acid

Gallic acid (3,4,5-trihydroxybenzoicacid, GA), is a polyhydroxyphenolic compound, which can be found in various natural products, like gallnuts, sumac, tea leaves, oak bark, green tea, apple-peels, grapes, strawberries, pineapples, bananas, lemons, and in red and white wine [212]. GA possesses cytotoxicity against cancer cells, and has anti-inflammatory and antimutagenic properties [213]. GA was described as an excellent free radical scavenger and as an inducer of differentiation and programmed cell death in a number of tumor cell lines [214-216]. Recently, it was revealed that GA from rose flowers exhibits antioxidative effects even in senescence accelerated mice and can reinstate the activities of catalase and gluthatione peroxidase [217]. Even though many reports revealed that gallic acid plays an important role in the prevention of malignant transformation and cancer development its effect on hepatocarcinogenesis.

In a study, pretreatment of the cultured cells with gallic acid, tea polyphenols or α-tocopherol could provide cytoprotective effect to the cells to improve cell viability, increase the content of reduced glutathione in cells, reduce lactate dehydrogenase leakage into culture medium and decrease the formation of malondialdehyde in the cells. It was shown that gallic acid and tea polyphenols displayed stronger cytoprotective effect against oxidative injury of the hepatocytes than α-tocopherol at same addition level and gallic acid was the most powerful compound [218]. To explore the effect of gallic acid extracted from leaves of *Phyllanthus emblica* on the apoptosis of BEL-7404 cells. Gallic acid could restrain the BEL-7404 cells proliferation at diffierent levels in a time and concentration dependent manner. The typical morphological changes of apoptosis were observed after BEL-7404 cells were treated with gallic acid. Annexin V/PI double label method and Tunel method showed that the viable apoptotic cell and apoptosis rates added as action time prolonged. Gallic acid can restrain the BEL-7404 cells proliferation and induce apoptosis, and its effect on apoptosis is time dependent [219]. Jagan et al. [220] investigated the antiproliferative effect of gallic acid during diethylnitrosamine (DEN)-induced HCC in male wistar albino rats. DEN treatment resulted in increased levels of aspartate transaminase, alanine transaminase, alkaline phosphatase, acid phosphatase, lactate dehydrogenase, gamma-glutamyltransferase, 50-nucleotidase, bilirubin, alpha-fetoprotein, carcinoembryonic antigen, argyophillic nucleolar organizing regions, and proliferating cell nuclear antigen. Gallic acid treatment significantly attenuated these alterations and decreased the levels of silver stained nucleolar organizer regions and tumor markers – proliferation.

## 6.6. Silymarin

Silymarin is a naturally available bioflavonoid, which is the main constituent of *Silybum marianum* (milk thistle, an European medicinal plant) and is a strong antioxidant with a capacity to inhibit the formation of tumors in several cancer models. Silymarin is composed mainly (80%, w/w) of silybin (also called silybinin, silybin, or silibinin) with smaller amounts of other stereoisomers such as isosilybin, dihydrosilybin, silydianin, and silychristin [221]. Silymarin has a strong antioxidant property and is able to scavenge both free radicals and reactive oxygen species [222]. Phamacological studies revealed that silymarin is non-toxic even at higher physiological doses, which suggests its safer use for the treatment of various diseases. Ramakrishnan et al. [223] observed that NDEA-induced rats showed severe hyperlipidemia along with upregulated expression of COX-2 as revealed by western blotting and immunohistochemistry. Dietary silymarin supplementation attenuated this hyperlipidemia and downregulated the expression of COX-2. Authors also concluded that compounds like silymarin with potent hypolipidemic effect are strong candidates as chemopreventive agents for the treatment of liver cancer. Silymarin exerted beneficial effects on liver carcinogenesis by attenuating the recruitment of mast cells and thereby decreased the expressions of MMP-2 and MMP-9 [224]. Silymarin inhibited population growth of the hepatocellular carcinoma cells in a dose-dependent manner, and the percentage of apoptotic cells. Silymarin treatment increased the proportion of cells with reduced DNA content (sub-$G(0)/G(1)$ or $A(0)$ peak), indicative of apoptosis with loss of cells in the $G(1)$ phase. Silymarin also decreased mitochondrial transmembrane potential of the cells, thereby increasing levels of cytosolic cytochrome c while up-regulating expression of pro-apoptotic proteins (such as p53, Bax, APAF-1 and caspase-3) with concomitant decrease in anti-apoptotic proteins (Bcl-2 and survivin) and proliferation-associated proteins (beta-catenin, cyclin D1, c-Myc and PCNA). These results demonstrated that silymarin treatment inhibited proliferation and induced apoptosis in the human hepatocellular carcinoma cell line HepG2 [224]. Silymarin treatment significantly attenuated the alteration of these markers and decreased the levels of MDA-DNA adduct formation. Silymarin could be developed as a promising chemotherapeutic adjuvant for the treatment of liver cancer. Silymarin treatment significantly attenuated the alteration of these markers and decreased the levels of MDA-DNA adduct formation. Silymarin could be developed as a promising chemotherapeutic adjuvant for the treatment of liver cancer. This drug exerts beneficial effects on the early stages of liver pathogenesis, preventing and delaying liver carcinogenesis [225]. Silymarin + NDEA treated groups 4 and 5 animals showed a significant decrease in the number of nodules with concomitant decrease in the lipid peroxidation status. The levels of GSH and the activities of antioxidant enzymes in both haemolysate and liver were improved when compared with hepatocellular carcinoma induced group 2 animals. The electron microscopy studies were also carried out which supports the chemopreventive action of the silymarin against NDEA administration during liver cancer progression [9]. These findings suggest that silymarin suppresses NDEA induced hepatocarcinogenesis by modulating the antioxidant defense status of the animals. Administration of garlic or silymarin significantly reduced the liver toxicity, combined administration was more effective in preventing the development of hepatotoxicity [226]. Altered enzyme levels were ameliorated significantly by administration of extract of *Terminalia arjuna* bark (EETA) at the concentration of 400 mg/kg in drug-treated animals [227]. This protective effect of EETA was associated with inhibition of LPO induced by DEN and to maintain the antioxidant enzyme levels. Our results show an antioxidant activity of *T. arjuna* bark against DEN-induced liver cancer might be presence of polyphenols.

## 6.7. Morin

Sivaramakrishnan and Devaraj [228] reported that the in vivo effect of morin (500ppm in diet) in fostering apoptosis in DEN (200mg/kg bodyweight) mediated experimental hepatocellular carcinogenesis model. We analyzed the expression of cytosolic protein Akt and their important apoptotic downstream targets like caspase-9, Bcl-2, Bax, GSK-3betain vivo, by immunoblot analysis. In silico docking studies indicated that morin could serve as a better inhibitor than the classical PI3K inhibitor LY294002. The results obtained from in vivo studies confirm this. We also demonstrate here that morin's interaction with a defined set of amino acids of PI3K p110gamma catalytic subunit resulted in the down-regulation of p-Akt(Ser473), p-Akt(Thr308) and total Akt causing the attenuation of its downstream targets in DEN-induced hepatocellular carcinoma. Further, morin caused the up-regulation of tumor suppressor PTEN, an important negative regulator of Akt, thus initiating apoptosis. Supplementation of morin to experimental animals modulated Bcl-2/Bax ratio causing the release of cyt C and up-regulation of caspase-3 and -9. Morin was also found to prevent the Akt-mediated suppression of GSK-3beta possibly causing cell cycle arrest at the G1/S phase. These observations were supported by the DNA fragmentation and transmission electron microscopy results, which showed the occurrence of apoptosis [228]. Reverse transcriptase polymerase chain reaction (RT-PCR) analysis revealed that administration of DEN (200 mg/kg bodyweight in drinking water) to experimental animals caused inflammation of the liver due to up-regulation of NF-kappaB-p65 and COX-2 [229]. RT-PCR and immunoblot analysis also revealed that the oral supplementation of morin (500 ppm in diet) to DEN-induced hepatocellular carcinoma rats down-regulated the expression of COX-2 and NF-kappaB-p65, thereby preventing inflammation and angiogenesis mediated hepatocellular carcinogenesis. Further, immunohistological analysis for NF-kappaB-p65 nuclear localization confirms the above observations. Gelatin zymography was performed for matrix metalloproteinase MMP-2 and MMP-9 expression to confirm their role in angiogenesis in DEN induced hepatocellular carcinoma and its modulation by morin [229]. Both MMP-2 and MMP-9 levels were found to be increased in DEN-induced animals when compared to control. MMP-2 and MMP-9 levels were down-regulated in morin post-treated animals when compared to DEN-induced animals favouring prevention of angiogenesis.

## 6.8. Others

*Ellagic acid* is a naturally occurring phenolic constituent in certain fruits and nuts. Research in the past decade confirms that Ellagic acid markedly inhibits the ability of other chemicals to cause mutations in bacteria. Ellagic acid from red raspberries has proven as an effective antimutagen and anticarcinogen as well as a inhibitor of cancer. Exposure to N-2-fluorenylacetamide (FAA) alone induced a substantial number of altered foci and at the end of experiment (week 36), the incidence of hepatocellular neoplasms was 100%. In the group receiving ellagic acid (EA) together with FAA, the number of altered foci was decreased at all time points and at termination, the final incidence of hepatocellular neoplasms (30%) was also reduced [230]. Thus, EA inhibited the hepatocarcinogenesis induced by FAA when it was administered concurrently with the carcinogen.

*Caffeic acid* (3,4-dihydroxycinnamic acid; CA) is a well-known phenolic phytochemical present in many foods, including coffee. Recent studies suggested that caffeic acid exerts anticarcinogenic effects, but little is known about the underlying molecular mechanisms and specific target proteins. CA, a strong and selective MMP-9 activity and transcription inhibitor, was isolated from the plant *Euonymus alatus* and its derivative, caffeic acid phenethyl ester (CAPE), was synthesized. CA and CAPE selectively inhibited MMP-2 and -9 but not -1, -3, -7, or cathepsin K. Treatment of HepG2 cells with CA (100 μg/mL) and CAPE (5 μg/mL) suppressed phorbol 12-myristate 13-acetate (PMA) -induced MMP-9 expression by inhibiting the function of NF-$\kappa$B, but not AP-1 [231]. Authors confirmed that CA and CAPE suppressed the growth of HepG2 tumor xenografts in nude mice in vivo. The subcutaneous and oral administrations of CA and CAPE significantly reduced the liver metastasis. These results confirm the therapeutic potential of the compounds and suggest that the anti-metastatic and anti-tumor effects of CA and CAPE are mediated through the selective suppression of MMP-9 enzyme activity and transcriptional down-regulation by the dual inhibition of NF-$\kappa$B as well as MMP-9 catalytic activity. CAPE, a natural component of propolis, shows anticarcinogenic properties in the modified resistant hepatocyte model when administered before initiation or promotion of hepatocarcinogenesis process. CAPE modifies the enzymatic activity of CYP isoforms involved in the activation of DEN, such as CYP1A1/2 and CYP2B1/2 [232]. These findings describe an alternative mechanism for understanding the ability of CAPE to protect against chemical hepatocarcinogenesis.

Administration of NDEA, 100 and 200 mg/kg of *Acacic nilotica* bark extract (ANBE) were administered orally once daily for 10 weeks. The levels of liver injury and liver cancer markers such as alanine transaminase (ALT), aspartate transaminase (AST), alkaline phosphatase (ALP), γ-glutamyl transferase (γ-GT), total bilirubin level (TBL), α-feto protein (AFP) and carcinoembryonic antigen (CEA) were substantially increased following NDEA treatment. However, ANBE treatment reduced liver injury and restored liver cancer markers [2]. ANBE also significantly prevented hepatic MDA formation and reduced GSH in NDEA-treated rats which was dose dependent. Additionally, ANBE also increased the activities of antioxidant enzymes viz., catalase (CAT), superoxide dismutase (SOD), glutathione peroxidase (GPx), and glutathione-*S*-transferase (GST) in the liver of NDEA-administered rats. Eventually, ANBE also significantly improved body weight and prevented increase of relative liver weight due to NDEA treatment [2]. Histological observations of liver tissues too correlated with the biochemical observations. HPLC analysis of ANBE showed the presence of gallic, protocatechuic, caffeic and ellagic acids, and also quercetin in ANBE. The results strongly support that *A. nilotica* bark prevents LPO and promote the enzymatic and non-enzymatic antioxidant defense system during NDEA-induced hepatocarcinogenesis which might be due to activities like scavenging of oxy radicals by the phytomolecules in ANBE [2].

*Thrombin* has been recently demonstrated to promote HCC cell migration by activation of the proteinase-activated receptor (PAR) subtypes PAR1 and PAR4 suggesting a role of these proteinase-receptor systems in HCC progression. In this study, we investigated the effect of (-)-EGCG, the major polyphenolic compound of green tea on thrombin-PAR1/PAR4-mediated hepatocellular carcinoma cell invasion and p42/p44 MAPKinase activation. Stimulation of HCC cells with thrombin, the PAR1-selective activating peptide, TFLLRN-NH2, and the PAR4-selective activating peptide, AYPGKF-NH2, increased cell invasion across a Matrigel-coated membrane barrier and stimulated activation of p42/p44 MAPK phosphorylation. Both the effects on p42/p44 MAPKs, and on cell invasiveness induced by thrombin and the PAR1/4 subtype-selective agonist peptides were effectively blocked by EGCG (Kaufmann et al., 2009). The results clearly identify EGCG as a potent inhibitor of the thrombin-PAR1/PAR4-p42/p44 MAPK invasive signaling axis in hepatocellular carcinoma cells as a previously unrecognized mode of action for EGCG in cancer cells. Moreover, the results suggest that (-)-epigal-locatechin-3-gallate might have therapeutic potential for hepatocellular carcinoma. Aldo-keto reductase family 1 B10 (AKR1B10) is a member of the NADPH-dependent aldo-keto reductase (AKR) superfamily, and has been considered to be a potential cancer therapeutic target. Total extract from the bark of *Rhus verniciflua* (*Toxicodendron vernicifluum* (Stokes)) showed AKR1B10 inhibitory activity [233]. To identify the active compounds from *R. verniciflua* responsible for AKR1B10 inhibition, nine compounds were isolated via bioactivity-guided isolation and tested for their effects against recombinant human AKR1B10 (rhAKR1B10). Results showed that butein, isolated from the ethyl acetate fraction, was most able to inhibit rhAKR1B10 [233].

The dietary administration of DAB induced well-differentiated HCC that showed increased expression of the markers of invasion, angiogenesis and epigenetic histone deacetylation compared with the controls [234]. The administration of Polyphenon-B significantly reduced the incidence of DAB-induced hepatomas as evidenced by modulation of the markers of invasion (matrix metalloproteinase, MMP-2, MMP-9, tissue inhibitor of matrix metalloproteinase, TIMP-2, and reversion-inducing cysteine rich protein with Kazal motifs RECK) and angiogenesis (hypoxia inducible factor 1α, HIF1α, vascular endothelial growth factor, VEGF, and VEGF receptor, VEGFR1) as well as the expression of histone deacetylase HDAC-1 [234]. Ginseng has been shown to enhance natural healing power and to improve general conditions and non-specific complaints due to the exhaustive and feverish illness through enhancement of natural healing power. Also, ginseng has been shown to inhibit carcinogenesis in animal models [235-237]. A recent case-control study in Korea demonstrated the prevention of cancer development in several organs by ginseng ingestion [238,239]. In the course of discussion, Fukushima and his colleagues who conducted animal carcinogenesis experiments, stated that ginseng did not increase or decrease the development of preneoplastic lesions in the liver. In an experiment found that red ginseng rather than white ginseng significantly inhibited the development of spontaneous liver tumors in mice. According to available data and studies, authors concluded that the intervention trial of ginseng on HCC could be applicable to the high risk group [240]. Background Dietary polyphenols have been reported to have a variety of biological actions, including anticarcinogenic and antioxidant activities. The polyphenols concentrations tested in presence or absence of Fpg (formamidopyrimidine-DNA glycosylase), or Endo III (Endonuclease III) caused DNA damage per se. Increasing concentrations of benzo(a)pyrene (BaP) (25-100 μM) induced a significant increase of DNA strand breaks, Fpg and Endo III sensitive sites in a dose dependent manner [241]. Myricetin and quercetin decreased DNA strand breaks and oxidized pyrimidines induced by NDEA, but not oxidized purines. However, both flavonoids reduced oxidized pyrimidines and purines induced by *N*-nitrosopyrrolidine (NPYR). DNA strand breaks induced by NPYR were prevented by quercetin, but not by myricetin. BaP-induced DNA strand breaks and oxidized pyrimidines were strongly reduced by myricetin and quercetin, respectively. While oxidized purines induced by BaP were reduced by quercetin, myricetin had no protective effect [241]. (+)-Catechin and (-)-epicatechin reduced DNA strand breaks, oxidized pyrimidines and oxidized purines induced by NDMA. DNA strand breaks, and oxidized purines induced by NPYR were also prevented by (+)-catechin and (-)-epicatechin, while the maximum reduction of oxidized pyrimidines was found by (+)-catechin and (-)-epicatechin at 10 µM. (+)-Catechin and (-)-epicatechin decreased also DNA strand breaks and oxidized pyrimidines but not oxidized purines induced by BaP [241]. These results clearly indicated that polyphenols protect human derived cells against DNA strand breaks and oxidative DNA damage effects of NDMA, NPYR or BaP, three carcinogenic compounds which occur in the environment.

# Conclusion

From this discussion it is clear that numerous polyphenolic compounds in fruits, vegetables, herbs and medicinal plants can interfere with multiple cell-signaling pathways. These compounds with strong antioxidant activity can be used either in their natural form for the prevention and perhaps in their pure form for the therapy for liver cancer, where large doses may be needed. While these polyphenolic compounds are pharmacologically safe in most situations, one of the concerns commonly expressed is the lack of bioavailability. Experience again indicates that these agents exhibit bioresponse at serum concentrations that are insufficient to demonstrate in vitro response; thus suggesting that their bioavailability should not be evaluated in the same manner as synthetic compounds. Most modern medicines currently available for treating liver cancers are very expensive, toxic, and less effective in treating the disease. Thus, one must investigate further in detail the agents derived from natural sources, described traditionally, for the prevention and treatment of liver cancer and disease. More clinical trials are also needed to validate the usefulness of these agents either alone or in combination with existing therapy.

# References

[1]   Plymoth S. Viviani and P. Hainaut. Control of hepatocellular carcinoma through Hepatitis B vaccination in areas of high endemicity: perspectives for global liver cancer prevention. *Cancer Letter*, 286(1),15–21, 2009.

[2]   N. Singh, B. R. Singh, B.K. Sarma, and H. B. Singh. Potential chemoprevention of N-nitrosodiethylamine-induced hepatocarcinogenesis by polyphenolics from Acacia nilotica bark. *Chemico-Biological Interactions*, 181,20–28, 2009a.

[3]   J. Ferlay, J. Bray, P. Pisani and D. M. Parkin. GLOBOCAN 2000: *Cancer incidence, Mortality and Prevalence Worldwide*. Version 1.0. IARC CancerBase No 5. International Agency for Research on Cancer, Lyon: IARC Press, 2001 [Limited version available from: *http://www-dep.iarc.fr/globocan/globocan.htm*].

[4]   H. B. Singh. B. N. Singh, S. P. Singh, and C. S. Nautiyal. Solid-state cultivation of Trichoderma harzianum NBRI-1055 for modulating natural antioxidants in soybean seed matrix. *Bioresource Technology, doi:10.1016/j.biortech.2010.03.057, (2010a).*

[5]  F. X. Bosch and J. Ribes. Chapter 1: Global Epidemiology. The Epidemiology of Primary Liver Cancer. In: Tabor E. (ed.) *Viruses and Liver Cancer. Rockville* (USA): Elsevier, 2002.

[6]  H. B. El-Serag and A. C. Mason. Risk factors for the rising rates of primary liver cancer in the United States. *Arch Intern Med*, 160,3227-3230, 2000.

[7]  G. J. Kapadia, M. A. Azuine, J. Takayasu, T. Konoshima, M. Takasaki, H. Nishino and H. Tokuda. Inhibition of Epstein-Barr virus early antigen activation promoted by 12-O-tetradecanoylphorbol-13-acetate by the non-steroidal anti-inflammatory drugs. *Cancer Letter* 161,221–229, 2000.

[8]  K. J. Jeena, K. L. Joy and R. Kuttan. Effect of Emblica officinalis, Phyllanthus amarus and Picrorrhiza kurroa on N-nitrosodiethylamine induced hepatocarcinogenesis. *Cancer Letter* 136,11–16, 1999.

[9]  G. Ramakrishnan, H. R. B. Raghavendran, R. Vinodhkumar and T. Devaki. Suppression of N-nitrosodiethylamine induced hepatocarcinogenesis by silymarin in rats. *Chemico-Biological Interactions*, 161,104–114, 2006.

[10]  B. B. Aggarwal and S. Shishodia. Molecular targets of dietary agents for prevention and therapy of cancer. *Biochemical Pharmacology*, 71,1397–1421, 2006.

[11]  H. Ch. Chang-qi K. sh., Qian R. Kilkuskie, Ch. Yung-chi and L. Kuo-Hsiung. Anti-AIDS agent, acacetin-7-O-β-D-galactopyranoside, an anti-HIV principle from Chrysanthemum morifolium and a structure–activity correlation with some related Flavonoids. *Journal of Natural Product*, 57,42–51, 1994.

[12]  F. Shahidi and M. Naczk. *Food Phenolics. Sources, Chemistry, Effects, Applications.* Lancaster, USA: Technomic Publishing Company, Inc. 1995.

[13]  J. B. Harborne. *The Flavonoids: Advances in Research Since 1986.* London, UK: Chapman & Hall, 1994.

[14]  D. Strack. Phenolic metabolism. In: Dey PM, Harborne JB, eds. *Plant Biochemistry.* London, UK: Academic Press, p. 387–416, 1997.

[15]  J. Kühnau. The Flavonoids: A Class of Semi –Essential Food Components; Their role in human nutrition. *World Review of Nutrition and Dietetics*, 24,117-191, 1976.

[16]  V. Di Matteo and E. Esposito. Biochemical and therapeutic effects of antioxidants in the treatment of Alzheimer's disease, Parkinson's disease, and amyotrophic lateral sclerosis, *Curr. Drug Targets-CNS Neurological Disorders*, 2,95–107, 2003.

[17]  S. N. Ames, M. K. Shigenaga and T. M. Hagen. Oxidants, antioxidants and degenerative diseases of aging. *The Procedings of National Acedemy of Sciences*, USA, 90,7915–7922, 1993.

[18]  D. Prakash, B. N. Singh, and G. Upadhyay. Antioxidant and free radical scavenging activities of phenols from onion (Allium cepa). *Food Chemistry*, 102,1389–1393, 2007a.

[19]  D. Prakash, S. Suri, G. Upadhyay and B. N. Singh. Total phenols, Antioxidant and Free radical scavenging activities of some medicinal plants. *International Journal of Food Science and Nutrition*, 58(1), 18–28, 2007b.

[20]  B. N. Singh, B. R. Singh, R. L. Singh, D. Prakash, R. Dhakarey, G. Upadhyay and H. B. Singh. Oxidative DNA damage protective activity, antioxidant and anti-quorum sensing potentials of Moringa oleifera. *Food and Chemical Toxicology*, 47(6),1109–1116, 2009b.

[21] K. L. Khanduja, R. Gandhi, K.V. Pathania and N. Syal. Prevention of N-nitrosodiethylamine-induced lung tumorigenesis by ellagic acid and quercetin in mice. *Food and Chemical Toxicology*, 37,313–318, 1999.

[22] V. R. Vásquez-Garzón, J. Arellanes-Robledo, R. Garcia-Román, D. I. Aparicio-Rautista and S. Villa-Trevino, Inhibition of reactive oxygen species and preneoplastic lesions by quercetin through an antioxidant defense mechanism. *Free Radical Research*, 43,128–137, 2009.

[23] T. Tanaka, T. Kojima, T. Kawamori, N. Yoshimi, H. Mori. Chemoprevention of diethylnitrosamine-induced hepatocarcinogenesis by a simple phenolic acid protocatechuic acid in rats. *Cancer Research*, 53,2775–2779, 1993.

[24] T. Tanaka, T. Kawamori, M. Ohnishi, K. Okamoto, H. Mori and A. Hara. Chemoprevention of 4-nitroquinoline 1-oxide-induced oral carcinogenesis by dietary protocatechuic acid during initiation and postinitiation phases. *Cancer Research*, 54,2359–2365, 1994.

[25] K. Polewski, S. Kniat and D. Slawinska. Gallic acid, a natural antioxidant, in aqueous and micellar environment: spectroscopic studies. *Current Topics in Biophysics*, 26,217–227, 2002.

[26] O. Beltrán-Ramírez, L. Alemán-Lazarini, M. Salcido-Neyoy, S.Hernández-García and S. Fattel-Fazenda et al. Evidence that the anticarcinogenic effect of caffeic acid phenethyl ester in the resistant hepatocyte model involves modifications of cytochrome P450. *Toxicological Science*, 10,100–106, 2008.

[27] R. Garcia-Closas, C. A. Gonzales, A. Agudo and E. Riboli. Intake of specific carotenoids and flavonoids and the risk of gastric cancer in Spain. Cancer Causes, 10,71–75, 1999.

[28] H. Bartsch, and R. Montesano. Relevance of nitrosoamines to human cancer. *Carcinogenesis*, 5,1381–1395, 1984.

[29] R. N. Loeppky. Nitrosamine and nitroso compound chemistry and biochemistry, in: *ACS Symposium Series*, vol. 553, American Chemical Society, Washington, DC, pp. 1–12, 1994.

[30] J. E. Klaunig and L. M. Kamendulis. The role of oxidative stress in carcinogenesis. *Annual Review of Pharmacology and Toxicology*, 44,239–267, 2004.

[31] M. Valko, C. J. Rhodes, J. Moncol, M. T. Cronin and M. Mazur. Free radicals, metals and antioxidants in oxidative stress-induced cancer. *Chemico-Biological Interactions*, 160,1–4, 2006.

[32] G. Fattovich and S. W. Schalm. Hepatitis C and cirrhosis. In: T. J. Liang, J. H. Hoofnagle eds. *Hepatitis C*. San Diego: Academic Press, 241-263, 2000.

[33] Z. Y. Tang. Hepatocellular Carcinoma-Cause, Treatment and Metastasis. *World Journal of Gastroenterology*, 7(4), 445-454, 2001.

[34] S. Bruno, E. Silini, A. Crosignani, F. Borzio, G Leandro, F. Bono et al. Hepatitis C virus genotypes and risk of hepatocellular carcinoma in cirrhosis: a prospective study. *Hepatology*, 25,754-758, 1997.

[35] H. Tanaka, H. Tsukuma, H. Yamano, Y. Okubo, A. Inoue, A. Kasahara and N. Hayashi. Hepatitis C virus 1b (II) infection and development of chronic hepatitis, liver cirrhosis and hepatocellular carcinoma: a case-control study in Japan. *Journal of Epidemiology* 8,244-249, 1998.

[36] J. F. Tsai, J. E. Jeng ,M. S. Ho, W. Y. Chang, M. Y. Hsieh, Z. Y. Lin and J. H. Tsai. Effect of hepatitis C and B virus infection on risk of hepatocellular carcinoma: a prospective study. *British Journal of Cancer*, 76,968-974, 1997.

[37] A. S. Abdulkarim, N. N. Zein, J. J. Germer, C. P. Kolbert, L. Kabbani, K. L. Krajnik, A. Hola, M. N. Agha, M. Tourogman and D. H. Persing. Hepatitis C virus genotypes and Hepatitis G virus in hemodialysis patients from Syria: identification of two novel hepatitis C virus subtypes. *American Journal of Tropical Medicine and Hygine*, 59,571–576, 1998.

[38] K. Tarao, Y. Rino, S. Ohkawa, A. Shimizu, S. Tamai, K. Miyakawa, H. Aoki, T. Imada K. Shindo, N. Okamoto, S. Totsuka. Association between high serum alanine aminotransferase levels and more rapid development and higher rate of incidence of hepatocellular carcinoma in patients with hepatitis C virus-associated cirrhosis. *Cancer*, 86,589-595, 1999.

[39] K. Moriya, H. Fujie, Y. Shintani, H. Yotsuyanagi ,T. Tsutsumi and K. Ishibashi. The core protein of hepatitis C virus induces hepatocellular carcinoma in transgenic mice. *Nature Medicine*, 4,1065-1067, 1998.

[40] J. I. Pitt and L. Tomaska. Are mycotoxins a health hazard in Australia? *Food Australia*, 53(12),545–559, 2001.

[41] J. D. Groopman, T W. Kensler and C. P. Wild. Protective interventions to prevent aflatoxin-induced carcinogenesis in developing countries. *Annual Review of Public Health*, 29,187–203, 2008.

[42] C. P. Wild and Y. Y. Gong. Mycotoxins and human disease: a largely ignored global health issue. *Carcinogenesis*, 31,71–82, 2010.

[43] A. Plymoth, S. Viviani and P. Hainaut. Control of hepatocellular carcinoma through Hepatitis B vaccination in areas of high endemicity: perspectives for global liver cancer prevention. *Cancer Letter*, 286(1),15–21, 2009.

[44] C. P. Wild, and R Montesano. A model of interaction: aflatoxins and hepatitis viruses in liver cancer aetiology and prevention. *Cancer Letter*, 286(1),22–28, 2009.

[45] G. D. Kirk, E. Bah and R. Montesano. Molecular epidemiology of human liver cancer: insights into etiology, pathogenesis and prevention from The Gambia, West Africa. *Carcinogenesis*, 27(10),2070–2082, 2006.

[46] M. Moriyama, H. Matsumura and H. Aoki et al. Long-term outcome, with monitoring of platelet counts, in patients with chronic hepatitis C and liver cirrhosis after interferon therapy. *Intervirology*, 46,296-307, 2003.

[47] M. M. Hassan, L. Y. Hwang, C. J. Hatten et al. Risk factors for hepatocellular carcinoma: synergism of alcohol with viral hepatitis and diabetes mellitus. *Hepatology*, 36,1206-1213, 2002.

[48] M. Schoniger-Hekele, C. Muller, M. Kutilek et al. Hepatocellular carcinoma in Austria: aetiological and clinical characteristics at presentation. *European Journal of Gastroenterology and Hepatology*, 12,941-948, 2000.

[49] Serag, H. B. and A. C. Mason. Risk factors for the rising rates of primary liver cancer in the United States. *Archives of Internal Medicine*, 160, 3227-3230, 2000.

[50] H. Kuper, A. Tzonou, E. Kaklamani, C. C. Hsieh, P. Lagiou, H. O. Adami, D. Trichopoulos and S. O. Stuver. Tobacco smoking, alcohol consumption and their interaction in the causation of hepatocellular carcinoma. *International Journal of Cancer*, 85,498-502, 2000.

[51] M. Mori, M. Hara, I. Wada, T. Hara, K. Yamamoto, M. Honda and J. Naramoto. Prospective study of hepatitis B and C viral infections, cigarette smoking, alcohol consumption, and other factors associated with hepatocellular carcinoma risk in Japan. *American Journal of Epidemiology*, 151,31-139, 2000.

[52] F. Donato, A. Tagger, R. Chiesa, M. L. Ribero, V. Tomasoni, M. Fasola, U. Gelatti, G. Portera, P. Boffetta and G. Nardi. Hepatitis B and C virus infection, alcohol drinking, and hepatocellular carcinoma: a case-control study in Italy. Brescia HCC Study. *Hepatology*, 26,579-584, 1997.

[53] A. Tagger, F. Donato, M. L. Ribero, R. Chiesa, G. Portera, U. Gelatti, A. Albertini, M. Fasola, P. Boffetta and G. Nardi. Case-control study on hepatitis C virus (HCV) as a risk factor for hepatocellular carcinoma: the role of HCV genotypes and the synergism with hepatitis B virus and alcohol. Brescia HCC Study. *International Journal of Cancer*, 81,695-699, 1999.

[54] E. Bugianesi, N. Leone and E. Vanni et al. Expanding the natural history of nonalcoholic steatohepatitis: from cryptogenic cirrhosis to hepatocellular carcinoma. *Gastroenterology*, 123,134-140, 2002.

[55] M. Elmberg, R. Hultcrantz and A. Ekbom et al. Cancer risk in patients with hereditary hemochromatosis and in their first-degree relatives. *Gastroenterology*, 125,1733-1741, 2003.

[56] H. O. Adami, W. H. Chow, and O. Nyren et al. Excess risk of primary liver cancer in patients with diabetes mellitus. *Journal of National Cancer Institute*, 88,1472-1477, 1996.

[57] N. Singh, T. Gayowski, V. L. Yu, and M. M. Wagener. Trimethoprim-sulfamethoxazole for the prevention of spontaneous bacterial peritonitis in cirrhosis: a randomized trial. *Annals of International Medicine*, 122,595-598, 1995.

[58] A. L. Fracanzani, D. Conte, and M. Fraquelli et al. Increased cancer risk in a cohort of 230 patients with hereditary hemochromatosis in comparison to matched control patients with non-iron-related chronic liver disease. Hepatology, 33,647-651, 2001.

[59] L. Caballeria, A. Pares, A. Castells, A. Gines, C. Bru and J. Rodes. Hepatocellular carcinoma in primary biliary cirrhosis: similar incidence to that in hepatitis C virus-related cirrhosis. *American Journal Gastroenterology*, 96,1160-1163, 2001.

[60] S. Sell and F. F. Beckar. Alpha feto protein. *National Cancer Institute*, 60,19–26, 1978.

[61] G. I. Abelev, S. D. Perova, N. I. Khramkova, Z. A. Postnikova and I. S. Irlin. Production of embryonal alpha-globulin by transplantable mouse hepatomas. *Transplantation*, 1,174–180, 1963.

[62] S. Gupta, S. Bent and J Kohlwes. Test characteristics of alpha-fetoprotein for detecting hepatocellular carcinoma in patients with hepatitis C. A systematic review and critical analysis. *Annals of Internal Medicine*, 139,46–50, 2003.

[63] K. Taketa, C. Sekiya, M. Namiki, K. Akamatsu, Y. Ohta, Y. Endo and K. Kosaka. Lectin-reactive profiles of alpha-fetoprotein characterizing hepatocellular carcinoma and related conditions. *Gastroenterology*, 99,508–518, 1990.

[64] A. Leerapun S. V. Suravarapu J. P. Bida R. J. Clark E. L. Sanders T. A. Mettler and L. M. Stadheim et al. The utility of Lens culinaris agglutinin-reactive alpha-fetoprotein in the diagnosis of hepatocellular carcinoma: evaluation in a United States referral population. *Clinical Gastroenterology and Hepatology,* 5,394–402, 2007.

[65] H. Oka, A. Saito, K. Ito, T. Kumada, S. Satomura, H. Kasugai, Y. Osaki, T. Seki M. Kudo and S. Nagataki. Multicenter prospective analysis of newly diagnosed hepatocellular carcinoma with respect to the percentage of Lens culinaris agglutinin-reactive alpha-fetoprotein. *Journal of Gastroenterology and Hepatology*, 16,1378–1383, 2001.

[66] Y. Sato, K. Nakata, Y. Kato, M. Shima, N. Ishii, T. Koji, K. Taketa, Y. Endo and S Nagataki. Early recognition of hepatocellular carcinoma based on altered profiles of alpha-fetoprotein. *New England Journal of Medicine*, 328,1802–1806, 1993.

[67] R. K. Sterling, L. Jeffers, F. Gordon, M. Sherman, A. P. Venook, K. R. Reddy, S. Satomura and M. E. Schwartz. Clinical utility of AFP-L3% measurement in North American patients with HCVrelated cirrhosis. *American Journal of Gastroenterology*, 102,2196–2205, 2007.

[68] S. S. Wang, R. H. Lu, F. Y. Lee, Y. Chao, Y. S. Huang C. C. Chen and S. D. Lee. Utility of lentil lectin affinity of alpha-fetoprotein in the diagnosis of hepatocellular carcinoma. *Journal of Hepatology*, 25,166–171, 1996.

[69] P. Gold and S. O. Freedman. Specific carcinoembryonic antigens of the human digestive system. *Journal of Experimental Medicine*, 122,467-481, 1965.

[70] M. Maeda, S. Tozuka, M. Kanayama and T. Uchida. Hepatocellular carcinoma producing carcinoembryonic antigen. *Digestive Diseases and Sciences*, 33(12),1629-163, 1983.

[71] M. Makuuchi, N. Kokudo and S. Arii et al. Development of evidencebased clinical guidelines for the diagnosis and treatment of hepatocellular carcinoma in Japan. *Hepatological Research*, 38,37–51, 2008.

[72] H. A. Liebman, B. C. Furie and M. J. Tong et al. Des-γ-carboxy (abnormal) prothrombin as a serum marker of primary hepatocellular carcinoma. *New England Journal of Medicine*, 310,1427–1431, 1984.

[73] M. Ishii, H. Gama, N. Chida, Y. Ueno, H. Shinzawa, T. Takagi, T. Toyota, T. Takahashi and R. Kasukawa. Simultaneous measurements of serum alpha-fetoprotein and protein induced by vitamin K absence for detecting hepatocellular carcinoma. South Tohoku District Study Group. *American Journal of Gastroenterology*, 95,1036–1040, 2000.

[74] Marrero, J. A,. G. L. Su, W. Wei, D. Emick, H. S. Conjeevaram, R. J. Fontana and AS Lok. Des-gamma carboxyprothrombin can differentiate hepatocellular carcinoma from nonmalignant chronic liver disease in American patients. *Hepatology*, 37,1114–1121, 2003.

[75] S. Nakamura, K. Nouso. K. Sakaguchi. Y. M. Ito. Y. Ohashi. Y. Kobayashi. N. Toshikuni. H. Tanaka. Y. Miyake. E. Matsumoto and Y. Shiratori. Sensitivity and specificity of des-gamma-carboxy prothrombin for diagnosis of patients with hepatocellular carcinomas varies according to tumor size. *American Journal of Gastroenterology*, 101,2038–2043, 2006.

[76] M. L. Volk. J. C. Hernandez. G. L. Su. A. S. Lok and J. A. Marrero. Risk factors for hepatocellular carcinoma may impair the performance of biomarkers: a comparison of AFP, DCP, and AFP-L3. *Cancer Biomark*, 3,79–87, 2007.

[77] H. C. Hsu. W. Cheng and P. L. Lai. Cloning and expression of a developmentally regulated transcript MXR7 in hepatocellular carcinoma:biological significance and temporospatial distribution. *Cancer Research*, 57,5179–5184, 1997.

[78] P. N. Grozdanov. M. I. Yovchev and M. D. Dabeva. The oncofetal protein glypican-3 is a novel marker of hepatic progenitor/oval cells. *Lab Investigation* 86,1272–1284, 2006.

[79] Y. Y. Xiang, V. Ladeda and J. Filmus. Glypican-3 expression is silenced in human breast cancer. *Oncogene*, 20,7408–12, 2001.

[80] H. Kim, G. L. Xu, A. C Borczuk, S. Busch, J. Filmus, M. Capurro et al. The heparan sulfate proteoglycan GPC3 is a potential lung tumour suppressor. American *Journal of Respiration and Cell Molecular Biology*, 29,694–701, 2003.

[81] X. B. Man, L. Tang, B. H. Zhang, S.J. Li, X. H. Qiu, M. C. Wu et al. Upregulation of Glypican-3 expression in hepatocellular carcinoma but downregulation in cholangiocarcinoma indicates its differential diagnosis value in primary liver cancers. *Liver International*, 25,962–6, 2005.

[82] Z. W. Zhu, H. Friess, L. Wang, M. Abou-Shady, A. Zimmermann and A. D. Lander et al. Enhanced glypican-3 expression differentiates the majority of hepatocellular carcinomas from benign hepatic disorders. *Gut*, 48,558–64 2001.

[83] Capurro M, Wanless IR, Sherman M, Deboer G, Shi W, Miyoshi E, Filmus J: Glypican-3: a novel serum and histochemical marker for hepatocellular carcinoma. *Gastroenterology*, 125,89–97, 2003.

[84] L. Di Tommaso, G. Franchi, Y. N. Park, B. Fiamengo, A. Destro, E. Morenghi et al. Diagnostic value of HSP70, glypican 3, and glutamine synthetase in hepatocellular nodules in cirrhosis. *Hepatology*, 45,725–734, 2007.

[85] Hippo Y, Watanabe K, Watanabe A, Midorikawa Y, Yamamoto S, Ihara S. et al. Identification of soluble NH2-terminal fragment of glypican-3 as a serological marker for early-stage hepatocellular carcinoma. *Cancer Research*, 64, 2418–2423, 2004.

[86] R. Iftikhar, R. D. Kladney, N. Havlioglu, A. Schmitt-Gräff, I. Gusmirovic H. and Solomon B. A. et al. Diseaseand cell-specific expression of GP73 in human liver disease. *American Journal of Gastroenterology*, 99,1087–1095, 2004.

[87] S. W. Johnson and J. A. Alhadeff. Mammalian alpha-L-fucosidases. *Comparative Biochemistry and Physiology Part-B*, 99,479–488, 1991.

[88] T. M. Block, M. A. Comunale, M. Lowman, L. F. Steel, P. R. Romano and C. Fimmel et al. Use of targeted glycoproteomics to identify serum glycoproteins that correlate with liver cancer in woodchucks and humans. *The Proccedings of the National Academy of Science*, USA, 102,779–784, 2005.

[89] J. A. Marrero, P. R. Romano, O. Nikolaeva, L. Steel, A. Mehta, C. J. Fimmel, M. A. Comunale, A. D'Amelio, A. S. Lok, T. M. Block. GP73, a resident Golgi glycoprotein, is a novel serum marker for hepatocellular carcinoma. *Journal of Hepatology*, 43,1007–1012, 2005.

[90] J. P. Annes, J. S. Munger and D. B. Rifkin. Making sense of latent TGF-activation. *Journal of Cell Science*, 116,217–224, 2003.

[91] B. C. Song, Y. H. Chung, J. A. Kim, W. B. Choi, D. D. Suh, S. I. Pyo, J. W. Shin, H. C. Lee, Y. S. Lee and D. J. Suh. Transforming growth factor-α1 as a useful serologic marker of small hepatocellular carcinoma. *Cancer*, 94,175–180, 2002.

[92] H. Yu and T. Rohan. Role of the insulin-like growth factor family in cancer development and progression. *Journal of National Cancer Institute*, 92, 1472–1489, 2000.

[93] J. F. Tsai, J. E. Jeng, L. Y. Chuang, H. L. You, M. S. Ho and C. S. Lai et al. Serum insulin-like growth factor-II and alpha-fetoprotein as tumor markers of hepatocellular carcinoma. *Tumor Biology,* 24,291–298, 2003.

[94] M. Howard A. O'Garra, H. Ishida R. de Waal Malefyt and J. de Vries. Biological properties of interleukin 10. *Journal of Clinical Immunology*, 12,239–247, 1992.

[95] G. Y. Chau, C. W. Wu, W. Y. Lui, T. J. Chang, H. L. Kao and L. H. Wu et al. Serum interleukin-10 but not interleukin-6 is related to clinical outcome in patients with resectable hepatocellular carcinoma. *Annals of Surgery*, 231,552–558, 2000.

[96] C. Y. Hsia, T. I. Huo, S. Y. Chiang, M. F. Lu, C. L. Sun, J. C. Wu et al. Evaluation of interleukin-6, interleukin-10 and human hepatocyte growth factor as tumor markers for hepatocellular carcinoma. *Eurpean Journal of Surgery Oncology*, 33,208–212, 2007.

[97] R. Cui, J. He, F. Zhang ,B. Wang, H. Ding, H. Shen, Y. Li and X. Chen. Diagnostic value of protein induced by vitamin K absence (PIVKAII) and hepatoma-specific band of serum gamma-glutamyl transferase (GGTII) as hepatocellular carcinoma markers complementary to alpha-fetoprotein. *British Journal of Cancer*, 88, 1878–1882, 2003.

[98] Y. Deugnier, V. David, P. Brissot, P. Mabo, D. Delamaire, M. Messner, M. Bourel and J. Y. Legall. Serum alpha-l-fucosidase: a new marker for the diagnosis of primary hepatic carcinoma? *Hepatology*, 4,889–892, 1984.

[99] M. G. Giardina, M. Matarazzo, R. Morante, A. Lucariello, A. Varriale, V. Guardasole and G. De Marco. Serum alpha-L-fucosidase activity and early detection of hepatocellular carcinoma: a prospective study of patients with cirrhosis. *Cancer*, 83,2468–2474, 1998.

[100] S. W. Johnson and J. A. Alhadeff. Mammalian alpha-L-fucosidases. *Comperative Biochemistry and Physiology* Part-B, 99,479–488, 1991.

[101] S. K. Yoon, N. K. Lim, S. A. Ha, Y. G. Park, J. Y. Choi, K. W. Chung and H. S. Sun et al. The human cervical cancer oncogene protein is a biomarker for human hepatocellular carcinoma. *Cancer Research*, 64,5434–5441, 2004.

[102] K. Masutomi, S. Kaneko, M. Yasukawa, K. Arai, S. Murakami and K. Kobayashi. Identification of serum anti-human telomerase reverse transcriptase (hTERT) auto-antibodies during progression to hepatocellular carcinoma. *Oncogene*, 21,5946–5950, 2002.

[103] H. W. Hann, J. Lee, A. Bussard, C. Liu, Y. R. Jin, K. Guha, M. M. Clayton, K. Ardlie, M. J. Pellini and M. A. Feitelson. Preneoplastic markers of hepatitis B virus-associated hepatocellular carcinoma. *Cancer Research,* 64,7329–7335, 2004.

[104] B.N. Singh, G. Zhang, Y. L. Hwa, J. Li, S. C. Dowdy and S. W. Jiang. Nonhistone protein acetylation as cancer therapy targets. *Expert Review of Anticancer Therapy*, (In press), (2010b).

[105] D. Prakash, G. Upadhyay, B. N. Singh, R. Dhakarey, S. Kumar and K. K. Singh. Free radical scavenging activities of Himalayan Rhododendrons. *Current Science*, 92(4),526–532, 2007c..

[106] D. Prakash G. Upadhyay B. N. Singh and H. B. Singh. Antioxidant and free radical-scavenging activities of seeds and agri-wastes of some varieties of soybean (Glycine max). *Food Chemistry*, 104,783–790, 2007d.

[107] B. N. Singh, B. R. Singh, R. L. Singh, D. Prakash, B. K. Sarma and H. B. Singh. Antioxidant and anti-quorum sensing activities of green pod of *Acacia nilotica L. Food and Chemical Toxicology*, 47(4),778–786, 2009c.

[108] B. N. Singh, B. R. Singh, R. L. Singh, D. Prakash, D. P. Singh, B. K. Sarma, G. Upadhyay, H.B. Singh. Polyphenolics from various extracts/fractions of red onion (Allium cepa) peel with potential antioxidant and antimutagenic activities. *Food and Chemical Toxicology*, 47(6),1161–1167, 2009d.

[109] A. Escarpa and M.C. Gonzalez. An overview of analytical chemistry of phenolic compounds in foods. *Critical Review of Analytical Chemistry*, 31,57-139, 2001.

[110] S. N. Nichenametla, T. G. Taruscio, D. L. Barney and J. H. Exon. A review of the effects and mechanisms of polyphenolics in cancer. Critical *Review of Food Science and Nutrition*, 46,161–183, 2006.

[111] T. P. Kondratyuk and J. M. Pezzuto. Natural Product Polyphenols of Relevance to Human Health. *Pharmaceutical Biology*, 42,46-63, 2004.

[112] J. J. Macheix, A. Fleuriet, J. Billot. *Fruit Phenolics*. Boca Raton, USA, CRC Press, 1990.

[113] J. B. Harborne. Plant phenolics. In: Dey PM, Harborne, JB, eds. *Methods in Plant Biochemistry*, Vol 1. London, UK: Academic Press, 1989.

[114] D. Amić, D. Davidović-amić, D Bešlo and N. Trinajstić. Structure-radical scavenging activity relationships of flavonoids. *Croatica Chemica Acta*, 76,55-61, 2003.

[115] I. M. C. M. Rietjens et al. The pro-oxidant chemistry of the natural antioxidants vitamin C, vitamin E, carotenoids and flavonoids. *Environmental Toxicology and Pharmacology*, 11,321–33, 2002.

[116] M. S. Hashim, S. Lincy, V. Remya, M. Teena and L. Anila. Effect of polyphenolic compounds from Coriandrum sativum on H2O2-induced oxidative stress in human lymphocytes. *Food Chemistry*, 92,653-60, 2005.

[117] A. Scalbert, and G. Williamson. Dietary intake and bioavailability of polyphenols. *Journal of Nutrition*, 130,2073-85, 2000.

[118] R. A. Larson. *Naturally occurring antioxidants*. Lewis Publishers, New York,83-186, 1997.

[119] P. Kris-etherton, K. Hecker, A. Bonanome, S. Coval, A. Binkoski, K. Hilpert. Bioactive compounds in foods: their role in the prevention of cardiovascular disease and cancer. *American Journal Medicine*, 113,71–8, 2002.

[120] B. B. Aggarwal. Nuclear factor-kappaB: the enemy within. *Cancer Cell* 6(3),203–8, 2004.

[121] S. Singh and B. B. Aggarwal. Activation of transcription factor NF-kappa B is suppressed by curcumin (diferuloylmethane). *Journal of Biology and Chemistry*, 270(42),24995–5000, 1995.

[122] S. K. Manna, A. Mukhopadhyay, B. B. Aggarwal. Resveratrol suppresses TNF-induced activation of nuclear transcription factors NF-kappa B, activator protein-1, and apoptosis: potential role of reactive oxygen intermediates and lipid peroxidation. *Journal of Immunology*, 164(12),6509–19, 2000.

[123] G. B. Chainy, S. K. Manna, M. M. Chaturvedi and B. B. Aggarwal. Anethole blocks both early and late cellular responses transduced by tumor necrosis factor: effect on NF-kappaB, AP-1, JNK, MAPKK and apoptosis. *Oncogene*, 19(25),2943–50, 2000.

[124] B. Sun, P. Zhang, W. Qu, X. Zhang, X. Zhuang and H. Yang. Study on effect of flavonoids from oil-removed seeds of Hippophae rhamnoides on inducing apoptosis of human hepatoma cell. *Zhong Yao Cai*, 26(12),875-7, 2003.

[125] D. Bohmann. T. J. Bos, A. Admon, T. Nishimura, P. K. Vogt and R. Tjian. Human proto-oncogene c-jun encodes a DNA binding protein with structural and functional properties of transcription factor AP-1. *Science*, 238(4832),1386–92, 1987.

[126] R. Eferl, E. F. Wagner. AP-1: a double-edged sword in tumorigenesis. *Nature Review of Cancer*, 3(11),859–68, 2003.

[127] Z. Dong. Effects of food factors on signal transduction pathways. *Biofactors*, 12(1–4),17–28, 2000.

[128] S. Lagarrigue, C. Chaumontet, C. Heberden, P. Martel and I. Gaillard-Sanchez. Suppression of oncogene-induced transformation by quercetin and retinoic acid in rat liver epithelial cells. *Cell and Molecular Biology Research*, 41(6), 551–60, 1995.

[129] W. Chen, Z. Dong, S. Valcic, B. N. Timmermann and G. T. Bowden. Inhibition of ultraviolet B-induced c-fos gene expression and p38 mitogen-activated protein kinase activation by (-)-epigallocatechin gallate in a human keratinocyte cell line. *Molecular Carcinogenesis*, 24(2),79–84, 1999.

[130] J. Y. Chung, J. O. Park, H. Phyu, Z. Dong and C. S. Yang. Mechanisms of inhibition of the Ras-MAP kinase signaling pathway in 30.7b Ras 12 cells by tea polyphenols (-)-epigallocatechin-3-gallate and theaflavin-3,30-digallate. *FASEB Journal*, 15(11), 2022–4, 2001.

[131] G. Y. Yang, J. Liao, C. Li, J. Chung, E. J. Yurkow, C. T. Ho et al. Effect of black and green tea polyphenols on c-jun phosphorylation and H2O2 production in transformed and non-transformed human bronchial cell lines: possible mechanisms of cell growth inhibition and apoptosis induction. *Carcinogenesis*, 21(11),2035–9, 2000.

[132] S. Balasubramanian, T. Efimova, and R. L. Eckert. Green tea polyphenol stimulates a Ras, MEKK1, MEK3, and p38 cascade to increase activator protein 1 factor-dependent involucrin gene expression in normal human keratinocytes. *Journal of Biology and Chemistry*, 277(3),1828–36, 2002.

[133] T. L. Wadsworth, T. L. McDonald and D. R. Koop. Effects of Ginkgo biloba extract (EGb 761) and quercetin on lipopolysaccharide-induced signaling pathways involved in the release of tumor necrosis factor-alpha. *Biochemical Pharmacology*, 62(7),963–74, 2001.

[134] V. Baldin, J. Lukas, M. J. Marcote, M. Pagano, G. Draetta. Cyclin D1 is a nuclear protein required for cell cycle progression in G1. *Genes Devlopment*, 7(5),812–21, 1993.

[135] J. A.Diehl. Cycling to cancer with cyclin D1. *Cancer Biology and Therapy*, 1(3),226–31, 2002.

[136] Z. Estrov, S. Shishodia, S. Faderl, D. Harris, Q. Van and H. M. Kantarjian et al. Resveratrol blocks interleukin-1beta-induced activation of the nuclear transcription factor NF-kappaB, inhibits proliferation, causes S-phase arrest, and induces apoptosis of acute myeloid leukemia cells. *Blood*, 102(3),987–95, 2003.

[137] M. Li, Z. Zhang, D. L. Hill, X. Chen, H. Wang and R. Zhang. Genistein, a dietary isoflavone, down-regulates the MDM2 oncogene at both transcriptional and posttranslational levels. *Cancer Research*, 65(18),8200–8, 2005.

[138] N. Takagaki, Y. Sowa, T. Oki, R. Nakanishi, S. Yogosawa and T. Sakai. Apigenin induces cell cycle arrest and p21/WAF1 expression in a p53-independent pathway. *International Journal of Oncology*, 26(1),185–9, 2005.

[139] A. K. Tyagi, R. P. Singh, C. Agarwal, D. C. Chan and R. Agarwal. Silibinin strongly synergizes human prostate carcinoma DU145 cells to doxorubicin-induced growth Inhibition, G2-M arrest, and apoptosis. *Clinical Cancer Research*, 8(11),3512–9, 2002.

[140] S. Gupta, N. Ahmad, A. L. Nieminen, and H Mukhtar. Growth inhibition, cell-cycle dysregulation, and induction of apoptosis by green tea constituent (-)-epigallocatechin-3-gallate in androgen-sensitive and androgen-insensitive human prostate carcinoma cells. *Toxicology and Applied Pharmacology*, 164(1),82–90, 2000.

[141] P. L. Kuo and C. C. Lin. Green tea constituent (-)-epigallocatechin-3-gallate inhibits Hep G2 cell proliferation and induces apoptosis through p53-dependent and Fas-mediated pathways. *Journal of Biomedical Science*, 10(2),219–27, 2003.

[142] O. N. Ozes, L. D. Mayo, J. A. Gustin, S. R. Pfeffer, L. M. Pfeffer and D. B. Donner. NF-kappaB activation by tumour necrosis factor requires the Akt serine-threonine kinase. *Nature*, 401(6748),82–5, 1999.

[143] A. Brunet, A. Bonni, M. J. Zigmond, M. Z. Lin, P. Juo, L. and S. Hu et al. Akt promotes cell survival by phosphorylating and inhibiting a Forkhead transcription factor. *Cell*, 96(6),857–68, 1999.

[144] Y Li and F. H. Sarkar. Inhibition of nuclear factor kappaB activation in PC3 cells by genistein is mediated via Akt signaling pathway. *Clinical Cancer Research*, 8(7),2369–77, 2002.

[145] F. Y. Tang, N. Nguyen, and M. Meydani. Green tea catechins inhibit VEGF-induced angiogenesis in vitro through suppression of VE-cadherin phosphorylation and inactivation of Akt molecule. *Internaltional Journal Cancer*, 106(6),871–8, 2003.

[146] W. S. el-Deiry, T. Tokino, V. E. Velculescu, D. B. Levy, R. Parsons and J. M. Trent et al. WAF1, a potential mediator of p53 tumor suppression. *Cell*, 75(4),817–25, 1993.

[147] C. Huang, W. Y. Ma, A. Goranson and Z Dong. Resveratrol suppresses cell transformation and induces apoptosis through a p53-dependent pathway. *Carcinogenesis*, 20(2),237–42, 1999.

[148] M. Gu, S. Dhanalakshmi, S. Mohan, R. P. Singh and R. Agarwal. Silibinin inhibits ultraviolet B radiation-induced mitogenic and survival signaling, and associated biological responses in SKH-1 mouse skin. *Carcinogenesis*, 26(8),1404–13, 2005.

[149] S. J. Baek, L. C. Wilson, T. E. Eling. Resveratrol enhances the expression of non-steroidal anti-inflammatory drugactivated gene (NAG-1) by increasing the expression of p53. *Carcinogenesis*, 23(3),425–34, 2002.

[150] P. - L. Kuo and C .- C. Lin Green Tea Constituent (-)-Epigallocatechin-3-Gallate Inhibits Hep G2 Cell Proliferation and Induces Apoptosis through p53-Dependent and Fas-Mediated Pathways. *Journal of Biomedical Sciences*, 10,219-227, 2003.

[151] M. Nachshon-Kedmi, S. Yannai, A. Haj, and F. A. Fares. Indole-3-carbinol and 3,30-diindolylmethane induce apoptosis in human prostate cancer cells. *Food and Chemical Toxicology*, 41(6),745–52, 2003.

[152] C. Hong, H. A. Kim, G. L. Firestone and L. F. Bjeldanes. 3,30-Diindolylmethane (DIM) induces a G(1) cell cycle arrest in human breast cancer cells that is accompanied by Sp1-mediated activation of p21(WAF1/CIP1) expression. *Carcinogenesis*, 23(8),1297–305, 2002.

[153] B. B. Aggarwal. Signalling pathways of the TNF superfamily: a double-edged sword. *Nature Review of Immunology*, 3(9),745–56, 2003.

[154] R. J. Moore, D. M. Owens, G. Stamp, C. Arnott, F. Burke and N. East et al. Mice deficient in tumor necrosis factor-alpha are resistant to skin carcinogenesis. *Natural Medicine*, 5(7),828–31, 1999.

[155] F. Yang, W. J. de Villiers, C. J. McClain and G. W. Varilek. Green tea polyphenols block endotoxin-induced tumor necrosis factor-production and lethality in a murine model. *Journal of Nutrition*, 128(12),2334–40, 1998.

[156] J. Kowalski, A. Samojedny, M. Paul, G. Pietsz and T. Wilczok. Effect of apigenin, kaempferol and resveratrol on the expression of interleukin-1beta and tumor necrosis factor-alpha genes in J774.2 macrophages. *Pharmacological Report*, 57(3),390–4, 2005.

[157] M. Hughes-Fulford, R. Tjandrawinata, R. Li Chai-Fei and S. Sayyah. Arachidonic acid, an omega-6 fatty acid, induces cytoplasmic phospholipase A2 in prostate carcinoma cells. *Carcinogenesis*, 26(9),1520-1526, 2005.

[158] K. Subbaramaiah and A. J. Dannenberg. Cyclooxygenase 2: a molecular target for cancer prevention and treatment. *Trends in Pharmacological Sciences*, 24(2),96–102, 2003.

[159] J. Baumann, F. von Bruchhausen, G. Wurm. Flavonoids and related compounds as inhibition of arachidonic acid peroxidation. *Prostaglandins*, 20(4),627–39, 1980.

[160] R. Landolfi, R. L. Mower and M. Steiner. Modification of platelet function and arachidonic acid metabolism by bioflavonoids. Structure–activity relations. *Biochemical Pharmacology*, 33(9),1525–30, 1984.

[161] C. A. W illiams, J. B. Harborne, H. Geiger and J. R. Hoult. The flavonoids of Tanacetum parthenium and T. vulgare and their anti-inflammatory properties. *Phytochemistry*, 51(3),417–23, 1999.

[162] M. Mutoh, M. Takahashi, K. Fukuda, Y. Matsushima-Hibiya, H. Mutoh and T. Sugimura et al. Suppression of cyclooxygenase-2 promoter-dependent transcriptional activity in colon cancer cells by chemopreventive agents with a resorcin-type structure. *Carcinogenesis*, 21(5),959–63, 2000.

[163] Y. C. Chen, S. C. Shen, L. G. Chen, T. J. Lee and L. L. Yang. Wogonin, baicalin, and baicalein inhibition of inducible nitric oxide synthase and cyclooxygenase-2 gene expressions induced by nitric oxide synthase inhibitors and lipopolysaccharide. *Biochemical Pharmacology*, 61(11),1417–27, 2001.

[164] C. Gerhauser, K. Klimo, E. Heiss, I. Neumann, A. Gamal-Eldeen and J. Knauft et al. Mechanism-based in vitro screening of potential cancer chemopreventive agents. *Mutation Research*, 523–524,163–72, 2003.

[165] K. Subbaramaiah, W. J. Chung, P. Michaluart, N. Telang, T. Tanabe and H. Inoue et al. Resveratrol inhibits cyclooxygenase-2 transcription and activity in phorbol ester-treated human mammary epithelial cells. *Journal of Biology and Chemical*, 273(34),21875–82, 1998.

[166] J. Hong, T. J. Smith, C. T. Ho, D. A. August and C. S. Yang. Effects of purified green and black tea polyphenols on cyclooxygenase- and lipoxygenase-dependent metabolism of arachidonic acid in human colon mucosa and colon tumor tissues. *Biochemical Pharmacology*, 62(9),1175–83, 2001.

[167] M. MacCarrone, T. Lorenzon, P. Guerrieri and A. F. Agro. Resveratrol prevents apoptosis in K562 cells by inhibiting lipoxygenase and cyclooxygenase activity. *European Journal of Biochemistry*, 265(1),27–34, 1999.

[168] M. J. Laughton, P. J. Evans, M. A. Moroney, J. R. Hoult and B. Halliwell. Inhibition of mammalian 5- lipoxygenase and cyclooxygenase by flavonoids and phenolic dietary additives. Relationship to antioxidant activity and to iron ionreducing ability. *Biochemical Pharmacology*, 42(9),1673–81, 1991.

[169] E. A. Eaton, U. K. Walle, A. J. Lewis, T. Hudson, A. A. Wilson and T. Walle. Flavonoids, potent inhibitors of the human P-form phenolsulfotransferase. Potential role in drug metabolism and chemoprevention. *Drug Metabolism and Disposition*, 24,232-237, 1996.

[170] B. J. Mounho and B. D. Thrall. The extracellular signal-regulated kinase pathway contributes to mitogenic and anti-apoptotic effects of peroxisome proliferators in vitro. *Toxicology and Applied Pharmacology*, 159,125-133, 1999.

[171] S. B. Yee, J. H. Lee, H. Y. Chung, K. S. Im, S. J. Bae, J. S. Choi and N. D. Kim. Inhibitory effects of luteolin isolated from Ixeris sonchifolia Hance on the proliferation of HepG2 human hepatocellular carcinoma cells. *Archives of Pharmacological Research*, 26,151-156, 2003.

[172] P. V. Jeyabal, M. B. Syed, M. Venkataraman, J. K. Sambandham and D. Sakthisekaran. Apigenin inhibits oxidative stress-induced macromolecular damage in N-nitrosodiethylamine (NDEA)-induced hepatocellular carcinogenesis in Wistar albino rats. *Molecular Carcinogenesis*, 44,11-20, 2005.

[173] B. Herrera, A. Alvarez, A. Sanchez, M. Fernandez, C. Roncero, M. Benito and I. Fabregat. Reactive oxygen species (ROS) mediates the mitochondrialdependent apopto sis induced by transforming growth factor (beta) in fetal hepatocytes. *FASEB Journal*, 15,741–51, 2001.

[174] G. Packham, R. Ashmun and J. Cleveland. Cytokines suppress apoptosis independent of increases in reactive oxygen levels. *Journal of Immunology*, 156,2792–800, 1996.

[175] S. Shen, Y. Chen, F. Hsu and W. Lee. Differential apoptosis-inducing effect of quercetin and its glycosides in human promyeloleukemic HL-60 cells by alternative activation of the caspase 3 cascade. *Journal of Cell Biochemistry*, 89,1044–55, 2003.

[176] T. Nguyen, E. Tran, T. Nguyen, P. Do, T. Huynh and H. Huynh. The role of activated MEK-ERK pathway in quercetin-induced growth inhibition and apoptosis in A549 lung cancer cells. *Carcinogenesis*, 25,647–59, 2004.

[177] P. Ferrer, M. Asensi, R. Segarra, A. Ortega, M. Benlloch, E. Obrador and M. T. Varea et al. Association between Pterostilbene and Quercetin Inhibits Metastatic Activity of B16 Melanoma. Neoplasia, 7(1),37–47, 2005.

[178] C. M. Rodrigue, F. Porteu, N. Navarro, E. Bruyneel, M. Bracke, P. H. Romeo, C. Gespach and M. C. Garel. The cancer chemopreventive agent resveratrol induces tensin, a cell-matrix adhesion protein with signaling and antitumor activities. *Oncogene*. 24,3274–3284, 2005.

[179] H. Mukhtar and N. Ahmad. Green tea in chemoprevention of cancer. *Toxicological Sciences*, 52,111–117, 1999.

[180] A. Yanagida, A. Shoji, Y. Shibusawa, H. Shindo, M. Tagashira, M. Ikeda and Y. Ito. Analytical separation of tea catechins and food-related polyphenols by high-speed counter-current chromatography. *Journal of Chromatography A*, 1112,195–201, 2006.

[181] N. T. Zaveri. Green tea and its polyphenolic catechins: medicinal uses in cancer and noncancer applications. *Life Sciences*, 78,2073–2080, 2006.

[182] S. Bastianetto, Z. X. Yao, V. Papadopoulos and R. Quirion. Neuroprotective effects of green and black teas and their catechin gallate esters against beta-amyloid-induced toxicity. *European Journal of Neuroscience*, 23,55–64, 2006.

[183] G. W. Dryden, M. Song and C. McClain. Polyphenols and gastrointestinal diseases. *Current Opinion of Gastroenterology*, 22,165–170, 2006.

[184] J. A. Vinson. Black and green tea and heart disease: a review. *Biofactors*, 13,127–132, 2000.

[185] L. N. Mu, X. F. Zhou, B. G. Ding, R. H. Wang ,Z. F. Zhang and C. W. Chen. et al. A case-control study on drinking green tea and decreasing risk of cancers in the alimentary canal among cigarette smokers and alcohol drinkers. *Zhonghua Liu Xing Bing Xue Za Zhi*, 24,192–195, 2003.

[186] J. D. Lambert and C. S. Yang. Mechanisms of cancer prevention by tea constituents. *Journal of Nutrition*, 133,3262–3267, 2003.

[187] T. T. Liu, N. S. Liang, Y. Li, F. Yang, Y. Lu, Zi.-Q. Meng and Li.-S. Zhang. Effects of long-term tea polyphenols consumption on hepatic microsomal drug-metabolizing enzymes and liver function in Wistar rats. *World Journal of Gastroenterology*, 9(12),2742-2744, 2003.

[188] S. Banerjee, S. Manna, P. Saha, C. K. Panda and S. Das. Black tea polyphenols suppress cell proliferation and induce apoptosis during benzo(a)pyrene-induced lung carcinogenesis. *European Journal of Cancer Prevention*, 14,215–221, 2005.

[189] G. W. Dryden, M. Song and C. McClain. Polyphenols and gastrointestinal diseases. *Current Opinion of Gastroenterology*, 22,165–170, 2006.

[190] N. Kalra, S. Prasad and Y. Shukla. Antioxidant potential of black tea against 7,12-dimethylbenz(a)anthracene-induced oxidative stress in Swiss albino mice. *Journal of Environmental Pathology, Toxicology and Oncology,* 24,105–114, 2009.

[191] P. P. Maliakal, P. F. Coville and S. Wanwimolruk. Tea consumption modulates hepatic drug metabolizing enzymes in Wistar rats. *Journal of Pharmacy and Pharmacology,* 53, 69–577, 2001.

[192] R. Krishnan, R. Raghunathan and G. B. Maru. Effect of polymeric black tea polyphenols on benzo(a)pyrene [B(a)P]-induced cytochrome P4501A1 and 1A2 in mice. Xenobiotica, 35,671–682, 2005.

[193] K. Imai and K. Nakachi. Cross sectional study of effects of drinking green tea on cardiovascular and liver diseases. *British Medical Journal*, 310,693–696, 1995.

[194] S. Srivastava, M. Singh, P. Roy, S. Prasad, J. George and Y. Shukla. Inhibitory effect of tea polyphenols on hepatic preneoplastic foci in Wistar rats. *Investigation of New Drugs*, 27,526–533, 2009.

[195] R. S. Murugan, K. Uchida, Y. Hara and S. Nagini. Black tea polyphenols modulate xenobiotic-metabolizing enzymes, oxidative stress and adduct formation in a rat hepatocarcinogenesis model. *Free Radical Research*, 42(10),873–884, 2008.

[196] N. Carbo, P. F. Costelli, M. Baccino, F. J. Lopez-Soriano and J. M. Argiles. Resveratrol, a natural product present in wine, decreases tumour growth in a rat tumour model. *Biochemical Biophysical Research and Communication*, 254,739-743, 1999.

[197] Sun ZJ, Pan CE, Liu HS and Wang GJ: Anti-hepatoma activity of resveratrol in vitro. World Journal Gastroenterology, 8,79-81, 2002.

[198] V. De Ledinghen A. Monvoisin, V. Neaud,S. Krisa, B. Payrastre and C. Bedin et al. trans-resveratrol, a grapevine-derived polyphenol, blocks hepatocyte growth factor-

induced invasion of hepatocellular carcinoma cells. *International Journal of Oncology*, 19,83-88, 2001.

[199] Y. Kozuki, Y. Miura and K. Yagasaki. Resveratrol suppresses hepatoma cell invasion independently of its anti-proliferative action. *Cancer Letter*, 167,151-156, 2001.

[200] H. P. Ciolino, and G. C. Yeh. The effects of resveratrol on CYP1A1 expression and aryl hydrocarbon receptor function in vitro. *Advances in Experimental Medicine and Biology*, 492,183-193, 2001.

[201] S. R. Beedanagari, I. Bebenek, P. Bui and O. Hankinson. Resveratrol Inhibits Dioxin-Induced Expression of Human CYP1A1 and CYP1B1 by Inhibiting Recruitment of the Aryl Hydrocarbon Receptor Complex and RNA Polymerase II to the Regulatory Regions of the Corresponding Genes. *Toxicological Sciences*, 110(1),61-67, 2009.

[202] H. P. Ciolino, P. J. Daschner and G. C. Yeh. Resveratrol inhibits transcription of CYP1A1 in vitro by preventing activation of the aryl hydrocarbon receptor. *Cancer Research*, 58,5707-5712, 1998.

[203] T. K. Chang, J. Chen and W. B. Lee. Differential inhibition and inactivation of human CYP1 enzymes by trans-esveratrol: evidence for mechanism-based inactivation of CYP1A2. *Journal of Pharmacology and Experimental Therapeutics*, 299,874-882, 2001.

[204] S. Godichaud, S. Krisa, B. Couronne, L. Dubuisson J. M. Merillon, A. Desmouliere, J. Rosenbaum. Deactivation of cultured human liver myofibroblasts by trans-resveratrol, a grapevine-derived polyphenol. *Hepatology*, 31,922–931, 2000.

[205] H. Nagase,K. Sasaki, H. Kito, A. Haga and T. Sato. Inhibitory effect of delphinidin from Solanum melongena on human fibrosarcoma HT-1080 invasiveness in vitro. *Planta Medicine*, 64,216–219, 1998.

[206] Y. T. Huang, J.-J. Hwang, P.-P. Lee, F.-C. Ke, J.-H. Huang, C.-J. Huang C. Kandaswami et al. Effects of luteolin and quercetin, inhibitors of tyrosine kinase, on cell growth and metastasis-associated properties in A431 cells overexpressing epidermal growth factor receptor. *British Journal of Pharmacology*, 128,999-1010.

[207] L. T. Lee, Y. T. Huang, J. J. Hwang, A. Y. Lee, F. C. Ke, C. J. Huang, C. Kandaswami, P. P. Lee and M. T. Lee. Transinactivation of the epidermal growth factor receptor tyrosine kinase and focal adhesion kinase phosphorylation by dietary flavonoids: effect on invasive potential of human carcinoma cells. *Biochemical Pharmacology*, 67,2103–2114, 2004.

[208] P. K. Vayalil A. Mittal and S. K. Katiyar. Proanthocyanidins from grape seeds inhibit expression of matrix metalloproteinases in human prostate carcinoma cells, which is associated with the inhibition of activation of MAPK and NF kappa B. *Carcinogenesis*, 25,987–995, 2004.

[209] T. K. Chang, W. B. Lee and H. H. Ko. trans-Resveratrol modulates the catalytic activity and mRNA expression of the procarcinogen-activating human cytochrome P450 1B1. *Candian Journal of Physiology and Pharmacology*, 78,874–881, 2000.

[210] B. Piver, F. Berthou, Y. Dreano and D. Lucas. Inhibition of CYP3A, CYP1A and CYP2E1 activities by resveratrol and other non volatile red wine components. *Toxicology Letter*, 125,83–91, 2001.

[211] T. Li W. Wang, and T. Li. The mechanism of resveratrol on anti-hepatoma Bel-7402 and modulating IL-8 in tumor model mice. *Zhong Yao Cai*, 31(5),697-702, 2008.

[212] S. Madlener, C. Illmer, and Z Horvath et al. Gallic acid inhibits ribonucleotide reductase and cyclooxygenases in human HL-60 promyelocytic leukemia cells. *Cancer Letter*, 245,156–162, 2007.

[213] G. Galati and P. J. O'Brien. Potential toxicity of flavonoids and other dietary phenolics: significance for their chemopreventive and anticancer properties. *Free Radical Biology and Medicine*, 37,287–303, 2004.

[214] M. Inoue, R. Suzuki, T. Koide, N. Sakaguchi, Y. Ogihara, Y. Yabu. Antioxidant, gallic acid, induces apoptosis in HL- 60RG cells. *Biochemical and Biophysical Research and Communication*, 204,898–904, 1994.

[215] M. Kawada, Y. Ohno, Y. Ri, T. Ikoma, H. Yuugetu and T. Asai. Anti-tumor effect of gallic acid on LL–2 lung cancer cells transplanted in mice. *Anticancer Drug*, 12,847–852, 2001.

[216] M. Salucci, L. A. Stivala, G. Maiani, R. Bugianesi and V. Vannini. Flavonoids uptake and their effect on cell cycle of human colon adenocarcinoma cells (Caco2). *British Journal of Cancer*, 86,1645–1651, 2002.

[217] L. Li, T. B. Ng, W. Gao, W. Li, M. Fu and S. M. Niu. Antioxidant activity of gallic acid from rose flowers in senescence accelerated mice. *Life Sciences*, 77,230–240, 2005.

[218] T. Li X. Zhang and X. Zhao. Powerful protective effects of gallic acid and tea polyphenols on human hepatocytes injury induced by hydrogen peroxide or carbon tetrachloride in vitro. *Journal of Medicinal Plants and Research*, 4(3),247-254, 2004.

[219] Z. G. Zhong, J. L. Huang, H. Liang, Y. N. Zhong, W. Y. Zhang, D. P. Wu, C. L. Zeng, J. S. Wang and Y. H. Wei . The effect of gallic acid extracted from leaves of Phyllanthus emblica on apoptosis of human hepatocellular carcinoma BEL-7404 cells. *Zhong Yao Cai*, 32(7),1097-101, 2009.

[220] S. Jagan, G. Ramakrishnan, P. Anandakumar, S. Kamaraj and T. Devaki Antiproliferative potential of gallic acid against diethylnitrosamine-induced rat hepatocellular carcinoma. *Molecular and Cellular Biochemistry,* 319,51–59, 2008.

[221] Y. Yanaida, H. Kohno and K. Yoshida et al. Dietary Silymarin suppresses 4-nitroquinoline 1-oxide induced tongue carcinogenesis in male F344 rats. *Carcinogenesis*, 23(5),787–794, 2002.

[222] K. Pradeep,C. V. R. Mohan, K Gobianand and S. Karthikeyan. Silymarin modulates the oxidant-antioxidant imbalance during diethylnitrosamine induced oxidative stress in rats. *European Journal of Pharmacology*, 560,110–116, 2007.

[223] G. Ramakrishnan, C. M. Elinos-Ba´ez, S. Jagan, T. A. Augustine, S. Kamaraj, P. Anandakumar and T. Devaki. Silymarin downregulates COX-2 expression and attenuates hyperlipidemia during NDEA-induced rat hepatocellular carcinoma. *Molecular and Cellular Biochemistry*, 313,53–61, 2008.

[224] G. Ramakrishnan, S. Jagan, S. Kamaraj, P. Anandakumar and T. Devaki. Silymarin attenuated mast cell recruitment thereby decreased the expressions of matrix metalloproteinases-2 and 9 in rat liver carcinogenesis. *Investigation of New Drugs*, 27,233–240, 2009.

[225] Y.-F. Wu, S.-L. Fu, C.-H. Kao, C.-W.Yang, C.-H. Lin, M.-T.Hsu, and T.-F. Tsai. Chemopreventive effect of silymarin on liver pathology in HBV X protein transgenic mice. *Cancer Research*, 68(6), 2033–42, 2008.

[226] S. M. Shaarawy, A. A. Tohamy, S. M. Elgendy, Z. Y. A. Elmageed, A. Bahnasy, M. S. Mohamed, E. Kandil and K. Matrougui. Protective Effects of Garlic and Silymarin on NDEA-Induced Rats Hepatotoxicity International Journal of Biological Sciences, 5,549-557, 2009.

[227] S. Sivalokanathan, M. Ilayaraja and M. P. Balasubramanian. Antioxidant activity of Terminalia arjuna bark extract on N-nitrosodiethylamine induced hepatocellular carcinoma in rats. *Molecular and Cellular Biochemistry*, 281(1-2),87-93, 2006.

[228] V. Sivaramakrishnan and S. N. Devaraj. Morin fosters apoptosis in experimental hepatocellular carcinogenesis model. *Chemico-Biological Interactions*, 183(2):284-92, 2010.

[229] V. Sivaramakrishnan and Niranjali S. Devaraj. Morin regulates the expression of NF-kappaB-p65, COX-2 and matrix metalloproteinases in diethylnitrosamine induced rat hepatocellular carcinoma. *Chemico-Biological Interactions*, 180(3),353-9, 2009.

[230] T. Tanaka,H. Iwata,K. Niwa,Y. Mori and H. Mori. Inhibitory effect of ellagic acid on N-2-fluorenylacetamide-induced liver carcinogenesis in male ACI/N rats. *Cancer Science*, 79(12),1297–1303, 1988.

[231] T.-W. Chung, S.-K. Moon, Y.-C. Chang, J.-H. Ko, Y.-C. Lee, Cho G. et al. Novel and therapeutic effect of caffeic acid and caffeic acid phenyl ester on hepatocarcinoma cells: complete regression of hepatoma growth and metastasis by dual mechanism. *The FASEB Journal*, 18,1670-1681, 2004.

[232] O. Beltrán-Ramírez, L. Alemán-Lazarini, M. Salcido-Neyoy and S. Hernández-García et al. Evidence that the anticarcinogenic effect of caffeic acid phenethyl ester in the resistant hepatocyte model involves modifications of cytochrome P450. *Toxicological Sciences*, 104(1),100-106, 2008.

[233] D.-G. Song, J.Y. Lee, E.H. Lee and S. H. Jung et al. Inhibitory effects of polyphenols isolated from Rhus verniciflua on Aldo-keto reductase family 1 B10. *BMB reports*, 43(4),268-272, 2010.

[234] R. S. Murugan, G.Vinothini, Y. Hara, S. Nagini. Black Tea Polyphenols Target Matrix Metalloproteinases, RECK, Proangiogenic Molecules and Histone Deacetylase in a Rat Hepatocarcinogenesis Model. *Anticancer Research*, 29(6),2301-2305, 2009.

[235] H. Nishino. Cancer chemoprevention by ginseng in mouse liver and other organs. *Proceeding of International Symposium on Cancer Chemoprevention of INSAM* (Ginseng) April 20, p. 20-1, 2001.

[236] T. K. Yun and S. Y. Choi. Preventive effect of ginseng intake against various human cancers: a case-control study on 1987 pairs. *Cancer Epidemiology Biomarkers and Prevention*, 4,401-8, 1995.

[237] T.Tode, Y. Kikuchi, T. Kita, J. Hirata, E. Imaizumi and I. Nagata. Inhibitory effects by oral administration of ginsenoside Rh2 on the growth of human ovarian cancer cells in nude mice. *Journal of Cancer Research and Clinical Oncology*, 120,24-6, 1993.

[238] T. K. Yun and S. Y. Choi. A case-control study of ginseng intake and cancer. *International Journal of Epidemiology*, 19,871-6, 1990.

[239] T.K. Yun. Experimental and epidemiological evidence of the cancerpreventive effects of Panax ginseng C.A. Mayer. *Nutrition Review*, 54,71-81, 1996.

[240] H. Ishikawa. Study on Chemoprevention of Hepatocellular Carcinoma by Ginseng: An Introduction to the Protocol. Journal of Korean Medical Science, 16(Suppl):70-4, 2001.

[241] D. M. Eugenia, H. A. Isabel, A. Niiria, G. Almudena and M. Paloma. Dietary polyphenols protect against N-nitrosamines and benzo(a)pyreneinduced DNA damage (strand breaks and oxidized purines/pyrimidines) in HepG2 human hepatoma cells. *European Journal of Nutrition*, 47,479-490, 2008.

In: Liver Cancer: Causes, Diagnosis and Treatment
Editor: Benjamin J. Valverde

ISBN: 978-1-61209-115-0
© 2011 Nova Science Publishers, Inc.

*Chapter II*

# Mechanisms of Hepatocarcinogenesis: A Dialogue Between Exogenous Factors and the Endogenous Response

### *Jordan C. Woodrick and Rabindra Roy*[*]
Lombardi Comprehensive Cancer Center,
Georgetown University, Washington, DC, USA

## Abstract

The World Health Organization (WHO) estimated in 2004 that primary liver cancer, claiming the lives of 610,000 people worldwide, is one of the top five cancers that contribute to the 7.4 million deaths due to cancer globally each year. In the United States, primary liver and bile duct cancers are the 6th and 9th leading causes of cancer death in men and women, respectively. In 2009 there were 22,620 newly diagnosed cases and 18,160 deaths of primary liver cancer, and the Surveillance, Epidemiology, and End Results (SEER) Program reported a dismal overall 5-year survival rate of primary liver cancers at 13.8% between 1999 and 2006. As is the case with many other diseases, understanding the underlying causes of liver cancers provides potentially useful information regarding prevention as well as diagnosis and treatment. This chapter will elucidate what is currently known concerning the causes of various types of hepatic malignancies. The major etiologic agents discussed here include infectious agents, such as hepatitis B and C viruses, Helicobacter, and liver flukes, as well as toxic agents, such as alcohol, metal accumulation, and Aflatoxin B. This chapter will also explore the role and known molecular mechanisms of inflammation in primary liver cancers, as it is one of the most influential risk factors for these diseases and plays a role in the carcinogenic effects of many of the etiologic agents. Liver cancers are heterogeneous in nature, so the multifactorial genetic and epigenetic alterations that drive hepatocarcinogenesis will be discussed. Finally, this chapter will also review current knowledge on the potential role of hepatic stem cells in the development of liver cancer.

---

[*] [2] Address Correspondence To: Dr. Rabindra Roy, Lombardi Comprehensive Cancer Center, Georgetown University, Washington, DC 20057-1468, telephone: 202-687-7390, e-mail: rr228@georgetown.edu.

**Keywords:** Liver cancer, hepatitis B virus, hepatitis C virus, chronic inflammation, DNA damage, DNA repair

# Abbreviations

ADH – alcohol dehydrogenase
AFB1 – aflatoxin B1
AKT - v-akt murine thymoma viral oncogene homolog 1
AP-1 – activator protein-1
ASL – angiosarcoma of the liver
BCP - basal core promoter
BER – base excision repair
CCA – cholangiocarcinoma
cccDNA – covalently closed circular DNA
COX2 - cyclooxygenase-2
COX2 - cyclooxygenase-2
CYP2E1 - cytochrome P450 2E1
DDB1 - UV-damaged DNA binding protein
DEN – diethylnitrosamine
DNMT – DNA methyltransferase
DSH – disheveled
EGF – epidermal growth factor
EGFR - epithelial growth factor receptor
ER - endoplasmic reticulum
FKHR - forkhead transcription factor
FZD – frizzled
GSH – glutathione
GSK3$\beta$ - glycogen synthase kinase 3 beta
GSTP1 – glutathione S-transferase P1
HBeAg - hepatitis B virus e antigen
HBV – hepatitis B virus
HBx – HBV X protein
HCA – hepatocellular adenoma
HCC – hepatocellular carcinoma
HCV – hepatitis C virus
HGF – hepatocyte growth factor
HH – hereditary hemochromatosis
HSC – hepatic stellate cell
hTERT – human telomerase reverse transcriptase
IGF – insulin-like growth factor
IGF2R – insulin-like growth factor 2 receptor
IKK - I$\kappa$B kinase
IL – interleukin
iNOS - inducible nitric oxide synthase

IR - insulin resistance
JAB1 - jun activation domain-binding protein 1
JAK - janus kinase
JNK - c-Jun NH2-terminal kinase
LTβ - lymphotoxin β
LXR – liver X receptor
MAPK – mitogen-activated protein kinase
MCF – monocyte-colony stimulating factor
miRNA – microRNA
MMP - matrix metalloproteinase
mTOR - mammalian target of rapamycin
NER – nucleotide excision repair
NF-κB - nuclear factor-κB
NO – nitric oxide
ORF – open reading frame
PDGF - platelet-derived growth factor
PI3K - phosphoinositide-3-kinase
PIN1 - peptidylprolyl cis/trans isomerase, NIMA-interacting 1
PKB – protein kinase B
PKC - protein kinase C
PPARα - peroxisome proliferator-activated receptor alpha
PPAR-γ - peroxisome proliferator-activated receptor gamma
Pre-C – pre-core
PYK2 - proline-rich tyrosine kinase 2
RANTES – chemokine (C-C motif) ligand 5; CCL5
RASSF1A – RAS association family 1
RB1 – retinoblastoma 1
RC-DNA – relaxed circular DNA
RONS - reactive oxygen-nitrogen species
ROS – reactive oxygen species
SAPK - stress-activated protein kinase
SOCS – suppressor of cytokine signaling
SRC - Rous sarcoma
SREBP1 - sterol regulatory element binding protein-1
STAT - signal transducer and activator of transcription
TGF - transforming growth factor
TIMP - tissue inhibitor of metalloproteinase
TLR – toll-like receptor
TNFR1 - tumor necrosis factor receptor 1
TNFα - tumor necrosis factor alpha
VCM - vinyl chloride monomer
VEGF - vascular endothelial growth factor
WD – Wilson's disease
WNT - wingless-type MMTV integration site

# Introduction

Primary liver cancer is the sixth most common cancer worldwide and the third most common cause of cancer death [1]. Incidence rates of liver cancer are higher in less-developed countries than more-developed countries, with 80% of hepatocellular carcinoma (HCC) cases occurring in southeast Asia and sub-Saharan Africa [2]. In the United States, a developed nation with relatively low incidence (3.2 per 100,000 persons in 2006), rates are increasing and are expected to double in the next 10-20 years. Moreover, the overall 5-year survival rate of primary liver cancers was shown to be 13.8% between 1999 and 2006 [2,3]. As is the case with many other diseases, understanding the underlying causes of liver cancers provides potentially useful information regarding prevention as well as diagnosis and treatment.

There are several different types of primary liver cancer. HCC which is a cancer of the hepatocytes, is the most common primary liver malignancy. Cancers of the bile ducts, called cholangiocarcinomas (CCAs), affect the cholangiocytes, which are the cells that comprise the bile ducts. When cancers form in the blood vessels of the liver, these malignancies are called angiosarcomas or hemangiosarcomas. Finally, hepatoblastomas are rare liver cancers that usually occur in children under 4 years of age.

This chapter will elucidate what is currently known concerning the causes of various types of hepatic malignancies. The major etiologic agents discussed here include infectious agents, such as hepatitis B and C viruses, Helicobacter, and liver flukes, as well as toxic agents, such as alcohol, metal accumulation, and Aflatoxin B. This chapter will also explore the role and known molecular mechanisms of inflammation in primary liver cancers, as it is one of the most influential risk factors for these diseases and plays a role in the carcinogenic effects of many of the etiologic agents. Liver cancers are heterogeneous in nature, so the multifactorial genetic and epigenetic alterations that drive hepatocarcinogenesis will be discussed. Finally, this chapter will also review current knowledge on the potential role of hepatic stem cells in the development of liver cancer.

# 1. Infectious Causes

The following section discusses two of the most prevalent and well-known etiologic agents in liver cancer: hepatitis B virus (HBV) and hepatitis C virus (HCV) infection. Important aspects of each virus will be reviewed, including virology, epidemiology, and direct and indirect modes of hepatocarcinogenesis. The role of other infectious agents in the development of liver cancer will also be explored, such as liver flukes and *Helicobacter* spp.

## 1.1. HBV

Globally, more than 2 billion people have been infected with HBV, and 350 million of those individuals suffer from chronic HBV infection [4]. It is estimated that approximately 53% of HCC cases worldwide are related to hepatitis B virus infection with chronically infected individuals having a 5-to 15-fold increased risk of HCC compared to the general population [2]. In fact, important risk factors for HCC are the viral load and levels of hepatitis B virus e antigen (HBeAg), which is a marker of active viral replication, in serum [4]. Furthermore, hepatitis B surface antigen (HBsAg) carriers have 25-37 times increased risk of developing HCC compared to non-infected individuals [5]. HBV is the most frequent underlying cause of HCC, and the following section will elucidate what is currently known regarding HBV-mediated hepatocarcinogenesis [2].

### 1.1.1. Virology

The HBV virion consists of an outer envelope that encloses an inner nucleocapsid. The outer envelope is formed by the hepatitis B surface antigen while the inner nucleocapsid is formed by the hepatitis B core antigen. Within the inner nucleocapsid lie the viral polymerase and genome, which is a partially double-stranded relaxed circular DNA molecule. The organization of the HBV genome consists of four partially overlapping open reading frames (ORFs) that encode the various viral structures and machinery [6]. The pre-S/S ORF encodes the envelope, the pre-core (pre-C)/core (C) ORF encodes the core, the P ORF encodes the viral polymerase and terminal protein, and the X ORF encodes the X protein, whose function is necessary for viral replication. When HBV enters the cell, the viral genome translocates to the nucleus and converts to a covalently closed circular conformation (cccDNA) [7]. This viral molecule becomes the template for viral RNA transcription, which subsequently leads to translation of viral proteins.

### 1.1.2. HBV Genomic Integration

Typically, HBV genomic integration precedes the development of HCC and is present in over 85-90% of HBV-related HCCs. Integration induces various genetic and chromosomal aberrations, such as chromosomal deletions, translocations, fusion transcript production, cellular DNA amplification, and genomic instability. It has been shown that HBV genomic integration often occurs at fragile sites and other regions of the human genome that are susceptible to instability in tumorigenesis. These regions are often sites that are responsible for the regulation of signaling, proliferation, and survival [6]. Specifically, early work has shown that cyclin A2, retinoic acid receptor β, human telomerase reverse transcriptase (hTERT), platelet-derived growth factor (PDGF) receptor, 60s ribosomal protein, calcium signaling-related, and mixed lineage leukemia genes are frequent HBV genomic integration targets [6]. Intriguingly, despite the collection of knowledge concerning cancer-related chromosomal and genetic targets of HBV genomic integration, a dominant viral oncogene has yet to be identified. In fact, the integration of the HBV genome into primary cells or transgenic mouse models has not shown strong evidence of transformation or liver tumorigenesis [7]. However, genomic integration is thought to provide the "first hit" by disrupting cellular genomic stability via large-scale chromosomal alterations or through the targeting of the aforementioned cellular genes during viral integration [7].

With regard to HBV virology, it must be noted, however, that viral DNA integration is not required for HBV replication. Pre-genomic RNA (pgRNA) is packaged into progeny capsids in the cytoplasm and is subsequently reverse-transcribed into viral minus-strand DNA. The cytoplasmic HBV DNA is then converted to relaxed circular DNA (RC-DNA), and these RC-DNA-containing capsids can be used for cccDNA amplification or for the assembly of viral particles that will inevitably be released from the cell [7].

## 1.1.3. HBV Proteins: HBx

### 1.1.3a. General

Many HCCs have integrated HBV sequences encoding HBx, the viral X protein that is required for viral replication and has also been shown to contribute to the development of HCC. HBx affects viral replication by transactivating cellular promoters and enhancers that are needed for persistent viral infection [6].

Additionally, the HBV X protein has been shown to activate important signaling cascades, particularly ones that promote tumorigenesis. It has been shown to activate transcription factors like activator protein-1 (AP-1), nuclear factor-κB (NF- κB), SP1, and Oct-1. Some studies suggest that HBx is able to activate AP-1 and NF- κB by activating protein kinase C (PKC), which subsequently activates the Raf-MEK-ERK pathway, also called the mitogen-activated protein kinase (MAPK) pathway. HBx is known to increase Ras/GTP complex formation by activating proline-rich tyrosine kinase 2 (PYK2.) PYK2 activates Rous sarcoma (Src) kinase enhancing the interaction between adaptor proteins Shc and Grb2, which recruit Sos. Sos is a guanine nucleotide exchange factor that activates Ras, which subsequently activates the Ras-Raf-ERK pathway [8]. Additionally, when localized in the nucleus, HBx is able to directly interact with cAMP response element binding (CREB) and activating transcription factor 2 (ATF-2), increasing their DNA binding affinity [5]. HBx can modulate gene expression by binding to TATA box binding protein (TBP) as well as increasing its expression [9]. The viral X protein can activate the phosphoinositide-3-kinase (PI3K) pathway, exerting an anti-apoptotic effect on hepatocytes, and this effect may be indirect through the activation of the janus kinase (JAK)/signal transducer and activator of transcription (STAT) signaling pathway [10,11]. HBx has also been shown to activate the stress-activated protein kinase (SAPK)/c-Jun NH2-terminal kinase (JNK) signaling pathway, which can lead to oncogenic phosphorylation of Smad (discussed in section 1.1.3d) [12]. Activation of the SAPK/JNK pathway by HBV X protein can also protect cells from Fas-mediated apoptosis. Finally, HBx has been shown to affect the wingless-type MMTV integration site (Wnt) pathway, possibly through activation of ERK (discussed in section 1.1.3b) [13].

### 1.1.3b. HBx & β-catenin

HBx has effects on the Wnt-β-catenin signaling pathway, which is a signaling pathway in which β-catenin, a transcription coactivator, is targeted for degradation by phosphorylation by glycogen synthase kinase 3 beta (GSK3β.) When unphosphorylated β-catenin accumulates in the cytoplasm, it can translocate to the nucleus to act as a coactivator for the Tcf/Lef transcription factor family. This results in the transcription of genes such as cyclin D1 and c-myc, which induce cell proliferation. Notably, there is a significant correlation between HBx expression and β-catenin accumulation in HCC tissue, and it has been shown that HBx inhibits the proteasomal degradation of β-catenin [13]. HBx may inactivate GSK3β via activation of ERK, which results in an inability of GSK3β to phosphorylate β-catenin, leaving it unable to be degraded. Pin1 is a peptidyl-propyl-isomerase that inhibits the interaction between β-catenin and adenomatous polyposis coli (APC), which also regulates the nuclear accumulation of β-catenin [14]. Overexpression of Pin1 has been shown to enhance HBx protein stability potentially by interacting with a serine-proline motif of the HBx protein [15].

### 1.1.3c. HBx & p53

p53, a known tumor suppressor, has been shown to be affected by HBx. The HBV X protein transcriptionally represses the p53 gene and, through interaction with p53, inactivates its important tumor suppressor activities, such as apoptosis, cell cycle regulation, and DNA repair [16]. HBx can bind to p53 and inhibit sequence-specific DNA binding as well as its transactivation activity. The HBx protein can also alter the association of p53 to excision repair cross complementing factor 3 (ERCC3/XPB) and other important NER factors like excision repair cross complementing factor 2 (ERCC2/XPD.) HBx can further inhibit NER by inactivating the UV-damaged DNA binding protein (DDB1.) The inhibition of DNA repair by HBx promotes mutations, specifically in cases of chemical carcinogen exposure in conjunction with HBV infection, and contributes to hepatocarcinogenesis [17,18]. Interestingly, p53 has also been shown to mediate HBx degradation, protecting cells from the potential oncogenic signaling by HBx [19].

### 1.1.3d. HBx & TGF-β

Transforming growth factor-β (TGF-β) has also been shown to be upregulated by viral HBx expression in HCC tissue. HBx transactivates transcription of TGF-β via early growth response 1 (EGR-1) binding sites [20]. Notably, TGF-β is known to have both tumor suppressive and oncogenic activity depending on the site of phosphorylation on its downstream signaling molecule, Smad3. When Smad3 is phosphorylated at the C-terminus (pSmad3C), the result is tumor suppressive signaling. However, when Smad3 is phosphorylated at its middle linker region (pSmad3L), the consequence is oncogenic signaling, such as cell proliferation and invasion. It has been shown that HBx expression in hepatocytes shifts the TGF-β signaling from tumor suppressive to oncogenic phosphorylation of Smad3 [12]. Interestingly, a similar TGF-β signaling switch is observed in HCV-related liver cancers, which will be discussed in more detail in section 1.2.

### 1.1.3e. HBx & Lipids

Fatty liver disease, or steatosis, is a condition where lipids abnormally accumulate in cells and is often associated with HCC. HBx has been shown to induce steatosis by transcriptionally activating the lipogenic transcription factor, sterol regulatory element binding protein-1 (SREBP1), and adipocyte differentiation transcription factor, peroxisome proliferator-activated receptor gamma (PPAR-γ.) Furthermore, HBx was also able to increase the transcriptional activity of PPAR-γ [21]. In addition, liver X receptor (LXR), an important regulator of cholesterol and lipid metabolism, has been shown to mediate HBx-induced lipogenesis in liver cancer. HBx enhances the binding of LXRα to LXR response elements (LXRE), resulting in increased transcription of SREBP1 and fatty acid synthase (FAS) [22]. This study also showed that HBx was able to recruit the transcription coactivator ASC2, a regulator of lipid metabolic pathways in the liver, to LXR and LXREs.

### 1.1.3f. Other Mechanisms

HBx may bind to DDB1, which leads to lagging chromosomes during mitosis. Lagging chromosomes during mitosis result in aberrant mitotic spindles and multi-nucleated cells, which enhance genomic instability [23]. The X protein may alter cellular and viral protein degradation by co-localizing with the proteasome and inhibiting serine protease inhibitors and proteasome complexes [24]. In addition, HBx has been shown to confer a survival benefit to cells under oxidative stress by converting reactive oxygen species (ROS) to less reactive molecules [25]. It also may promote the mitochrondrial localization of c-Raf, which protects cells from stress-induced apoptosis, by inducing oxidative stress [26]. Other mechanisms of hepatocarcinogenesis mediated by HBx include upregulation of beclin 1 followed by starvation-induced autophagy [27]. Finally, HBx has been shown to interact with DNA methyltransferase (DNMT) and confer epigenetic modifications by recruiting DNMT to certain loci or preventing DNMT from localizing to specific regions [28].

### 1.1.4. HBV Proteins: Pre-S/S Protein

While the HBx protein seems to have an important role in HBV-mediated hepatocarcinogenesis, the pre-S/S protein that comprises the viral envelope may also be significant in liver tumorigenesis. The pre-S2/S product in its truncated form is known to be regulatory and to transactivate some cancer-related cellular genes such as c-myc, c-fos, and c-Ha-ras [5]. This class of regulatory proteins is designated pre-S2 activator and can activate PKC-dependent activation of the c-Raf-1/MEK/ERK signaling pathway [29]. Pre-S2 has also been shown to upregulate hTERT and induce telomerase activation, enhancing malignant transformation in human HCC cell lines [30]. Additionally, the pre-S2 activator is able to induce endoplasmic reticulum (ER) stress and subsequent oxidative DNA damage and genomic instability [31]. Cell cycle progression and proliferation of hepatocytes can be increased by the pre-S2 activator via its ability to upregulate cyclooxygenase-2 (COX2) and cyclin A [31]. The pre-S2 activator has been shown to interact with Jun activation domain-binding protein 1 (JAB1), which allows JAB1 to cause the degradation of p27(Kip1), a Cdk inhibitor [32]. This results in an increase of Cdk2, which is regulated by p27(Kip1), and subsequent hyperphosphorylation of tumor suppressor retinoblastoma 1 (Rb.) This deactivates the cell cycle inhibitory action of Rb, and suggests a mechanism for oncogenic activity of the pre-S2 activator. Finally, the pre-S2 activator has been shown to activate the v-akt murine thymoma viral oncogene homolog 1 (Akt)/mammalian target of rapamycin (mTOR) signaling pathway via upregulation of vascular endothelial growth factor-A (VEGF-A), resulting in enhanced hepatocyte growth advantage in the transition from preneoplasia to HCC [33]

### 1.1.5. HCC & HBV Genotypes and Other Variations

There are eight identified genotypes of HBV (A-H) that have distinct geographic and ethnic distributions. Furthermore, hybrid viral strains arise from the genomic recombination between different HBV genotypes. Importantly, the observed genotypic variance in HBV seems to have a prognostic role in determining the risk and progression of HCC. In one study researchers found a 5-fold increase in risk of HCC in patients infected with HBV genotype C compared to patients infected with genotypes A or B [34]. Genotype and viral load were shown to be additive in their association with HCC risk, and genotype C was associated with a higher viral load. In a second study, genotype C carriers' HCC incidence rate per 100,000 person-years was more than twice as high as the genotype B carrier's incidence rate [4]. For genotype C vs genotype B, the multi-variable adjusted hazard ratio for developing HCC was 1.76 (95% CI = 1.19-2.61.) Beyond genotypic differences mutations in the pre-C region of the viral genome and in the basal core promoter (BCP) are common in the HBV genome. Pre-core mutations were the first to be discovered, and a G to A substitution at nucleotide 1896

(G1896A) is the most common mutation observed. Interestingly, the study referenced above also found that the multi-variable-adjusted hazard ratio of developing HCC was 0.34 (95% CI = 0.21-0.57) for precore G1896A vs wild type, indicating that the mutation may have a protective effect against hepatocarcinogenesis [4]. The most common variant in the BCP is a double mutation where there is an A to T substitution at nucleotide 1762 and a G to A substitution at nucleotide 1764 (BCP A1762T/G1764A), which results in increased viral genome replication. Notably, the aforementioned study found an increase in risk of HCC in individuals infected with this HBV variant with a multi-variable adjusted hazard ratio of 1.73 (95% CI = 1.13-2.67) indicating an increase in the oncogenicity of the double mutant variant [4].

## 1.2. HCV

HCV, like HBV, is a major risk factor for the development of HCC and has been shown to be linked to the development of intrahepatic cholangiocarcinoma (ICC) [35,36]. In fact, 27%-80% of HCC patients harbor markers of HCV infection. Moreover, there is a 17-fold increase in HCC risk in patients infected with HCV compared with non-infected individuals. Unfortunately, the molecular mechanisms of HCV-induced hepatocarcinogenesis remain elusive. HCV, in contrast to HBV, does not integrate into its host genome and primarily has a cytoplasmic life cycle. These attributes of the virus indicate that its role in hepatocarcinogenesis must involve indirect mechanisms, including chronic inflammation, steatosis, fibrosis and oxidative stress. Thus, establishing a correlation between gene expression patterns and HCC in HCV-related liver cancers is difficult. However, some HCV proteins may exert direct oncogenic effects and induce cellular mitogenic processes. The viral infection may also increase cell proliferation due to oxidative stress in infected hepatocytes, which may lead to the accumulation of DNA damage and subsequent genomic instability, promoting malignant transformation. This section will provide a brief overview of the virology of HCV and address the aforementioned mechanisms of HCV-induced hepatocarcinogenesis [37].

### 1.2.1. Virology

The HCV genome is a single-stranded, positive sense RNA that has short non-coding regions (NCR) at each end. The 5'-region of the viral genome encodes the nucleocapsid protein (core) and two envelope glycoproteins (E1 and E2) [37]. The core, E1, and E2 proteins comprise the viral particle, which interacts with cellular surface receptors and is internalized. The 3'-region of the viral genome encodes nonstructural proteins (p7, NS2, NS3, NS4A, NS4B, NS5A, and NS5B) [6]. Once the virus is internalized, its genome is released into the cytoplasm, at which point it acts as mRNA for the translation of viral proteins or as a template for RNA replication. The viral genome may also be packaged into new particles [6].

Acute infection with HCV usually progresses to chronic infection, with only 10-40% of acute infections resolving spontaneously. Chronic disease progresses to cirrhosis and liver cancer at a variable rate depending on other factors. Alcohol intake, HIV and/or HBV infection, obesity, male sex, and older age appear to increase the rate of progression to severe liver disease [37].

## 1.2.2. HCV Proteins: Core Protein

The HCV core protein has been shown to be involved in several cellular processes, such as apoptosis, signal transduction, ROS formation, lipid metabolism, transcriptional activation, transformation, and immune system alterations [6].

### 1.2.2a. Apoptosis & Cell Cycle Arrest

The viral core protein affects apoptosis and cellular growth arrest mechanisms by interacting with tumor suppressors, such as p53, p73, and pRb. The regulatory domain of the core protein repressed p53 promoter transcriptional activity and thus the transcription of the p53 tumor suppressor [38]. The viral core protein is able to bind to p73α and inhibit its growth arrest activities in a p53-dependent manner [39]. The HCV core protein has also been shown to decrease levels of pRb, resulting in increased rates of cell proliferation [40]. Interestingly, this decrease in pRb seemed to simultaneously sensitize cells to apoptosis, which may benefit the virus by helping to spread virus progeny to other cells. Furthermore, the core protein has been shown to inhibit the expression of the p21, a Cdk inhibitor, when it is in its mature form (amino acids 1-173.) However, when the viral core protein is in its innate form (amino acids 1-191), it increases the levels of p21 [41]. Finally, the HCV core protein may be able to modulate cellular apoptosis by activating NF-κB [42]. It is able to activate NF-κB by interacting with the intracellular domain of tumor necrosis factor receptor 1 (TNFR1) and the lymphotoxin β (LTβ) receptor, which differs from the manner in which HBx activates NF-κB (via the MAPK pathway.)

### 1.2.2b. Cellular Signaling Pathways

The HCV core protein has been shown to be involved in several cellular signaling pathways. It is able to induce activation of the Raf1/MAPK pathway as well as the Wnt/β-catenin pathway, which are both important oncogenic signaling cascades. Additionally, the core protein has been shown to modulate the TGF-β pathway and androgen receptor signaling. The core protein's ability to activate the Raf1/MAPK signaling pathway is dependent on its binding to 14-3-3 protein family members [43]. The viral core protein has been shown to affect the Wnt/β-catenin pathway by upregulation of Wnt-1 and a downstream target of Wnt-1, WISP-2 [44]. While cases of HCV show increased levels of TGF-β, the HCV core protein has an inhibitory effect on TGF-β signaling [45]. As discussed in section 1.1.3d, TGF-β signaling can be tumor suppressive or oncogenic. Interestingly, it has been shown that some variants of the HCV core protein can bind to and inhibit the DNA binding activity of Smad3, an important downstream effector of TGF-β, resulting in a decrease in TGF-β signaling [46]. It should be noted that other oncogenic viruses, such as Epstein-Barr virus (EBV), human T-cell lymphotropic virus (HTLV-1), human papilloma virus (HPV), and adenovirus, exhibit a similar inhibition of TGF-β signaling, indicating that the inhibition may be important for some virally-induced cancers [46]. Another study has shown that the core protein's ability to decrease Smad3 activation switches the TGF-β tumor suppressive effects to tumor promoting and epithelial-mesenchymal transition (EMT) effects [47] Finally, the viral core protein has been shown to increase VEGF expression by inducing androgen receptor signaling, indicating a potential role for the viral protein in angiogenesis, tumor progression, and metastasis [48].

### 1.2.3. HCV Proteins: Envelope Protein

The E2 protein exerts several oncogenic effects. First, it has been shown to inhibit natural killer (NK) cells via the E2 protein's CD81 receptor, which is an important mechanism of evading the immune system in order to maintain infection and progress to chronic infection and subsequent HCC [49]. The E2 protein has also been shown to promote survival and growth of hepatocytes by activating the MAPK/ERK pathway and the downstream transcription factor ATF-2 [50]. Interestingly, this effect of the E2 protein also relies on CD81 because MAPK activation by E2 was decreased by blocking the CD81 receptor.

### 1.2.4 .HCV Proteins: Non-Structural Proteins

#### 1.2.4a. NS3 Protein

The HCV NS3 protein may be influential in the early stages of hepatocarcinogenesis in HCV-infected individuals. The NS3 protein has been shown to inhibit the activity of the p21 promoter possibly via modulation of p53 [51]. The NS3 protein may also interact with and suppress the transactivation activities of p53 in an NS3 sequence-specific manner, which may contribute to HCV-related hepatocarcinogenesis [52] In addition, NS3 expression increases JNK activation and the DNA-binding activities of AP-1 and ATF-2 transcription factors as well as promotes cell growth [53] Finally, by activating AP-1 and NF-κB, the HCV NS3 protein is able to induce tumor necrosis factor alpha (TNFα) levels, promoting inflammatory processes in the liver, which contribute to tumor promotion [53].

#### 1.2.4b. NS5A Protein

The HCV NS5A protein plays a role in multiple cellular functions, such as apoptosis, signaling pathways, transcription, transformation, and the production of ROS. NS5A is able to bind to p53 tumor suppressor, inhibiting its transactivation activity, including its transcriptional activation of the growth arrest gene p21, as well as the ability of p53 to induce apoptosis [54]. Notably, NS5A can inhibit apoptosis independently of its effect on p53. It has been shown to interact with the pro-apoptotic protein Bax and prevent apoptosis via Bcl-2 homology domains (BH3, BH1, and BH2) [55]. TNFα-induced apoptosis of hepatocytes may also be blocked by NS5A. The viral protein is able to inhibit activation of the pro-apoptotic initiator caspase, caspase-3, and inhibit cleavage of the death substrate poly (ADP-ribose) polymerase (PARP) [56]. Finally, the NS5A protein was shown to be able to activate the NF-κB pathway, which could potentially inhibit apoptosis in HCV-infected hepatocytes [57]. Overexpression of NS5A activates STAT-3, and specifically, it has been shown to activate the STAT-3 and NF-κB transcription factors by inducing oxidative stress and increasing intracellular calcium levels. The increase in calcium promotes the generation of ROS in the mitochondria, which results in the nuclear translocation of both STAT-3 and NF-κB [58]. The viral protein may also activate STAT-3 signaling via activation of Src-family kinases, such as Fyn, Hck, Lck, and Lyn [59]. NS5A further promotes survival by binding to the p85 regulatory subunit of PI3K, activating the pathway and exhibiting a potential mechanism for HCV-induced HCC [60].

Interestingly, unlike HBV proteins, NS5A is known to inhibit ERK signaling. This is probably due to the ability of NS5A to bind to Grb2, preventing its translocation to growth factor receptors and ability to activate the Ras pathway [59]. However, like the HBV X and

HCV core proteins, NS5A plays a role in modulating the Wnt/β-catenin pathway. NS5A expression via activation of the PI3K/Akt pathway inhibits Forkhead transcription factor (FKHR), a substrate of activated Akt. The inhibition of FKHR induces phosphorylation of GSK-3β, which leads to the stabilization of β-catenin and the transcription of β-catenin-responsive genes [61]. The NS5A protein also plays a role in TGF-β signaling, like both HBV and HCV core proteins. In fact, like the HCV core protein, the NS5A protein inhibits TGF-β signaling by interacting with the TGF-β receptor 1 and inhibiting the nuclear translocation of Smad proteins, downstream effectors of the TGF-β signaling pathway [62]. This study also showed that NS5A had the ability to decrease Smad2 phosphorylation and inhibit the heterodimerization of Smad3 and Smad4.

Finally, NS5A plays a role in chromosome instability, which may be a mechanism of HCV-induced hepatocarcinogenesis. The viral protein has been shown to downregulate the mitotic spindle protein ASPM via the double-stranded RNA-activated protein kinase R (PKR)-p38 signaling pathway, which results in aberrations in mitosis and chromosome instability [63].

### 1.2.5. Oxidative Stress, Steatosis & Insulin Resistance

While the modulation of cellular growth signaling pathways by HCV viral proteins has been shown to be sufficient to induce HCC, there seems to be a synergism between the indirect oncogenic effects of viral proteins and the chronic inflammation associated with long-term HCV infection [37]. Chronic HCV infection is associated with increased oxidative stress, demonstrated by the increased lipid peroxidation and oxidative DNA damage in patients infected with HCV. Some of the events occurring during HCV infection that contribute to oxidative stress include mitochondrial dysfunction, ER stress, and immune-cell-mediated oxidative bursts, which generate ROS. The increased formation of ROS has several effects on the cell, including modulation of gene expression, cell adhesion, cell metabolism, cell cycle and apoptosis, and the generation of oxidative DNA damage. This DNA damage can result in the development of mutations and subsequent hepatocyte transformation. Furthermore, ROS can activate several important pathways involved in cancer, including MAPK, PI3K, p53, Wnt/β-catenin, and angiogenesis signaling pathways [6].

For example, as mentioned in section 1.2.4b, by inducing oxidative stress and increasing intracellular calcium levels, NS5A is able to activate transcription factors like NF-κB and STAT-3 [58]. Furthermore, another HCV nonstructural protein, NS3, can activate NADPH oxidase 2 (NOX2), generating ROS [64]. The HCV core protein is also involved in oxidative stress in HCV-infected hepatocytes. The viral core protein decreases levels of glutathione (GSH) and mitochondrial NADPH, resulting in an increase in intracellular calcium levels. This increase in calcium leads to increased calcium uptake and generation of ROS by the mitochondria, similarly to the previously discussed effect of NS5A on ROS levels [65]. The HCV core protein contributes to increased oxidative stress and cellular levels of ROS by inducing ER stress and modulating expression of inducible nitric oxide synthase (iNOS) and cyclooxygenase-2 (COX2.) In fact, because of the NF-κB binding sites on the iNOS promoter, the core protein is able to activate the iNOS gene via activation of NF-κB [66]. The ability of the core protein to activate COX2 transcription may be attributable to its ability to transactivate peroxisome proliferator-activated receptor alpha (PPARα) ligands [67]. Notably, ER stress generated by the HCV core protein results in the induction of apoptosis in hepatocytes [68].

Furthermore, HCV-related steatosis and insulin resistance (IR) act as pro-carcinogenic cofactors. Approximately 30-70% of patients with chronic HCV infection exhibit steatosis, which is associated with a more severe fibrosis and the development of HCC [6]. It is generally believed that HCV induces steatosis by altering lipid metabolism, including lipid secretion, degradation, and synthesis. The HCV core protein may play a role in altering lipid metabolism via its constant activation of PPARα [69]. Additionally, HCV infection may result in the inhibition of assembly and/or secretion of very low density lipoprotein (VLDL), providing a potential mechanism of HCV-induced steatosis [70]. Both steatosis and ER/oxidative stress can cause IR, and steatosis is itself aggravated by IR. These processes promote chronic liver inflammation, apoptosis, and fibrogenesis and contribute to the development of HCC in HCV-infected patients [37].

## 1.3. Liver Flukes

Infection with liver flukes is the strongest risk factor for CCA, primary cancer of the epithelial cells in the bile ducts [71]. The liver flukes Clonorchis sinensis (C. sinensis) and Opisthorchis viverrini (O. viverrini) are foodborne trematodes that chronically infect the bile ducts. Infections with both species are classified as Group I carcinogens, meaning they are "carcinogenic to humans." C. sinensis is found primarily in Asian countries, including China, Japan, Korea, and Vietnam while O. viverrinni is geographically distributed in Thailand, Laos, Cambodia, and Vietnam. In fact, in Thailand approximately 6 million people are infected with O. viverrinn, while 15 million people are infected with C. sinensis in China [72]. The following section will discuss what is known about the parasitology and oncogenecity of liver flukes.

### 1.3.1. Parasitology

C. sinensis and O. viverrini infections cause clonorchiasis and opisthorchiasis, respectively. Generally, individuals acquire the infection by eating raw or uncooked cyprinoid fish products. The fluke eggs are ingested by snails, and the flukes eventually can swim to reside in the flesh or skin of fresh water fish. Then, when the fish is ingested by the human host, the flukes move to the liver from the duodenum via the ampulla of Vater. In the liver they enter the bile ducts and mature to adult worms. These flukes can remain in the intrahepatic bile ducts, or they can reside in the extrahepatic bile ducts, gallbladder, and pancreatic duct. They obstruct the biliary tract, causing severe inflammation, which underlies most of the disease manifestations [72].

### 1.3.2. Mechanisms of Liver Fluke-Induced Hepatocarcinogenesis

Since C. sinensis has only recently been placed as a Group I carcinogen, the mechanism of hepatocarcinogenesis with this fluke species specifically has not been explored in detail. Several mechanisms for the hepatocarcinogenesis of the liver flukes O. viverrini have been proposed, however, and the following will focus on the carcinogenic mechanisms proposed for O. viverrini. In the case of this fluke species, some have suggested that the mechanical injury from the oral and ventral suckers of the fluke when they hook onto the biliary epithelium is significant to the development of damage and inflammation. The attachment of the fluke results in a lesion that ulcerates as the parasite grows and matures [73]. In addition, the flukes secrete metabolic byproducts that are immunogenic, inducing a host immune response, which may contribute to carcinogenesis (See section 3.) These secretions may also be toxic to the biliary epithelium, inducing damage to the tissue. Furthermore, when human CCA cells were stimulated with excretory/secretory products from *O. viverrini*, the cells exhibited a dramatic increase in proliferation, indicating that the metabolic products of the fluke may act as mitogens [73]. During the infection inflammation, periductal fibrosis, and proliferative responses are observed. These proliferative responses include epithelial hyperplasia, goblet cell metaplasia, and adenomatous hyperplasia, which may promote pre-cancerous lesions [74]. One study showed that murine fibroblasts co-cultured with *O. viverrini* overexpressed growth-promoting genes, and results indicated a role in fluke-induced HCC for the TGFβ and EGF pathways [75].

Generally speaking, chronic inflammation induced by long-term liver fluke infection promotes CCA. Nitric oxide (NO) and ROS are produced by inflammatory cells. When NO reacts with ROS, reactive oxygen-nitrogen species (RONS) are formed, including peroxynitrite, and these ROS and RONS can induce DNA damage. In hamsters infected with *O. viverrini*, nitrative and oxidative DNA damage (8-nitroguanine and 8-oxoguanine) and increased iNOS expression have been reported in the biliary epithelium [76]. These lesions persisted in the cells for at least 180 days post-infection, and were shown to be induced by inflammatory processes. Furthermore, NO may play a role in inhibiting DNA repair and apoptosis, contributing to hepatocarcinogenesis [73]. In fact, in human cases of *O. viverrini* infection, higher endogenous nitrosation have been observed as compared to uninfected individuals [77,78]. N-nitroso compounds from exogenous sources may act in concert with the inflammatory response. Finally, opisthorchiasis is associated with increased bile acids, which are tumor promoters and can block degradation of the Bcl-2 family anti-apoptotic protein myeloid cell leukemia protein 1 (MCL-1) through the activation of the epithelial growth factor receptor (EGFR) signaling pathway [79].

The specific carcinogenic mechanisms of *C. sinensis* are only beginning to be explored. In a recent study, cells treated with E/S products from *C. sinensis* and a small amount of carcinogen, dimethylnitrosamine (DMN), exhibited uncontrolled cellular proliferation and the increased expression of cell cycle-related proteins, such as E2F1, hyperphosphorylated Rb (p-pRb), and cyclin B [22]. Like *O. viverrini*, chronic inflammation from infection with *C. sinensis* is able to induce hyperplasia and adenomatous changes of the biliary epithelium [80]. These hyperplastic changes make cells vulnerable to DNA damaging agents that can induce transformation. Also, the *C. sinensis* infection, like *O. viverrini*, can cause endogenous nitrosation and the formation of *N*-nitroso compounds that may lead to carcinogenesis [80].

## 1.4. Helicobacter spp

*Helicobacter* spp infect almost every vertebrate species and can reside in many areas of the digestive tract, including the choledochus, gallbladder, intrahepatic bile ducts, and liver. The bacteria *Helicobacter hepaticus* (*H. hepaticus*) was first discovered in laboratory mice that exhibited a novel form of chronic active hepatitis. Currently, the association between *Helicobacter* spp and HCC in humans remains debatable. Ten case-control studies have been performed to investigate whether or not the presence of *Helicobacter* spp in the liver is associated with the development of HCC [81]. All but one of the studies found an association, but a meta-analysis could be performed because of the level of clinical heterogeneity among the studies in areas such as patient/control selection criteria and the methods used. The central argument against an association between the bacterium and liver cancer is the inability to culture the bacterium in the liver. It has not been shown if *Helicobacter* spp DNA obtained in the liver indicates a true colonization or simply enterohepatic circulation of the bacterium. Others suggest that the failure to culture the bacteria from liver specimens is due to the low bacterial load [81].

Interestingly, other evidence indicates *Helicobacter* spp may have tumorigenic effects in the liver. *H. hepaticus* upregulates H19 fetal liver mRNA and intestinal trefoil factor 3, two supposed tumor markers, in mice [82]. Infected mice also exhibit hepatocellular dysplasia and increased proliferation of hepatocytes [83]. *Helicobacter* spp also produce toxins that can damage hepatocytes, such as cytolethal distending toxin (Cdt) from *H hepaticus* and VacA from *H pylori*. Finally, it has been suggested that *Helicobacter* spp induce pro-inflammatory cytokines by activating the NF-κB pathway. In doing so, the liver may undergo chronic inflammation, which is an important risk factor for developing HCC (see section 3) [84].

## Sectional Summary

Multiple infectious agents have been implicated in hepatocarcinogenesis, including viral, bacterial, and parasitic agents. HBV and HCV infections are two of the most prevalent and widely known risk factors for HCC. HBV can promote genomic instability by genomic integration and can affect cellular signaling pathways via its viral proteins. These proteins, such as HBx and pre-S2/S, are able to activate several pathways involved in cancer, including NF-κB, Ras-Raf-Erk, and PI3K/Akt. Furthermore, these HBV proteins can affect the TGF-β and Wnt/ β-catenin pathways and p53 activity. HCV can exert some of the same effects as HBV although the virus cannot directly affect genomic stability by genomic integration. Instead, HCV proteins, such as the core, envelope, and non-structural proteins, are able to affect cellular signaling in several ways. These HCV proteins can activate several transcription factors, as well as both the TGF-β and Wnt/ β-catenin pathways. They can also interact with and inhibit tumor suppressors, such as p53, p73, and pRb. Both viruses can cause significant oxidative stress and inflammation in the liver, which can also promote hepatocarcinogenesis.

While the mechanisms by which liver flukes and Helicobacter spp. induce tumorigenesis are unknown, several pathways have been suggested. Liver flukes may secrete metabolic products that act as mitogens, and Helicobacter spp. secrete damaging toxins. Both liver flukes and Helicobacter spp. induce chronic inflammation and the generation of NO and ROS, which can damage DNA and promote tumorigenesis.

# 2. Toxic Causes

## 2.1. Alcohol Consumption

While HCC is a rare cancer in the United States, with an incidence rate of 1-2.5/100,000, HCC incidence in America has been rising over the past 20 years. This phenomenon may be due to increased HCV infection, but the alcohol-associated risk for developing HCC is still considered a major risk factor [85]. The majority of consumed alcohol is metabolized in the liver, specifically by the enzyme alcohol dehydrogenase (ADH.) Another important enzyme involved in the metabolism of alcohol is the cytochrome P450 2E1 (CYP2E1) enzyme, which is found predominantly in hepatocytes and mucosal cells of the gastrointestinal tract. CYP2E1 seems to be induced in cases of sustained alcohol consumption or chronic alcohol abuse while ADH quickly metabolizes alcohol to acetate in situations of mild to moderate alcohol intake.

Both ADH and CYP2E1 enzymes convert alcohol to acetaldehyde, which is a toxic and mutagenic compound. Furthermore, when CYP2E1 is induced, hepatocytes undergo increased oxidative stress due to ROS generation from the reaction between CYP2E1 and molecular oxygen. ROS can promote lipid peroxidation, which results in the formation of other reactive aldehydes, such as 4-hydroxynonenal (HNE) and malondialdehyde (MDA.) Acetaldehyde and aldehyde compounds associated with alcohol metabolism are reactive and can form DNA adducts. Acetaldehyde induces $N^2$-ethyl-2'-deoxyguanosine ($N^2$-ethyl-dG) while the aldehydes or enals generate cyclic $N^2$-propano-2'-deoxyguanosine ($N^2$-PdG) DNA adducts. The enals are also able to form more complex DNA lesions, such as DNA-protein and DNA-DNA cross-links [85]. Acetaldehyde and aldehydes can also form adducts with cellular proteins, including important DNA repair proteins. Additionally, these alcohol metabolites have been shown to induce collagen synthesis in hepatic stellate cells (HSCs), which is critical to fibrosis [86].

While alcohol metabolism and its generation of mutagenic acetaldehyde and harmful ROS contribute to the hepatocarcinogenic process, there are other mechanisms that may play a role in promoting alcohol-related liver cancer. For instance, CYP2E1 induction during chronic alcohol consumption and abuse may have other roles in promoting liver cancer. Importantly, CYP2E1 converts some procarcinogens, such as nitrosamines and azo-compounds, to carcinogens, and many of these compounds can also be found in alcoholic beverages and tobacco smoke [87]. Secondly, during cellular respiration, the mitochondria generate high levels of ROS, which are antagonized and kept to physiologically acceptable levels by the endogenous mitochondrial antioxidant, GSH. However, alcoholic liver disease and cirrhosis are associated with GSH depletion and oxidation [88], which can result in an increase in ROS. This increase can lead to lipid, protein, and DNA adduct formation, which damages the cell and can promote mutagenesis.

Overall intrahepatic events are important to the carcinogenicity of alcohol consumption as well. Increased alcohol consumption alters the delicate balance of bacteria in the GI tract, and increases its permeability to lipopolysaccharide (LPS) [89]. This increases LPS levels in the liver, activating Kupffer cells, which are the macrophages of the liver. Kupffer cells release pro-inflammatory cytokines to signal organ damage and to activate HSCs, which induce fibrosis and cirrhosis. Interestingly, ethanol can also induce HSC activation via ROS production and increased oxidative stress [85]. Furthermore, the increased rate of regeneration due to damage in the alcoholic liver results in more inflammatory cytokine signaling in replicating cells, which has been shown to be associated with liver cancer (see section 3), and may lead to genetic mutation due to susceptibility of the dividing cells and mutagenic metabolites.

## 2.2. Aflatoxin-B1

Aflatoxin B1 (AFB1) is a toxin produced by the fungus *Aspergillus* spp, which is often found in Asia and sub-Saharan Africa. A humid climate and poor storage techniques promote growth of the fungus, so it is a frequent food contaminant, usually in grain, corn, peanuts and legumes. AFB1 can be metabolized into AFB1-8, 9-epoxide, which can intercalate into DNA and alkylate bases. These adducts, if not repaired, can lead to mutations. Furthermore, AFB1 can induce the formation of ROS and cause oxidative stress, which can also damage DNA and lead to mutagenesis [90]. Thus, high exposure to the toxin is associated with high prevalence of HCC, and, interestingly, the areas where AFB1 exposure is elevated are also areas with endemic HBV infection [91]. It was shown that both HBV and AFB1 exposures together conferred the highest risk of developing HCC [91]. This synergistic effect may be due to cytochrome P450 induction by chronic HBV infection, which may lead to the metabolism of AFB1 into its mutagenic metabolite. Furthermore, the HBV X protein inhibits NER, which is the DNA repair pathway that removes AFB1-DNA adducts and prevents mutations [92]. Notably, AFB1 exposure has been shown to be associated with a mutation at codon 249 of the p53 tumor suppressor gene in HCCs [93].

## 2.3. Transition Metal Accumulation

### 2.3.1. Hereditary Hemochromatosis

HCC is one of the major complications of hereditary hemochromatosis (HH), and in affected individuals, it is the most common cause of premature death. Hemochromatosis is characterized by toxic accumulation of iron in parenchymal cells of organs. The syndrome is caused by genetic mutations in any gene that limits iron entry into the blood [94]. There are 5 different types of hereditary hemochromatosis that are classified by mutation, with type 1 being the most common: type 1 (hereditary hemochromatosis, HFE), type 2a (hemojuvelin, HJV or HFE2), type 2b (hepcidin, HAMP), type 3 (transferring receptor 2, TFR2), and type 4 (ferroportin, FPN or SLC40A1) [95].

Individuals with HH have iron accumulation in the liver that culminates in cirrhosis and HCC. Notably, non-cirrhotic HCC has been reported in individuals with HH, suggesting that hepatic iron accumulation can directly induce hepatocarcinogenesis [96,97]. This mechanism of liver tumorigenesis could be attributable to the generation of ROS and oxidative damage by free hepatic iron, which could produce mutations [98]. However, other iron overload conditions have not been shown to promote the development of HCC, indicating that a complex network of genetic factors may be involved in non-cirrhotic hereditary hemochromatosis-related HCC [95].

HH seems to have genetic and epigenetic effects that may be relevant to the development of HCC in these patients. Interestingly, p53 is mutated in 71% of HCCs from individuals with HH. Other alterations in HCCs seen often in HH patients are epigenetic defects, specifically increased methylation. Interestingly, these methylation changes are even seen in non-neoplastic tissue in HH patients. One study showed that the majority of liver biopsies sampled from normal tissue of HH patients displayed methylation silencing of at least one of the six genes most frequently hypermethylated in HCC: RASSF1A, cyclin D2, p16, GSTP1, SOCS1, and APC. This study showed that changes in DNA methylation patterns were early events that preceded malignant transformation in HH patients [99].

### 2.3.2. Wilson's Disease

Wilson's disease (WD) is an autosomal recessive disorder caused by a mutation in the ATP7B gene, which encodes a protein that regulates Cu transport. Affected individuals have defective copper metabolism due to the ATP7B mutation which results in a decreased ability of the liver to secrete excess copper into the bile for elimination. The result is copper (and iron) accumulation in the liver, eyes, central nervous system (CNS), and kidneys and severe liver injury. Notably, affected individuals have an increased risk for liver cancer and other intra-abdominal malignancies, but some studies convey inconclusive results regarding the association between WD and HCC due to the rarity of the disease and the lengthy follow-up [100]. It should be noted, however, that there have been at least 20 reported cases of HCC associated with WD despite its rarity. In an unusual case of an HCC diagnosis prior to diagnosis of WD, the non-tumorous liver tissue was found to be cirrhotic with abnormal nodules, suggesting that the mechanism of WD-related hepatocarcinogenesis may be chronic inflammation leading to cirrhosis [101].

### 2.3.3 .Transition Metal Accumulation and Hepatocarcinogenesis

It has been shown that both HH and WD patients harbor significantly increased levels of DNA damage as a result of persistent oxidative stress and lipid peroxidation induced by the accumulation of transition metals in the liver [102,103]. DNA damage can lead to mutations, and mutations in certain genes relevant to cancer can increase genomic instability, promoting liver carcinogenesis. In fact, non-tumorous liver tissues of both WD and HH patients display high levels of p53 mutations and sometimes increased iNOS expression, which may be a source of increased oxidative stress and DNA damage [104].

## 2.4. Vinyl Chloride

Vinyl chloride monomer (VCM) is used in the plastics industry to produce its polymerized form, polyvinyl chloride (PVC.) VCM is found exclusively in factories as it does not occur naturally, but it is also found in cigarette smoke. It is causally associated with angiosarcoma of the liver (ASL) and has recently been suggested to cause HCC as well. The relationship between VCM and liver cancer has been especially described in the population of workers in factories that produce VCM. Before the establishment of environmental controls, worker exposure levels to VCM were extremely high (approximately 7800 mg/m$^3$.) Now, in countries where exposure limits are enforced, VCM exposure levels in factory employees are less than 1 mg/m$^3$ [105].

VCM is metabolized by the liver to chloroethylene oxide, which is a reactive intermediate that is detoxified by glutathione conjugation or aldehyde dehydrogenase. Chloroethylene oxide is able to form mutagenic DNA adducts and induces DNA strand breaks, sister chromatid exchanges, micronucleus formation, and other chromosomal alterations. The DNA adducts formed include 7-(2-oxyethyl) guanine (7OEG), 3,N$^4$-ethenocytosine (εC), 1,N$^6$-ethenoadenne (εA), and N$^2$,3-ethenoguanine (N$^2$,3-εG) [106].

VCM is mutagenic, but whether or not some mutations associated with ASL are due to VCM exposure is unclear. For example, mutations in K-ras have been shown in ASL (two G to A transversions at codons 13 and 12), but some of the same mutations have been observed in ASL in the absence of VCM exposure [105]. Furthermore, VCM has been shown to induce liver injury with fibrosis and endothelial cell hyperplasia. In fact, endothelial cell nuclei become enlarged and display irregular morphology and hyperchromatism, which may indicate pre-neoplastic changes.

There is some debate over whether or not VCM can cause HCC. Some retrospective studies have shown a dose-response relationship between the amount of VCM exposure and mortality due to HCC. Additionally, some retrospective studies show similar results with increased mortality from a liver cancer other than ASL being associated with VCM exposure. Unfortunately, one cannot be sure that the liver cancer was diagnosed correctly because of certain biases. For example, in Taiwan, where one such mortality study was performed, patients who die a cancer death with a liver mass are assumed to have HCC, which makes results of the study unclear. Also, some participants in the retrospective studies were diagnosed in the 1960s and 1970s when less reliable methods of detecting HCC were used. Again, patients who displayed liver failure and a mass in the liver were more likely to be diagnosed as HCC than ASL since ASL is a rarer liver tumor type [107,108].

## Sectional Summary

Several toxic materials display a causal relationship to liver cancer. Many of these agents or conditions, while diverse in nature, seem to exert similar effects on hepatocytes and other cells present in the liver that result in hepatocarcinogenesis. Generally, the generation of oxidative stress can induce DNA damage, promoting transformation and tumorigenesis. Alcohol consumption, a well-known risk factor for HCC, can generate oxidative stress via the formation of reactive acetaldehyde and other aldehydes (enals) or by the induction of a key metabolizing enzyme CYP2E1. Both hereditary hemochromatosis and Wilson's disease are conditions of transition metal accumulation in the liver and are associated with a higher susceptibility to liver cancer. These transition metals, iron and copper, cause increased lipid peroxidation and generate reactive oxygen and nitrogen species (RONS), which can damage DNA. Finally, both aflatoxin B1 and vinyl chloride can be metabolized to reactive intermediates that can form DNA adducts and other types of DNA damage that may lead to tumorigenic mutations.

# 3. Inflammation-mediated Hepatocarcinogenesis

Rudolph Virchow first suggested a link between inflammation and malignancy in the early nineteenth century. Currently, it is known that approximately 25% of human malignancies are attributable to an underlying chronic inflammatory condition. At this point several etiologies of liver cancer have been explored in this chapter, including hepatitis viruses, bacterial and parasitic infections, metal accumulation, and alcohol consumption. While in some ways these etiologic agents are varied in their proposed methods of oncogenecity, a common thread that runs through these seemingly separate and distinct agents is each one's ability to induce the organ wound-healing process and the resulting inflammatory response. In fact, HCC, the most common liver malignancy, almost always develops as the culmination of chronic hepatitis and cirrhosis.

## 3.1. Regeneration, Fibrosis, & Cirrhosis

A unique and fascinating characteristic of the liver is its ability to regenerate. Liver regeneration is a compensatory hyperplasia and hypertrophy that occurs in response to hepatic injury, whether due to viral or toxic exposures [109]. Liver regeneration is a tightly controlled process that requires many signaling pathways that are necessary to repair damage to the organ. In the context of chronic hepatitis, the prolonged activation of the regenerative pathways is believed to contribute to the development of HCC. Furthermore, the sustained disease state results in a constant inflammatory response, which creates a microenvironment that favors the survival of preneoplastic cells, promoting tumorigenesis [110].

After prolonged disease and hepatic regeneration, the wound-healing response becomes fibrogenic, resulting in liver scarring that is associated with the accumulation of matrix proteins. Acute injury may sometimes activate fibrogenic processes, but the extended period of chronic liver disease due to infection, metabolic disorders, and other toxicities are required for the accumulation of significant scarring [111]. The principal cells directing fibrosis are the hepatic stellate cells (HSCs), a population of cells found in the liver. In the normal liver, HSCs are quiescent and function as the body's vitamin A storage cells. When damage to the liver occurs, these quiescent HSCs are activated and transdifferentiate into a myofibroblast phenotype [112]. An important inflammatory stimulus that activates stellate cells is the apoptosis of parenchymal cells as a result of injury. ROS and cytokines also provide activation stimuli for hepatic stellate cells. Activated HSCs secrete several chemokines to recruit inflammatory cells [111]. The activation of stellate cells results in autocrine secretion of mitogens and cytokines, such as TGF-α and epidermal growth factor (EGF), hepatocyte growth factor (HGF), stem cell factor, insulin-like growth factor I/II (IGF1/2), and platelet-derived growth factor (PDGF.) Activated HSCs have also been shown to be involved in the inflammatory response by recruiting neutrophils and secreting pro-inflammatory cytokines, including interleukin-6 (IL-6), monocyte-colony stimulating factor (MCF), and RANTES. MCF promotes macrophage accumulation while RANTES is a chemotactic protein for T cells. The autocrine secretion of TGF-β1 by HSCs has the most impact on the secretion and accumulation of extracellular matrix molecules [113]. Furthermore, HSCs overproduce tissue inhibitor of metalloproteinase-1, -2 (TIMP-1,2), which inhibit collagen degradation and promote fibrosis [114].

Cirrhosis is the most advanced stage of fibrosis. It is characterized by fibrotic scarring, but it is the distorted parenchymal architecture caused by excessive collagen deposition that distinguishes cirrhosis from fibrosis [111]. The scar tissue septa enclose nodules of regenerating and partially dedifferentiated hepatocytes. Interestingly, cirrhosis is also characterized by telomere shortening, while telomerase reactivation has been shown in HCC. The shortening of the telomeres during chronic liver disease is due to high hepatocyte turnover, and it has been suggested that this telomere shortening promotes chromosome instability [115]. It has been shown that telomere dysfunction may be required for genomic instability and the initiation of preneoplastic lesions [116]. However, for the lesion to progress to malignant HCC, telomerase must be reactivated to restore genomic stability to a level that will promote the viability of cancer cells.

## 3.2. Molecular Mechanisms of Inflammation-Mediated Hepatocarcinogenesis

In general, several inflammatory mediators and intracellular signal transducers have been implicated in the development of liver cancer on a background of chronic disease and inflammation. The following subsections elucidate what is known regarding several key molecular links between inflammation and HCC.

### 3.2.1. TNFα

TNFα and its receptor TNFR1 have been shown to be important both in liver regeneration and in the promotion of HCC. HCC is induced in mice administered a choline-deficient and ethionine-supplemented diet. When these mice are deficient for TNFR1, the development of HCC is attenuated, indicating an important role for TNFα in promoting liver malignancy [117]. Additionally, an Mdr2-knockout mouse model that spontaneously develops HCC after a period of cholestatic hepatitis has been used to explore the role of inflammation and cancer. In this model it was shown that treatment with anti- TNFα antibody could lead to apoptosis in transformed hepatocytes and prevent the progression to HCC [118].

### 3.2.2. NF-κB

Importantly, TNFα signaling activates NF-κB, a transcription factor that is a key regulator of the inflammatory response and has been shown to be a potential link between chronic inflammation and HCC. Interestingly, there seem to be conflicting observations regarding the specific role NF-κB plays in the development of HCC, whether it is protective or tumorigenic. In one study, hepatocyte-specific deletion of IκB kinase β-subunit (IKK-β), a kinase that is essential for the activation of NF-κB, in a diethylnitrosamine (DEN)-induced hepatocarcinogenesis mouse model led to increased incidence of HCC [119]. The IKK-β regulatory subunit NEMO/IKKγ is also necessary for the activation of NF-κB. Similiarly to the previous study, conditional ablation of NEMO/IKKγ and thus the NF-κB pathway resulted in spontaneous steatohepatitis and hepatocarcinogenesis [120]. On the other hand, it has been demonstrated that NF-κB inhibition in liver parenchymal cells during later stages of HCC development results in a slower rate of tumor progression [118].

One might be able to reconcile these opposing reports by examining the timing and cell specificity in targeting the NF-κB pathway. Early inactivation of NF-κB sensitizes hepatocytes to apoptosis, resulting in a loss of parenchymal cells. This tissue loss instigates the regenerative process, which places proliferative pressure on the surviving hepatocytes that exist under inflammatory and oxidative stress conditions. These cells, including their DNA, may be damaged and their proliferation increases the risk of malignant transformation of the hepatocytes. On the other hand, NF-κB activity may act to promote survival during late stages of hepatocarcinogenesis, so inactivation of the transcription factor at this stage results in an inhibition of tumor progression [110]. It was then shown in a DEN model of hepatocarcinogenesis that NF-κB activity loss led to enhanced chemical carcinogenesis via JNK1 activation. Without NF-κB activity, the DEN-induced TNFα levels promote the sustained activation of JNK1, which results in apoptosis and necrosis of hepatocytes. The loss of organ mass then triggers compensatory proliferation of the surviving cells, potentially promoting the transformation of hepatocytes. When JNK1 is deleted, these effects are not observed; and the development of HCC is impaired [121].

Notably, the role of NF-κB in hepatocarcinogenesis becomes even more complex when one examines its activity in immune cells. The number and size of DEN-induced tumors were demonstrated to be reduced when IKK-β was inactivated in both hepatocytes and immune cells, including Kupffer cells, which are the liver macrophages [119]. When IKK-β was deleted in Kupffer cells, levels of inflammatory cytokines and mitogens, such as TNFα, IL-6, and HGF, were significantly decreased; and DEN-induced hepatocyte proliferation was inhibited [119].

### 3.2.3. IL-6

Since a reduction in inflammatory molecules and mitogens was coupled with a reduction in hepatocyte proliferation, when NF-κB activity was suppressed in Kupffer cells, it is clear that the dialogue occurring between inflammatory cells and hepatocytes is critical to the development of inflammation-mediated HCC. A key inflammatory mediator that warrants attention is IL-6. Notably it has been shown that many inflammatory conditions of the liver, such as chronic alcohol consumption, viral infections, or hepatic metal accumulation, are associated with elevated circulating levels of IL-6. In patients diagnosed with HCC following a chronic inflammatory condition, levels of circulating IL-6 were even higher [122]. Interestingly, in a DEN-induced hepatocarcinogenesis model, IL-6-knockout mice severely inhibited the formation of HCC [123]. The DEN mouse model, as well as human epidemiological studies, show that males are more susceptible to liver cancers than females. The previous study also showed that levels of IL-6 were higher in the DEN-treated wild-type (WT) male mice than in the DEN-treated WT female mice. Interestingly, deletion of IL-6 could eliminate the gender disparity in susceptibility to HCC in the IL-6-knockout mice, but this was due to a decrease in the incidence of HCC in male mice, not an increase in HCC incidence in female mice. Estrogen inhibits IL-6 promoter activity via its ability to decrease the activity of transcription factors such as NF-κB and C/EBPβ. Therefore, DEN-treated WT male mice that were administered an estrogen receptor agonist displayed levels of IL-6 comparable to those of DEN-treated WT female mice. These observations from this study indicate that estrogen in females exerts a protective effect against liver cancer via decreased activation of the IL-6 promoter compared to males [123].

Furthermore, the previously referenced study elucidated the importance of MyD88, a TLR (toll-like receptor) adaptor protein, in the role of IL-6 in hepatocarcinogenesis after DEN treatment. The study showed that IL-6 production through the TLR-MyD88-NF-κB pathway was critical for the development of HCC [123]. It was suggested that the necrosis of hepatocytes activated TLR-MyD88 signaling and the production of IL-6, showing a potential role for this pathway in promoting the regenerative process and compensatory proliferation. It should be noted that IL-6 appears to contribute to other inflammation-related cancers, such as colitis-associated cancer and possibly other intestinal cancers [122].

### 3.2.4. STAT3

IL-6 is able to exert its effects on hepatocytes via its activation of the transcription factor STAT3. The IL-6 receptor (IL-6R) is associated with two subunits of gp130, and when activated by IL-6, a gp130 subunit activates JAK1. JAK1 subsequently phosphorylates a tyrosine residue on a gp130 subunit and STAT3, which results in the dimerization of STAT3. The STAT3 dimer then translocates to the nucleus to activate transcription of target genes involved in cell proliferation and survival [124]. The JAK-STAT pathway has been demonstrated to be induced in liver inflammation as well as in HCC, and these conditions are associated with a downregulation of JAK-STAT pathway suppressors, such as SOCS3 [125]. It has been shown that loss of SOCS3 expression can be attributed to methylation or other methods of silencing [126], and hypermethylation of SOCS3 was demonstrated to result in increased focal adhesion kinase (FAK) phosphorylation and enhanced cell migration [127]. These studies show that without SOCS3 expression, the regenerative response in hepatocytes is enhanced, and the cells become more susceptible to transformation. These studies indicate and support an important role for Il-6-STAT3 signaling aberrations in inflammation-mediated hepatocarcinogenesis.

### 3.2.5. IL-1

Recently, it has been shown that the release of IL-1α from damaged hepatocytes is critical for the stimulation of regenerative proliferation. In the DEN-induced hepatocarcinogenesis model, compensatory proliferation and liver regeneration are necessary for the development of HCC. In this model, it was demonstrated that inhibition of IL-1 receptor (IL-1R) activation results in reduced IL-6 production, proliferation, and tumorigenesis [121]. It was also demonstrated that, as in the IL-6 pathway, MyD88 plays an essential role in IL-1R activation of downstream pathways. Notably, IL-1β has been implicated in the development of HCC in HBV and HCV-infected patients. Patients infected with HCV, both with and without HCC, were evaluated for a genetic polymorphism in IL-1β, and it was demonstrated that a polymorphism at position 511 (IL1B-511) was a risk factor for developing HCC [128]. In a second study, a different IL-1β polymorphism at the same position in patients infected with HBV was shown to be associated with high levels of IL-1β in the liver and associated with development of HCC in these patients [129]. IL-1β may be able to affect hepatocarcinogenesis via its activation of NF-κB (see section 3.2.2) [130]. NF-κB has been shown to activate iNOS which generates nitric oxide NO, a chronic inflammatory mediator that may play a role in tumorigenesis by regulating proliferation, survival, angiogenesis, DNA repair, and other processes [131].

### 3.2.6. Growth Signaling

While the inflammatory cytokine signaling that occurs during chronic hepatitis appears to be important in the development of HCC, the mitogenic growth factor signaling occurring during liver regeneration is also critical. These important growth pathways include IGF, HGF, Wnt, TGFβ, and EGFR signaling.

### 3.2.6a. IGF Signaling

IGF signaling dysregulation in HCC seems mostly to occur with IGF-II overexpression and maximal autocrine signaling in hepatocytes. IGF-II is highly expressed in the fetal liver, but after birth its expression is strongly abrogated. It has been shown to exert anti-apoptotic, proliferative, and angiogenic effects during hepatocarcinogenesis and is overexpressed in 16-40% of human HCCs [132]. When IGF-II activates the IGF-1R, insulin receptor substrates (IRS) are activated, which lead to the activation of PI3K, AKT/protein kinase B (PKB), and MAPK signaling pathways. These pathways transcriptionally activate many target genes, including p27, MYC, FOS, cyclin B, and VEGF [132]. The increased levels of IGF-II may be due to downregulation or deletion of IGF2R, which is the IGF receptor that directs IGFs to degradation. In fact, 63% of HCCs exhibit reduced expression of this receptor while 70% show loss of heterozygosity at the gene locus with 25% having inactivating mutations in the remaining allele [133,134]. Furthermore, circulating IGF-II levels can be reduced by IGF binding proteins (IGFBPs), and it has been shown that IGFBP1, -3, and -4 are frequently downregulated in HCCs, indicating yet another possible mechanism of IGF-II overexpression in human liver cancer [135].

### 3.2.6b. HGF Signaling

HGF is a growth factor for hepatocytes that binds to its only known receptor, MET, which is a receptor tyrosine kinase. MET is known to be expressed on epithelial and endothelial cells and regulates proliferation, migration, cell survival, morphogenesis, angiogenesis, and tissue regeneration. When HGF binds to MET and the receptor multimerizes, auto- and para-phosphorylation occur in the cytoplasmic domain of the receptor. These phosphorylation events result in the activation of phospholipase C (PLC)$\gamma$, STATs, PI3K, and ERK1/2. Transcription factors, such as Ets-1 and AP-1 are activated, and proceed to transactivate target genes, including matrix metalloproteinases (MMPs) and urokinase-type plasminogen activator (uPA), which are involved in tissue remodeling. While MET is detected in approximately 70% of HCCs, overexpression of the receptor is only observed in 20-48% of samples. This increased expression may be due to tumor hypoxia, which has been shown to activate transcription of MET, sensitizing tumor cells to HGF [136]. HGF is also able to transcriptionally activate MET via activation of AP-1 [137]. HGF has been shown to be over-represented in liver malignancies, but this expression is in the hepatic stellate cells, which are induced to secrete HGF during organ damage and inflammation and by tumor cell products (See section 3.1.)

### 3.2.6c. Wnt/ $\beta$-catenin Signaling

The Wnt/$\beta$-catenin pathway is an important cell growth and proliferation pathway that plays a role in several cancer types. When the canonical pathway is not being activated, GSK3$\beta$, Axin1/2, and APC form a complex with the transcriptional co-activator $\beta$-catenin in the cytoplasm, which results in its phosphorylation by GSK3$\beta$ and subsequent degradation. On the other hand, when the Wnt ligand activates its transmembrane receptor frizzled (FZD), dishevelled (DSH) is phophorylated and activated, resulting in the inhibition of the GSK3$\beta$, Axin1/2, and APC complex. $\beta$-catenin is not phosphorylated and remains stabilized and is able to translocate and accumulate in the nucleus. Once in the nucleus, $\beta$-catenin forms complexes with TCF-LEF transcription factors and acts as a co-activator of transcription of several target genes, including Myc, survivin, MMPs, and VEGF. In human HCCs, the dysregulation of the Wnt/$\beta$-catenin pathway is due to abnormal $\beta$-catenin accumulation in the nucleus, leading to tumor growth and progression. Approximately 17-40% of human HCCs display nuclear accumulation of $\beta$-catenin [132]. This accumulation is generally due to stabilizing mutations and deletions in the N-terminal phosphorylation domain of β-catenin. Additionally, mutational inactivation has been observed in Axin-1 and Axin-2, in which the mutations generally found are at binding sites for GSK3β and β-catenin [138]. Another mechanism of aberrant β-catenin accumulation is the upregulation of PIN1, a negative regulator of the β-catenin/APC interaction. In fact, 50% of all HCCs display upregulation of PIN1 with nuclear accumulation of β-catenin [139]. Many other alterations in the Wnt/β-catenin pathway have been observed in human HCC, including FZD-7 overexpression, downregulation of DSH inhibitors, as dysregulation of DKK-3, which inhibits Wnt signaling [32,140-142].

### 3.2.6d. TGFβ Signaling

The TGFβ signaling pathway is activated when TGFβ binds to TGFβ receptor type II (TβR-II), which recruits and transphosphorylates TβR-I. Then the receptor complex phosphorylates Smad2 and Smad3, activating them and releasing them from the receptor. These activated Smads heterodimerize with Smad4 and form complexes with transcriptional regulators, including CBP/p300, FAST-1, and SKI/SNO. In hepatocytes, TGFβ acts as a growth inhibitor, but interestingly, TGFβ levels in HCC patients are increased [117]. In fact, TGFβ is upregulated in approximately 40% of HCCs, and, generally speaking, up to 70% of HCCs exhibit reduction in TGFβ receptors [132,143]. It has been suggested that the differential roles of TGFβ could be due to the presence of oncogenic Ras [144], and that in the presence of oncogenic Ras, TGFβ could induce an epithelial to fibroblastoid conversion (EFC.) The EFC was characterized by an altered morphology in the hepatocytes and autocrine secretion of TGFβ [144]. Additionally, the Smad proteins have been investigated for alterations in HCC, but the Smad-mediated cascade has been shown to be generally intact. However, some reports have shown that the inhibitory Smad7 is upregulated in approximately 60% of advanced HCCs but not dysplastic nodules and early HCCs, potentially acting as a resistance mechanism to any growth inhibitory effects of TGFβ [145].

### 3.2.6e. EGFR Signaling

Finally, EGFR signaling occurs through the tyrosine kinase receptors of the EGFR family: ErbB-1 (EGFR), ErbB-2, ErbB-3, and ErbB-4. The ligands of these growth factor receptors commonly observed to be important in HCC are TGFα and EGF, which are potent mitogens for hepatocytes. In fact, many human HCCs exhibit overexpression of TGFα, which has been shown to act during early hepatocarcinogenesis and to correlate with tumor differentiation and proliferation [146,147]. Overexpression of EGFR has also been demonstrated in human HCCs, but, unlike other cancers, amplification of the ErbB-2 gene is not common [148,149]. Interestingly, it has been shown that EGFR activation is important for the activation of the NF-κB pathway [150]. EGFR activation, like other receptor tyrosine kinases, can activate multiple cell proliferation, growth, and survival pathways, including Ras-MAPK and PI3K-Akt. Therefore, while EGFR activation has been demonstrated to be critical to the hepatocyte proliferation and regeneration after damage, chronic EGFR activation may contribute to hepatocyte transformation [148,151].

### 3.2.7. Inflammation, DNA Damage, & Repair

Chronic inflammation may exert carcinogenic effects via dysregulated cytokine and regenerative (growth factor) signaling. Interestingly, however, there is another possibly effective avenue of tumorigenesis in the DNA damage produced from inflammation-related free radicals, such as RONS. RONS are released by neutrophils and macrophages and can directly oxidize and deaminate DNA bases. Additionally, via lipid peroxidation, RONS can induce etheno and propano DNA adduct formation [152,153]. Furthermore, chronic inflammation has been known to induce DNA double strand breaks as well [154]. Typically, DNA damage is recognized, and the DNA damage response pathway is activated, which can lead to cell cycle arrest and DNA repair or even apoptosis. This response protects cells from replicating damaged DNA that can lead to mutations and ultimately transformation and tumorigenesis.

Interestingly, some models of inflammation-mediated carcinogenesis indicate a role for the inflammatory response in abrogating DNA repair, which provides a potential mechanism for tumorigenesis with a background of chronic inflammation. Generally, RONS-damaged bases, such as those produced by immune cell respiratory burst, are repaired by the base excision repair (BER) pathway, which is a DNA repair pathway that repairs non-helix-distorting lesions in the DNA. It has been demonstrated that the repair of RONS-related DNA damage is important for the suppression of inflammation-mediated colorectal carcinoma and gastric cancer [155]. Moreover, a study performed in a rat model of spontaneous inflammation-mediated hepatocarcinogenesis, the Long Evans Cinnamon rat, which mimics Wilson's disease in humans, showed that acute hepatitis was able to impair BER of oxidative DNA damage, and this reduction in repair was shown to precede the appearance of preneoplastic foci based on results from a second study in the same animal model [156,157]. The regulatory mechanisms of BER and alterations in those mechanisms specifically during inflammation remain to be investigated and may indicate a direct mechanism of hepatocarcinogenesis via un-repaired inflammation-induced DNA damage.

## Sectional Summary

Chronic inflammation has been shown to be one of the most important underlying factors in liver tumorigenesis. Chronic liver damage induces the regenerative response of the liver, which can lead to fibrosis after long periods of time. Cirrhosis, which is end-stage fibrosis, is a significant risk factor for the development of HCC. Cirrhosis is known to be associated with hyperplastic nodules and telomere dysfunction, which may promote hepatocarcinogenesis. Several inflammatory mediators have been implicated in the development of liver cancer, including NF-κB, TNFα, IL-6, STAT3, and IL-1. Furthermore, growth factor signaling, which is involved in liver regeneration in response to wounding, plays a role in tumor progression. These growth factor pathways include IGF, HGF, Wnt/β-catenin, TGFβ, and EGFR signaling. Importantly, chronic inflammation induces free radical formation, which can directly oxidize and deaminate DNA bases. RONS can induce cyclic etheno and propano DNA base adducts via lipid peroxidation. Generally, oxidative DNA damage is repaired by DNA repair mechanisms like the BER pathway. Notably, some acute inflammatory conditions may suppress DNA repair. This suppression, coupled with continuous generation of inflammation-associated damage, can directly promote mutagenesis and lead to tumorigenesis.

# 4. Genetic & Epigenetic Alterations in Liver Cancer

HCC is a particularly heterogeneous tumor with diverse genetic and epigenetic alterations, especially since many genetic alterations accumulate during the lengthy process of hepatocarcinogenesis [158]. Comprehensive analyses of genetic and epigenetic aberrations in HCC have been beneficial in identifying potential molecular classifications of liver malignancies in order to better predict response to current therapies and to possibly determine new therapy targets for these tumors [159]. The following will discuss what is currently understood about genetic mutations in tumor suppressor genes and oncogenes as well as epigenetic alterations and microRNA (miRNA) expressional changes in HCC.

## 4.1. Genetic Mutations

### 4.1.1. Wnt/ β-catenin Pathway

Twenty to 40% of HCCs possess mutations activating the oncogene β-catenin, making it the most frequent activating mutation in HCC. Notably, the Wnt/β-catenin pathway is involved in several physiological functions in the liver, including lineage specification, differentiation, stem cell renewal, epithelial-mesenchymal transition, zonation, proliferation, cell adhesion, and liver regeneration [159]. The mutations in β-catenin are predominantly found within the N-terminus, and they usually lead to the loss of phosphorylation sites necessary for the negative regulation of β-catenin by the GSK3β/APC/Axin complex [160]. It has been shown that mutations in β-catenin seem to occur more frequently in patients without HBV infection and are associated with chromosome stability [161,162]. Interestingly, one study demonstrated that these mutations often develop in non-cirrhotic liver, which is particularly unusual since cirrhosis is a common risk factor for the development of HCC [163]. This study also found that liver tumors that exhibited β-catenin mutations were more histologically aggressive than liver tumors that did not harbor these alterations. Clinically, however, it is debated whether or not mutations and expression alterations in β-catenin confer good or bad prognoses [161,163,164].

Axin1 is another important member of the Wnt/β-catenin pathway that is involved in the negative regulation of β-catenin and has been shown to be mutated in HCC. However, the proportion of mutations in this gene is less than that of β-catenin as biallelic inactivating mutations of Axin1 are found in less than 10% of cases [165,166]. Liver malignancies with Axin1 mutations also exhibit a different phenotype than those with β-catenin mutations. They are generally associated with chromosome instability and are more related to HBV infections [167].

### 4.1.2. p53

The tumor suppressor gene most frequently mutated in HCC is p53. These mutations are frequently associated with HCCs in geographic areas with high aflatoxin-B1 (AFB1) exposure and are not commonly found in regions without the exposure. In the areas of high levels of exposure to AFB1, a G→T transversion at codon 249 leading to an amino acid substitution (R249S) is present in more than 50% of HCC cases [93,168]. In areas that have no exposure to AFB1, p53 mutations are found in less than 20% of HCC cases, and there is no specific mutational hotspot although there is some debate concerning a potential mutational hotspot at codon 220 in hereditary hemochromatosis-related HCC [167,169]. Some studies have demonstrated a relationship between p53 mutations and poorly differentiated HCCs. p53 mutations were also associated with chromosome instability and poor prognosis [167,170,171].

### 4.1.3. Rare Mutations

Other mutations that are rarely observed in HCC include IL6ST (gp130) and HNF1A, which are frequently mutated in hepatocellular adenoma (HCA) [172,173]. It has been suggested the HCC harboring these mutations may arise of a nondiagnosed HCA that underwent malignant transformation [159]. Additionally, some oncogenes and tumor suppressor gene that are frequently mutated in other tumor types are infrequently mutated in HCC, including PIK3CA (PI3K), RB1, KRAS, and HRAS. Mutations in PIK3CA were observed in less than 3% of HCC cases while frameshift mutations in RB1were observed in less than 11% of HCCs (alterations in RB1 are discussed below) [174-176]. Mutations in the Ras proto-oncogene were observed in 3-5% of HCCs. In fact, KRAS mutations are associated with exposure to the carcinogen vinyl chloride, specifically the carcinogenic metabolite of vinyl chloride, chloroethylene oxide [158]. However, vinyl chloride is only rarely associated with the development of HCC, which may explain the observed infrequency of KRAS mutations in HCC cases. Furthermore, mutations in PTEN, a tumor suppressor in the PI3K pathway, have been observed in 5-10% of HCC cases while mutations in IGF2R have been observed in 0-13% of HCCs [177-181]. CDKN2A (p16), a cell cycle inhibitor, has been shown to display point mutations and large deletions in HCC, but these alterations are rare [182,183].

## 4.2. Chromosomal Aberrations

HCC is known to have a complex karyotype and accumulate many chromosomal rearrangements, demonstrating the fact that multi-stage hepatocarcinogenesis is the result of multiple aberrations. The most commonly deleted chromosome arms in HCC are 17p, 16q, 16p, 4q, 9p, 13q, 1p, and 6q while the most frequent gains are 1q, 7q, 8q, and 17q [158]. The tumor suppressor genes that exhibit loss of heterozygosity (LOH) in HCC are found at 17p, 13q, 16p, 9p, and 6q, corresponding to the inactivation of TP53, RB1, Axin1, CDKN2A, and IGF2R, respectively [158]. However, on the other frequently deleted chromosome arms, no tumor suppressor gene targets have been identified.

Approximately 30% of HCC cases display a loss of chromosome 13 which encodes the tumor suppressor gene RB1 [184]. LOH was observed at this locus with very few HCCs exhibiting mutations in the second allele, suggesting that the second allele may be inactivated by epigenetic mechanisms [185]. Additionally, LOH at chromosome arm 9p, the region encoding the CDK-inhibitor p16, which is a tumor suppressor in the retinoblastoma pathway, was observed in about 20% of HCC cases [167,184]. Other, epigenetic aberrations in p16 discussed in section 4.3.

## 4.3. Epigenetics

Epigenetic alterations, such as DNA methylation have been reported in cases of HCC. While DNA methylation does not change genetic information, it does inhibit the readability of the DNA by transcription machinery, resulting in inactivation of genes, specifically tumor suppressor genes in cancer. In HCCs the genes frequently inactivated via methylation, specifically promoter hypermethylation, include genes related to proliferation and apoptosis, cell adhesion and invasion, DNA repair, and inflammatory signaling. The overexpression of DNMT, the enzyme that catalyzes hypermethylation, has been observed in HCC compared to normal liver tissue, which may be the causative factor in observed epigenetic silencing of these tumor suppressor genes [186]. Interestingly, some of the following epigenetically modified genes in HCC are observed to be altered in premalignant conditions, such as chronic hepatitis and cirrhosis, indicating they may be potentially useful biomarkers of early neoplastic changes.

### 4.3.1. Proliferation

As indicated in section 4.2, the retinoblastoma pathway, including RB1 and p16 are important altered pathways in HCC. CDKN2A not only codes for p16 but also p14$^{ARF}$, which are both genes that negatively regulate the cell cycle. P16 binds to CDK4, inhibiting its ability to interact with cyclin D1, a major driver of cell proliferation while p14$^{ARF}$ binds to Mdm2 to prevent the degradation of p53, inducing cell cycle arrest. As mentioned in section 4.2, inactivation of p16 observed in HCC can be due to LOH at chromosome arm 9p. However, CpG island promoter methylation at the p16 locus has been observed in 55-73% of HCC cases [187,188]. Notably, these changes were observed in premalignant conditions, such as chronic hepatitis and liver cirrhosis as well. P14$^{ARF}$ promoter methylation was described less frequently (8-20%), and its inactivation in HCC may be due to homozygous deletions.

### 4.3.2. Apoptosis

Caspase 8 (CASP8) is an initiator caspase that is an important apoptotic gene involved in both extrinsic and intrinsic mechanisms of apoptosis. The gene has been reported to be silenced by promoter methylation in up to 72% of HCC cases [189]. Promoter methylation of another pro-apoptotic gene, TMS1/ASC, has been observed in 80% of HCCs [190]. The TMS1 gene is a negative regulator of NF-κB that inhibits transcription of survival genes [191].

### 4.3.3. Cell Adhesion & Invasion

An important adhesion molecule, E-cadherin, is expressed in all epithelial cells. Loss of E-cadherin expression in tumors leads to tumor progression, cell invasion, and metastasis.

Thirty-three to 67% of HCCs display reduced or null E-cadherin expression due to CpG island methylation [192,193]. Silencing of another cadherin, M-cadherin, was observed in 55% of HCCs while 21% of cases exhibited methylation of H-cadherin [191,194].

TIMP3 inhibits cell migration and angiogenesis, and its overexpression can even induce apoptosis [195]. It is not often methylated in HCC, only occurring in 13-19% of cases. Interestingly, in cases of hepatocellular cancer emboli in portal veins, methylation of TIMP3 was observed at a frequency of 25% [196]. Another gene that inhibits invasion in tumors is TFPI-2, which suppresses the activation of MMP1 and MMP3. Loss of the mRNA transcript expression was observed in 90% of HCCs sampled, and 47% exhibited methylation at the TFPI-2 locus [197].

### 4.3.4. DNA Repair

Promoter methylation of DNA repair genes in HCC is frequently observed in the mismatch repair system, which corrects DNA replication errors. For the mismatch repair gene hMLH1, promoter methylation occurred in 5-13% of cases while methylation of hMSH2 and hMSH3 were observed more frequently, occurring in 68% and 75% of HCC cases, respectively [198]. MGMT (O6-methylguanine DNA methyltransferase) is a DNA repair gene that repairs alkylation at O6-guanine and exhibits its highest activity in the liver. Loss of MGMT due to methylation occurred in 22-39% of HCC cases sampled, and that frequency was higher in chronic viral hepatitis-associated HCC [199,200].

### 4.3.5. Other Methylated Genes Associated with HCC

In HCC tissue methylation of the detoxifying GSTP1 gene was observed in 41-85% of cases [201-203]. Interestingly, this epigenetic alteration of GSTP1 was associated with higher levels of AFB1-DNA adducts and could be detected in the serum of HCC patients well [202,204].

As discussed in section 3, inflammatory cytokine signaling is highly important in the development of HCC. Specifically, the JAK/STAT signaling pathway was mentioned to have a significant role in cell proliferation and survival in liver cancer. SOCS1 and SOCS3 are negative regulators of this pathway that bind to JAK and inhibit the phosphorylation and activation of STATs and their downstream target genes. In cases of HCC, promoter methylation of SOCS-1 was observed with a frequency of 60% while SOCS3 methylation occurred less frequently, with a frequency of 33%. Interestingly, promoter methylation of SOCS1 was detected even in HCV-induced chronic hepatitis and cirrhosis, and the methylation frequency increased with stage of fibrosis [127,205,206].

Finally, RASSF1A is a tumor suppressor gene that is one of the most frequently methylated genes at the methylation hotspot, chromosome arm 3p. Specifically, hypermethylation was observed in 54-95% of HCCs. Notably, these epigenetic changes were observed even in cirrhotic liver and chronic hepatitis. Furthermore, HBV-related HCCs exhibited higher levels of RASSF1A methylation compared to HCCs without risk factors [207].

## 4.4. MicroRNAs as Tumor Suppressors and Oncogenes in HCC

MicroRNAs (miRNAs) are precursor transcripts produced by RNA polymerase II that are processed by several mechanisms. Once mature, miRNAs bind to imperfect complementary target sequences on mRNA, resulting in the negative regulation of gene expression either by mRNA degradation or translation [208]. MiR-122, the most abundant known miRNA in the liver, is involved in the cellular stress response and hepatocarcinogenesis. Its downregulation has been shown to correlate with the development of HCC in rats and could be a potential biomarker for liver cancer [209]. This study also showed that the miRNAs let-7a, miR-21, miR-23, miR-130, miR-190, and miR-17-92 were upregulated in HCC in rats. Interestingly, increased cyclin G1 expression is associated with a higher incidence of primary liver malignancy, and another study showed miR-122a regulation of cyclin G1 expression [210]. Another miRNA, miR-21, has been demonstrated to be overexpressed in HCC tumors and cell lines. Notably, when miR-21 was suppressed, PTEN, a tumor suppressor of the PI3K pathway, showed increased expression. This resulted in a decrease in tumor cell proliferation, migration, and invasion. It was subsequently found that PTEN is a direct target of miR-21, and that miR-21 was also able to modulate focal adhesion kinase phosphorylation and MMP-2/-9 expression [211].

## Sectional Summary

HCC is a highly heterogeneous tumor that can have several genetic and epigenetic alterations. Furthermore, liver cancer develops over an extended period of time, which leads to the accumulation of many genetic mutations and aberrations. The Wnt/$\beta$-catenin pathway is commonly altered via mutations in $\beta$-catenin or Axin1. Mutations in the tumor suppressor p53 have also been found in liver malignancies, specifically those associated with aflatoxin B1 exposure. Other alterations include LOH at several important loci that encode tumor suppressor genes, such as p53, Rb, and p16. Epigenetic silencing via promoter methylation is a fairly frequent event in HCC. For example, p16, a cell cycle inhibitor, and pro-apoptotic genes such as caspase 8 are often silenced, which can promote tumorigenesis. Furthermore, mismatch repair genes have also been shown to be hypermethylated, including hMLH1, hMSH2, and hMSH3. JAK/STAT signaling is important in many liver cancers, so the methylation silencing of negative regulators of this pathway, SOCS1 and SOCS3, can affect the progression of liver malignancies. Finally, miRNAs, such as miR—122 and miR-21, have been shown to be downregulated and overexpressed, respectively, in HCC tumors, pointing to their potential roles in hepatocarcinogenesis.

# 5. Stem Cell Theory & Liver Cancer

The idea that states that only a small population of cells within a tumor is capable of generating tumors is not a new proposal, but research on "cancer stem cells" (CSC) in tumors has risen in the last ten years. The CSC theory states that tumors arise from a subpopulation of cells that have stem cell-like qualities and undergo epigenetic and genetic changes, resulting in transformation. In the liver the three primary hepatocellular targets for malignant transformation are the hepatocytes, cholangiocytes, and adult stem/progenitor cells [212].

Regarding the stem cell theory, even mature hepatocytes could act as cancer stem cells because of their regenerative properties. Hepatocytes have intrinsic "stemness" and could be the liver cancer stem cells that originate tumor formation. Hepatic stem/progenitor cells, which are often called oval cells, give rise to both cholangiocytes and hepatocytes. These oval cells may be a source of CSC in liver cancer and they have been shown to activate and proliferate in precancerous, chronic inflammatory conditions of the liver, including hepatitis B and C, alcoholic hepatitis, and steatohepatitis [213,214]. Finally, bone marrow-derived stem cells have been implicated in hepatocarcinogenesis, but convincing evidence has not yet been shown. However, these cells have been shown to be involved in liver regeneration, so further studies are needed in order to elucidate their potential role in liver malignancies.

Some evidence that adult liver stem cells are the cells of origin in liver cancer has been shown. Preoplastic conditions in the liver, such as chronic inflammation, show ductular reaction, which refers to the massive proliferation of stem/progenitor cells [215]. In fact, there is a correlation between the extent of ductular reaction and the severity of liver disease [216]. Interestingly, the markers present on liver tumor cells point to a potential hepatic stem cell origin of liver cancer. Many HCCs display bipotential characteristics, such as the coexpression of biliary and hepatocyte markers. These markers include cytokeratin 7 (CK7), CK19, OV6, $\alpha$-fetoprotein (AFP), and albumin, and are associated with a more aggressive phenotype and poor prognosis [217,218]. Finally, other studies demonstrate a possible role for alterations in IL-6 and TGF-$\beta$ signaling in the transformation of stem cells [219]. Furthermore, it was shown that transformation with a background of chronic liver injury often occurred in proliferating liver progenitor cells with c-KIT expression, which is a proto-oncogenic receptor tyrosine kinase [220].

Interestingly, many of the molecular signatures found in HCC as well as during regeneration are involved in stem cell maintenance and self-renewal. These important pathways in HCC and regeneration include Wnt/$\beta$-catenin, TGF-$\beta$, Met, and Hedgehog (Hh). Also, the Myc oncogene has been shown to be an important gene involved in the transition from preneoplasia to malignancy. This gene is also a key factor in the reactivation of an embryonic stem cell-like program in both normal and tumor cells. Furthermore, Bmi1, a polycomb group protein, is another protein that is involved in stem cell self-renewal and may have a role in liver cancer.

## Sectional Summary

Currently, there is no conclusive evidence that hepatic stem cells are, in fact, the cells of origin in liver cancer. However, several studies have provided clues that point to the possibility that liver cancer may be a cancer that follows the cancer stem cell theory. Several pathways and genes that are involved in stem cell maintenance and self-renewal are also critical during hepatocarcinogenesis. Additionally, cells from liver tumors have been known to coexpress biliary and hepatocyte markers, providing some evidence that these malignant cells arise from bipotential stem cells.

# Conclusion

Liver cancer is a heterogeneous disease with multiple etiologies that include several infectious and toxic agents. Chronic inflammation is one of the most influential risk factors for liver malignancy and plays a role in the carcinogenic effects of many of the etiologic agents. Both HBV and HCV proteins seem to exert some direct action on the members of important cancer signaling pathways, but the role of the chronic inflammatory response in hepatocarcinogenesis with a background of viral infection cannot be ignored, especially in cases of HCV infection. As is depicted *in Figure 1*, chronic inflammation, induced by apparently every known etiologic agent, plays a central role in the development of liver cancer.

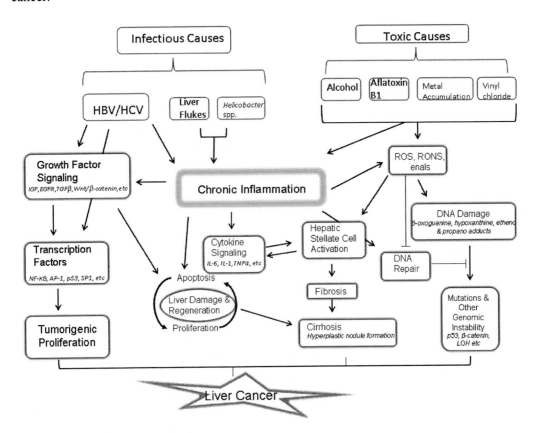

Figure 1.

Toxic agents, such as transition metals or alcohol metabolites, can generate free radicals, either directly or via the cellular inflammatory response to these agents. Liver infections also induce inflammation, leading to the release of free radicals. These free radicals can cause damage to cellular DNA, leading to tumorigenic mutations if not repaired by DNA repair mechanisms, which themselves can be suppressed by inflammation. Importantly, inflammation also causes severe damage to hepatocytes, which the liver repairs via the regenerative process, where damaged cells undergo apoptosis and are replaced by the proliferation of other hepatocytes, restoring the organ. Generally, during chronic inflammation the sustained exposure to cytokines and other stimulants in the liver microenvironment activates hepatic stellate cells, which secrete extracellular matrix proteins, resulting in hepatic fibrosis. After an extended period of time, fibrosis culminates in cirrhosis, which is characterized by abnormal nodules and hyperplasia. The proliferative pressure generated by the regenerative process, combined with tumorigenic mutations and hyperplastic changes in cells, results in the development of liver cancer.

Future studies in hepatocarcinogenesis must focus on the mechanisms of hyperplastic changes in pre-cancerous cirrhosis. It is true that some liver cancers develop in a non-cirrhotic liver, so mechanisms in the development of liver cancer without the predisposing condition of cirrhosis must be investigated. Furthermore, understanding the suppressive role of inflammation on DNA repair is important to establishing direct tumorigenic effects of inflammatory signaling, so studies in this particular area of research are needed. Mechanistic studies in the regulation of apoptosis and proliferation during liver regeneration may also be useful in understanding the hyperplasia that probably contributes to hepatocarcinogenesis. In general, treating chronic inflammatory processes as the hub of liver cancer development could be beneficial to a variety of studies on specific etiologic agents. Finally, studies that specifically direct and sharpen the focus on chronic inflammation as the chief etiologic factor in the development of liver cancer may provide the much-needed background information necessary for the development of preventive and therapeutic tools that could be used for a variety of liver malignancies.

# Acknowledgments

The authors' research is supported by US Public Health Services Research grants R01 CA92306, RO1 CA113447 (RR). The authors thank the Roy laboratory members for scientific discussions. Finally, we apologize for the omission of many relevant publications because of space limitation.

# References

[1] Kamangar,F; Dores,GM; Anderson,WF. Patterns of cancer incidence, mortality, and prevalence across five continents: defining priorities to reduce cancer disparities in different geographic regions of the world. *J Clin Oncol,* 2006 *24*, 2137-2150.

[2] El Serag,HB; Rudolph,KL. Hepatocellular carcinoma: epidemiology and molecular carcinogenesis. *Gastroenterology,* 2007 *132*, 2557-2576.

[3] Altekruse SF; Kosary CL; Krapcho M; Neyman N; Aminou R; Waldron W; Ruhl J; Howlader N; Tatalovich Z; Cho H; Mariotto A; Eisner MP; Lewis DR; Cronin K; Chen HS; Feuer EJ; Stinchcomb DG; Edwards BK . SEER Cancer Statistics Review,1975-2007. 2009.

[4] Yang,HI; Yeh,SH; Chen,PJ; Iloeje,UH; Jen,CL; Su,J; Wang,LY; Lu,SN; You,SL; Chen,DS; Liaw,YF; Chen,CJ; REVEAL-HBV Study Group. Associations between

hepatitis B virus genotype and mutants and the risk of hepatocellular carcinoma. *J Natl Cancer Inst,* 2008 *100*, 1134-1143.

[5] Lupberger,J; Hildt,E. Hepatitis B virus-induced oncogenesis. *World J Gastroenterol,* 2007 *13*, 74-81.

[6] Tsai,WL; Chung,RT. Viral hepatocarcinogenesis. *Oncogene,* 2010 *29*, 2309-2324.

[7] Neuveut,C; Wei,Y; Buendia,MA. Mechanisms of HBV-related hepatocarcinogenesis. *J Hepatol.,* 2010 *52*, 594-604.

[8] Diao,J; Khine,AA; Sarangi,F; Hsu,E; Iorio,C; Tibbles,LA; Woodgett,JR; Penninger,J; Richardson,CD. X protein of hepatitis B virus inhibits Fas-mediated apoptosis and is associated with up-regulation of the SAPK/JNK pathway. *J Biol Chem,* 2001 *276*, 8328-8340.

[9] Diao,J; Garces,R; Richardson,CD. X protein of hepatitis B virus modulates cytokine and growth factor related signal transduction pathways during the course of viral infections and hepatocarcinogenesis. *Cytokine Growth Factor Rev,* 2001 *12*, 189-205.

[10] Lee,YH; Yun,Y. HBx protein of hepatitis B virus activates Jak1-STAT signaling. *J Biol Chem,* 1998 *273*, 25510-25515.

[11] Shih,WL; Kuo,ML; Chuang,SE; Cheng,AL; Doong,SL. Hepatitis B virus X protein inhibits transforming growth factor-beta -induced apoptosis through the activation of phosphatidylinositol 3-kinase pathway. *J Biol Chem,* 2000 *275*, 25858-25864.

[12] Murata,M; Matsuzaki,K; Yoshida,K; Sekimoto,G; Tahashi,Y; Mori,S; Uemura,Y; Sakaida,N; Fujisawa,J; Seki,T; Kobayashi,K; Yokote,K; Koike,K; Okazaki,K. Hepatitis B virus X protein shifts human hepatic transforming growth factor (TGF)-beta signaling from tumor suppression to oncogenesis in early chronic hepatitis B. *Hepatology,* 2009 *49*, 1203-1217.

[13] Ding,Q; Xia,W; Liu,JC; Yang,JY; Lee,DF; Xia,J; Bartholomeusz,G; Li,Y; Pan,Y; Li,Z; Bargou,RC; Qin,J; Lai,CC; Tsai,FJ; Tsai,CH; Hung,MC. Erk associates with and primes GSK-3beta for its inactivation resulting in upregulation of beta-catenin. *Mol Cell,* 2005 *19*, 159-170.

[14] Ryo,A; Nakamura,M; Wulf,G; Liou,YC; Lu,KP. Pin1 regulates turnover and subcellular localization of beta-catenin by inhibiting its interaction with APC. *Nat Cell Biol,* 2001 *3*, 793-801.

[15] Pang,R; Lee,TK; Poon,RT; Fan,ST; Wong,KB; Kwong,YL; Tse,E. Pin1 interacts with a specific serine-proline motif of hepatitis B virus X-protein to enhance hepatocarcinogenesis. *Gastroenterology,* 2007 *132*, 1088-1103.

[16] Lee,SG; Rho,HM. Transcriptional repression of the human p53 gene by hepatitis B viral X protein. *Oncogene,* 2000 *19*, 468-471.

[17] Jia,L; Wang,XW; Harris,CC. Hepatitis B virus X protein inhibits nucleotide excision repair. *Int J Cancer,* 1999 *80*, 875-879.

[18] Wang,XW; Forrester,K; Yeh,H; Feitelson,MA; Gu,JR; Harris,CC. Hepatitis B virus X protein inhibits p53 sequence-specific DNA binding, transcriptional activity, and association with transcription factor ERCC3. *Proc Natl Acad Sci U.S A,* 1994 *91*, 2230-2234.

[19] Park,SG; Min,JY; Chung,C; Hsieh,A; Jung,G. Tumor suppressor protein p53 induces degradation of the oncogenic protein HBx. *Cancer Lett,* 2009 *282*, 229-237.

[20] Yoo,YD; Ueda,H; Park,K; Flanders,KC; Lee,YI; Jay,G; Kim,SJ. Regulation of transforming growth factor-beta 1 expression by the hepatitis B virus (HBV) X transactivator. Role in HBV pathogenesis. *J Clin Invest,* 1996 *97,* 388-395.

[21] Kim,KH; Shin,HJ; Kim,K; Choi,HM; Rhee,SH; Moon,HB; Kim,HH; Yang,US; Yu,DY; Cheong,J. Hepatitis B virus X protein induces hepatic steatosis via transcriptional activation of SREBP1 and PPARgamma. *Gastroenterology,* 2007 *132,* 1955-1967.

[22] Kim,EM; Kim,JS; Choi,MH; Hong,ST; Bae,YM. Effects of excretory/secretory products from Clonorchis sinensis and the carcinogen dimethylnitrosamine on the proliferation and cell cycle modulation of human epithelial HEK293T cells. *Korean J Parasitol.,* 2008 *46,* 127-132.

[23] Martin-Lluesma,S; Schaeffer,C; Robert,EI; van Breugel,PC; Leupin,O; Hantz,O; Strubin,M. Hepatitis B virus X protein affects S phase progression leading to chromosome segregation defects by binding to damaged DNA binding protein 1. *Hepatology,* 2008 *48,* 1467-1476.

[24] Sirma,H; Weil,R; Rosmorduc,O; Urban,S; Israel,A; Kremsdorf,D; Brechot,C. Cytosol is the prime compartment of hepatitis B virus X protein where it colocalizes with the proteasome. *Oncogene,* 1998 *16,* 2051-2063.

[25] Severi,T; Vander,BS; Libbrecht,L; VanAelst,L; Nevens,F; Roskams,T; Cassiman,D; Fevery,J; Verslype,C; van Pelt,JF. HBx or HCV core gene expression in HepG2 human liver cells results in a survival benefit against oxidative stress with possible implications for HCC development. *Chem Biol Interact.,* 2007 *168,* 128-134.

[26] Chen,J; Siddiqui,A. Hepatitis B virus X protein stimulates the mitochondrial translocation of Raf-1 via oxidative stress. *J Virol.,* 2007 *81,* 6757-6760.

[27] Tang,H; Da,L; Mao,Y; Li,Y; Li,D; Xu,Z; Li,F; Wang,Y; Tiollais,P; Li,T; Zhao,M. Hepatitis B virus X protein sensitizes cells to starvation-induced autophagy via up-regulation of beclin 1 expression. *Hepatology,* 2009 *49,* 60-71.

[28] Zheng,DL; Zhang,L; Cheng,N; Xu,X; Deng,Q; Teng,XM; Wang,KS; Zhang,X; Huang,J; Han,ZG. Epigenetic modification induced by hepatitis B virus X protein via interaction with de novo DNA methyltransferase DNMT3A. *J Hepatol.,* 2009 *50,* 377-387.

[29] Hildt,E; Munz,B; Saher,G; Reifenberg,K; Hofschneider,PH. The PreS2 activator MHBs(t) of hepatitis B virus activates c-raf-1/Erk2 signaling in transgenic mice. *EMBO J,* 2002 *21,* 525-535.

[30] Liu,H; Luan,F; Ju,Y; Shen,H; Gao,L; Wang,X; Liu,S; Zhang,L; Sun,W; Ma,C. In vitro transfection of the hepatitis B virus PreS2 gene into the human hepatocarcinoma cell line HepG2 induces upregulation of human telomerase reverse transcriptase. *Biochem Biophys.Res Commun,* 2007 *355,* 379-384.

[31] Wang,HC; Huang,W; Lai,MD; Su,IJ. Hepatitis B virus pre-S mutants, endoplasmic reticulum stress and hepatocarcinogenesis. *Cancer Sci,* 2006 *97,* 683-688.

[32] Hsieh,SY; Hsieh,PS; Chiu,CT; Chen,WY. Dickkopf-3/REIC functions as a suppressor gene of tumor growth. *Oncogene,* 2004 *23,* 9183-9189.

[33] Yang,JC; Teng,CF; Wu,HC; Tsai,HW; Chuang,HC; Tsai,TF; Hsu,YH; Huang,W; Wu,LW; Su,IJ. Enhanced expression of vascular endothelial growth factor-A in ground

glass hepatocytes and its implication in hepatitis B virus hepatocarcinogenesis. *Hepatology,* 2009 *49*, 1962-1971.

[34] Yu,MW; Yeh,SH; Chen,PJ; Liaw,YF; Lin,CL; Liu,CJ; Shih,WL; Kao,JH; Chen,DS; Chen,CJ. Hepatitis B virus genotype and DNA level and hepatocellular carcinoma: a prospective study in men. *J Natl Cancer Inst,* 2005 *97*, 265-272.

[35] Kobayashi,M; Ikeda,K; Saitoh,S; Suzuki,F; Tsubota,A; Suzuki,Y; Arase,Y; Murashima,N; Chayama,K; Kumada,H. Incidence of primary cholangiocellular carcinoma of the liver in japanese patients with hepatitis C virus-related cirrhosis. *Cancer,* 2000 *88*, 2471-2477.

[36] Shaib,YH; El Serag,HB; Nooka,AK; Thomas,M; Brown,TD; Patt,YZ; Hassan,MM. Risk factors for intrahepatic and extrahepatic cholangiocarcinoma: a hospital-based case-control study. *Am J Gastroenterol,* 2007 *102*, 1016-1021.

[37] Bartosch,B; Thimme,R; Blum,HE; Zoulim,F. Hepatitis C virus-induced hepatocarcino-genesis. *J Hepatol.,* 2009 *51*, 810-820.

[38] Ray,RB; Steele,R; Meyer,K; Ray,R. Transcriptional repression of p53 promoter by hepatitis C virus core protein. *J Biol Chem,* 1997 *272*, 10983-10986.

[39] Alisi,A; Giambartolomei,S; Cupelli,F; Merlo,P; Fontemaggi,G; Spaziani,A; Balsano,C. Physical and functional interaction between HCV core protein and the different p73 isoforms. *Oncogene,* 2003 *22*, 2573-2580.

[40] Cho,J; Baek,W; Yang,S; Chang,J; Sung,YC; Suh,M. HCV core protein modulates Rb pathway through pRb down-regulation and E2F-1 up-regulation. *Biochim.Biophys. Acta,* 2001 *1538*, 59-66.

[41] Anzola,M. Hepatocellular carcinoma: role of hepatitis B and hepatitis C viruses proteins in hepatocarcinogenesis. *J Viral Hepat.,* 2004 *11*, 383-393.

[42] Tai,DI; Tsai,SL; Chang,YH; Huang,SN; Chen,TC; Chang,KS; Liaw,YF. Constitutive activation of nuclear factor kappaB in hepatocellular carcinoma. *Cancer,* 2000 *89*, 2274-2281.

[43] Aoki,H; Hayashi,J; Moriyama,M; Arakawa,Y; Hino,O. Hepatitis C virus core protein interacts with 14-3-3 protein and activates the kinase Raf-1. *J Virol.,* 2000 *74*, 1736-1741.

[44] Fukutomi,T; Zhou,Y; Kawai,S; Eguchi,H; Wands,JR; Li,J. Hepatitis C virus core protein stimulates hepatocyte growth: correlation with upregulation of wnt-1 expression. *Hepatology,* 2005 *41*, 1096-1105.

[45] Nelson,DR; Gonzalez-Peralta,RP; Qian,K; Xu,Y; Marousis,CG; Davis,GL; Lau,JY. Transforming growth factor-beta 1 in chronic hepatitis C. *J Viral Hepat.,* 1997 *4*, 29-35.

[46] Pavio,N; Battaglia,S; Boucreux,D; Arnulf,B; Sobesky,R; Hermine,O; Brechot,C. Hepatitis C virus core variants isolated from liver tumor but not from adjacent non-tumor tissue interact with Smad3 and inhibit the TGF-beta pathway. *Oncogene,* 2005 *24*, 6119-6132.

[47] Battaglia,S; Benzoubir,N; Nobilet,S; Charneau,P; Samuel,D; Zignego,AL; Atfi,A; Brechot,C; Bourgeade,MF. Liver cancer-derived hepatitis C virus core proteins shift TGF-beta responses from tumor suppression to epithelial-mesenchymal transition. *PLoS One.,* 2009 *4*, e4355.

[48] Kanda,T; Steele,R; Ray,R; Ray,RB. Hepatitis C virus core protein augments androgen receptor-mediated signaling. *J Virol.*, 2008 *82*, 11066-11072.

[49] Crotta,S; Stilla,A; Wack,A; D'Andrea,A; Nuti,S; D'Oro,U; Mosca,M; Filliponi,F; Brunetto,RM; Bonino,F; Abrignani,S; Valiante,NM. Inhibition of natural killer cells through engagement of CD81 by the major hepatitis C virus envelope protein. *J Exp Med,* 2002 *195*, 35-41.

[50] Zhao,LJ; Wang,L; Ren,H; Cao,J; Li,L; Ke,JS; Qi,ZT. Hepatitis C virus E2 protein promotes human hepatoma cell proliferation through the MAPK/ERK signaling pathway via cellular receptors. *Exp Cell Res,* 2005 *305*, 23-32.

[51] Kwun,HJ; Jung,EY; Ahn,JY; Lee,MN; Jang,KL. p53-dependent transcriptional repression of p21(waf1) by hepatitis C virus NS3. *J Gen Virol.*, 2001 *82*, 2235-2241.

[52] Deng,L; Nagano-Fujii,M; Tanaka,M; Nomura-Takigawa,Y; Ikeda,M; Kato,N; Sada,K; Hotta,H. NS3 protein of Hepatitis C virus associates with the tumour suppressor p53 and inhibits its function in an NS3 sequence-dependent manner. *J Gen Virol.*, 2006 *87*, 1703-1713.

[53] Hassan,M; Selimovic,D; Ghozlan,H; Abdel-Kader,O. Induction of high-molecular-weight (HMW) tumor necrosis factor(TNF) alpha by hepatitis C virus (HCV) non-structural protein 3 (NS3) in liver cells is AP-1 and NF-kappaB-dependent activation. *Cell Signal,* 2007 *19*, 301-311.

[54] Majumder,M; Ghosh,AK; Steele,R; Ray,R; Ray,RB. Hepatitis C virus NS5A physically associates with p53 and regulates p21/waf1 gene expression in a p53-dependent manner. *J Virol.*, 2001 *75*, 1401-1407.

[55] Chung,YL; Sheu,ML; Yen,SH. Hepatitis C virus NS5A as a potential viral Bcl-2 homologue interacts with Bax and inhibits apoptosis in hepatocellular carcinoma. *Int J Cancer,* 2003 *107*, 65-73.

[56] Ghosh,AK; Majumder,M; Steele,R; Meyer,K; Ray,R; Ray,RB. Hepatitis C virus NS5A protein protects against TNF-alpha mediated apoptotic cell death. *Virus Res,* 2000 *67*, 173-178.

[57] Bonte,D; Francois,C; Castelain,S; Wychowski,C; Dubuisson,J; Meurs,EF; Duverlie,G. Positive effect of the hepatitis C virus nonstructural 5A protein on viral multiplication. *Arch Virol.*, 2004 *149*, 1353-1371.

[58] Gong,G; Waris,G; Tanveer,R; Siddiqui,A. Human hepatitis C virus NS5A protein alters intracellular calcium levels, induces oxidative stress, and activates STAT-3 and NF-kappa B. *Proc Natl Acad Sci U.S A,* 2001 *98*, 9599-9604.

[59] Macdonald,A; Harris,M. Hepatitis C virus NS5A: tales of a promiscuous protein. *J Gen Virol.*, 2004 *85*, 2485-2502.

[60] Street,A; Macdonald,A; Crowder,K; Harris,M. The Hepatitis C virus NS5A protein activates a phosphoinositide 3-kinase-dependent survival signaling cascade. *J Biol Chem,* 2004 *279*, 12232-12241.

[61] Street,A; Macdonald,A; McCormick,C; Harris,M. Hepatitis C virus NS5A-mediated activation of phosphoinositide 3-kinase results in stabilization of cellular beta-catenin and stimulation of beta-catenin-responsive transcription. *J Virol.*, 2005 *79*, 5006-5016.

[62] Choi,SH; Hwang,SB. Modulation of the transforming growth factor-beta signal transduction pathway by hepatitis C virus nonstructural 5A protein. *J Biol Chem,* 2006 *281,* 7468-7478.

[63] Wu,SC; Chang,SC; Wu,HY; Liao,PJ; Chang,MF. Hepatitis C virus NS5A protein down-regulates the expression of spindle gene Aspm through PKR-p38 signaling pathway. *J Biol Chem,* 2008 *283,* 29396-29404.

[64] Bureau,C; Bernad,J; Chaouche,N; Orfila,C; Beraud,M; Gonindard,C; Alric,L; Vinel,JP; Pipy,B. Nonstructural 3 protein of hepatitis C virus triggers an oxidative burst in human monocytes via activation of NADPH oxidase. *J Biol Chem,* 2001 *276,* 23077-23083.

[65] Korenaga,M; Wang,T; Li,Y; Showalter,LA; Chan,T; Sun,J; Weinman,SA. Hepatitis C virus core protein inhibits mitochondrial electron transport and increases reactive oxygen species (ROS) production. *J Biol Chem,* 2005 *280,* 37481-37488.

[66] de Lucas,S; Bartolome,J; Amaro,MJ; Carreno,V. Hepatitis C virus core protein transactivates the inducible nitric oxide synthase promoter via NF-kappaB activation. *Antiviral Res,* 2003 *60,* 117-124.

[67] Nunez,O; Fernandez-Martinez,A; Majano,PL; Apolinario,A; Gomez-Gonzalo,M; Benedicto,I; Lopez-Cabrera,M; Bosca,L; Clemente,G; Garcia-Monzon,C; Martin-Sanz,P. Increased intrahepatic cyclooxygenase 2, matrix metalloproteinase 2, and matrix metalloproteinase 9 expression is associated with progressive liver disease in chronic hepatitis C virus infection: role of viral core and NS5A proteins. *Gut,* 2004 *53,* 1665-1672.

[68] Benali-Furet,NL; Chami,M; Houel,L; De Giorgi,F; Vernejoul,F; Lagorce,D; Buscail,L; Bartenschlager,R; Ichas,F; Rizzuto,R; Paterlini-Brechot,P. Hepatitis C virus core triggers apoptosis in liver cells by inducing ER stress and ER calcium depletion. *Oncogene,* 2005 *24,* 4921-4933.

[69] Tanaka,N; Moriya,K; Kiyosawa,K; Koike,K; Aoyama,T. Hepatitis C virus core protein induces spontaneous and persistent activation of peroxisome proliferator-activated receptor alpha in transgenic mice: implications for HCV-associated hepatocarcinogenesis. *Int J Cancer,* 2008 *122,* 124-131.

[70] Negro,F. Mechanisms and significance of liver steatosis in hepatitis C virus infection. *World J Gastroenterol,* 2006 *12,* 6756-6765.

[71] Shin,HR; Oh,JK; Masuyer,E; Curado,MP; Bouvard,V; Fang,YY; Wiangnon,S; Sripa,B; Hong,ST. Epidemiology of cholangiocarcinoma: an update focusing on risk factors. *Cancer Sci,* 2010 *101,* 579-585.

[72] Marcos,LA; Terashima,A; Gotuzzo,E. Update on hepatobiliary flukes: fascioliasis, opisthorchiasis and clonorchiasis. *Curr Opin.Infect.Dis,* 2008 *21,* 523-530.

[73] Sripa,B; Kaewkes,S; Sithithaworn,P; Mairiang,E; Laha,T; Smout,M; Pairojkul,C; Bhudhisawasdi,V; Tesana,S; Thinkamrop,B; Bethony,JM; Loukas,A; Brindley,PJ. Liver fluke induces cholangiocarcinoma. *PLoS Med,* 2007 *4,* e201.

[74] Kaewpitoon,N; Kaewpitoon,SJ; Pengsaa,P; Sripa,B. Opisthorchis viverrini: the carcinogenic human liver fluke. *World J Gastroenterol,* 2008 *14,* 666-674.

[75] Thuwajit,C; Thuwajit,P; Uchida,K; Daorueang,D; Kaewkes,S; Wongkham,S; Miwa,M. Gene expression profiling defined pathways correlated with fibroblast cell proliferation

induced by Opisthorchis viverrini excretory/secretory product. *World J Gastroenterol,* 2006 *12*, 3585-3592.

[76] Pinlaor,S; Ma,N; Hiraku,Y; Yongvanit,P; Semba,R; Oikawa,S; Murata,M; Sripa,B; Sithithaworn,P; Kawanishi,S. Repeated infection with Opisthorchis viverrini induces accumulation of 8-nitroguanine and 8-oxo-7,8-dihydro-2'-deoxyguanine in the bile duct of hamsters via inducible nitric oxide synthase. *Carcinogenesis,* 2004 *25*, 1535-1542.

[77] Srivatanakul,P; Ohshima,H; Khlat,M; Parkin,M; Sukaryodhin,S; Brouet,I; Bartsch,H. Opisthorchis viverrini infestation and endogenous nitrosamines as risk factors for cholangiocarcinoma in Thailand. *Int J Cancer,* 1991 *48*, 821-825.

[78] Srivatanakul,P; Ohshima,H; Khlat,M; Parkin,M; Sukarayodhin,S; Brouet,I; Bartsch,H. Endogenous nitrosamines and liver fluke as risk factors for cholangiocarcinoma in Thailand. *IARC Sci Publ.,* 1991, 88-95.

[79] Yoon,JH; Werneburg,NW; Higuchi,H; Canbay,AE; Kaufmann,SH; Akgul,C; Edwards,SW; Gores,GJ. Bile acids inhibit Mcl-1 protein turnover via an epidermal growth factor receptor/Raf-1-dependent mechanism. *Cancer Res,* 2002 *62*, 6500-6505.

[80] Papachristou,GI; Schoedel,KE; Ramanathan,R; Rabinovitz,M. Clonorchis sinensis-associated cholangiocarcinoma: a case report and review of the literature. *Dig.Dis Sci,* 2005 *50*, 2159-2162.

[81] Pellicano,R; Menard,A; Rizzetto,M; Megraud,F. Helicobacter species and liver diseases: association or causation? *Lancet Infect.Dis,* 2008 *8*, 254-260.

[82] Boutin,SR; Rogers,AB; Shen,Z; Fry,RC; Love,JA; Nambiar,PR; Suerbaum,S; Fox,JG. Hepatic temporal gene expression profiling in Helicobacter hepaticus-infected A/JCr mice. *Toxicol Pathol.,* 2004 *32*, 678-693.

[83] Fox,JG; Li,X; Yan,L; Cahill,RJ; Hurley,R; Lewis,R; Murphy,JC. Chronic proliferative hepatitis in A/JCr mice associated with persistent Helicobacter hepaticus infection: a model of helicobacter-induced carcinogenesis. *Infect.Immun.,* 1996 *64*, 1548-1558.

[84] Pikarsky,E; Porat,RM; Stein,I; Abramovitch,R; Amit,S; Kasem,S; Gutkovich-Pyest,E; Urieli-Shoval,S; Galun,E; Ben Neriah,Y. NF-kappaB functions as a tumour promoter in inflammation-associated cancer. *Nature,* 2004 *431*, 461-466.

[85] McKillop,IH; Schrum,LW. Role of alcohol in liver carcinogenesis. *Semin Liver Dis,* 2009 *29*, 222-232.

[86] Casini,A; Cunningham,M; Rojkind,M; Lieber,CS. Acetaldehyde increases procollagen type I and fibronectin gene transcription in cultured rat fat-storing cells through a protein synthesis-dependent mechanism. *Hepatology,* 1991 *13*, 758-765.

[87] Guengerich,FP; Shimada,T; Yun,CH; Yamazaki,H; Raney,KD; Thier,R; Coles,B; Harris,TM. Interactions of ingested food, beverage, and tobacco components involving human cytochrome P4501A2, 2A6, 2E1, and 3A4 enzymes. *Environ Health Perspect.,* 1994 *102 Suppl 9*, 49-53.

[88] Lash,LH. Mitochondrial glutathione transport: physiological, pathological and toxicological implications. *Chem Biol Interact.,* 2006 *163*, 54-67.

[89] Thurman,RG. II. Alcoholic liver injury involves activation of Kupffer cells by endotoxin. *Am J Physiol,* 1998 *275*, G605-G611.

[90] Bedard,LL; Massey,TE. Aflatoxin B1-induced DNA damage and its repair. *Cancer Lett,* 2006 *241*, 174-183.

[91] Gomaa,AI; Khan,SA; Toledano,MB; Waked,I; Taylor-Robinson,SD. Hepatocellular carcinoma: epidemiology, risk factors and pathogenesis. *World J Gastroenterol,* 2008 *14*, 4300-4308.

[92] Kew,MC. Synergistic interaction between aflatoxin B1 and hepatitis B virus in hepatocarcinogenesis. *Liver Int,* 2003 *23*, 405-409.

[93] Bressac,B; Kew,M; Wands,J; Ozturk,M. Selective G to T mutations of p53 gene in hepatocellular carcinoma from southern Africa. *Nature,* 1991 *350*, 429-431.

[94] Pietrangelo,A. Hereditary hemochromatosis: pathogenesis, diagnosis, and treatment. *Gastroenterology,* 2010 *139*, 393-408, 408.

[95] Chen,J; Chloupkova,M. Abnormal iron uptake and liver cancer. *Cancer Biol Ther,* 2009 *8*, 1699-1708.

[96] Harrison,SA; Bacon,BR. Relation of hemochromatosis with hepatocellular carcinoma: epidemiology, natural history, pathophysiology, screening, treatment, and prevention. *Med Clin North Am,* 2005 *89*, 391-409.

[97] Hiatt,T; Trotter,JF; Kam,I. Hepatocellular carcinoma in a noncirrhotic patient with hereditary hemochromatosis. *Am J Med Sci,* 2007 *334*, 228-230.

[98] Asare,GA; Mossanda,KS; Kew,MC; Paterson,AC; Kahler-Venter,CP; Siziba,K. Hepatocellular carcinoma caused by iron overload: a possible mechanism of direct hepatocarcinogenicity. *Toxicology,* 2006 *219*, 41-52.

[99] Lehmann,U; Wingen,LU; Brakensiek,K; Wedemeyer,H; Becker,T; Heim,A; Metzig,K; Hasemeier,B; Kreipe,H; Flemming,P. Epigenetic defects of hepatocellular carcinoma are already found in non-neoplastic liver cells from patients with hereditary haemochromatosis. *Hum Mol Genet,* 2007 *16*, 1335-1342.

[100] Walshe,JM; Waldenstrom,E; Sams,V; Nordlinder,H; Westermark,K. Abdominal malignancies in patients with Wilson's disease. *QJM.,* 2003 *96*, 657-662.

[101] Xu,R; Bu-Ghanim,M; Fiel,MI; Schiano,T; Cohen,E; Thung,SN. Hepatocellular carcinoma associated with an atypical presentation of Wilson's disease. *Semin Liver Dis,* 2007 *27*, 122-127.

[102] Bartsch,H; Nair,J. Oxidative stress and lipid peroxidation-derived DNA-lesions in inflammation driven carcinogenesis. *Cancer Detect Prev,* 2004 *28*, 385-391.

[103] Nair,J; Carmichael,PL; Fernando,RC; Phillips,DH; Strain,AJ; Bartsch,H. Lipid peroxidation-induced etheno-DNA adducts in the liver of patients with the genetic metal storage disorders Wilson's disease and primary hemochromatosis. *Cancer Epidemiol Biomarkers Prev,* 1998 *7*, 435-440.

[104] Hussain,SP; Raja,K; Amstad,PA; Sawyer,M; Trudel,LJ; Wogan,GN; Hofseth,LJ; Shields,PG; Billiar,TR; Trautwein,C; Hohler,T; Galle,PR; Phillips,DH; Markin,R; Marrogi,AJ; Harris,CC. Increased p53 mutation load in nontumorous human liver of wilson disease and hemochromatosis: oxyradical overload diseases. *Proc Natl Acad Sci U.S A,* 2000 *97*, 12770-12775.

[105] Sherman,M. Vinyl chloride and the liver. *J Hepatol.,* 2009 *51*, 1074-1081.

[106] WHO . Vinyl Chloride. Environmental health criteria 215 . 1999.

[107] Wong,RH; Chen,PC; Du,CL; Wang,JD; Cheng,TJ. An increased standardised mortality ratio for liver cancer among polyvinyl chloride workers in Taiwan. *Occup.Environ Med,* 2002 *59*, 405-409.

[108] Wong,RH; Chen,PC; Wang,JD; Du,CL; Cheng,TJ. Interaction of vinyl chloride monomer exposure and hepatitis B viral infection on liver cancer. *J Occup.Environ Med,* 2003 *45*, 379-383.

[109] Markiewski,MM; DeAngelis,RA; Lambris,JD. Liver inflammation and regeneration: two distinct biological phenomena or parallel pathophysiologic processes? *Mol Immunol.,* 2006 *43*, 45-56.

[110] Berasain,C; Castillo,J; Perugorria,MJ; Latasa,MU; Prieto,J; Avila,MA. Inflammation and liver cancer: new molecular links. *Ann N Y Acad Sci,* 2009 *1155*, 206-221.

[111] Friedman,SL. Mechanisms of hepatic fibrogenesis. *Gastroenterology,* 2008 *134*, 1655-1669.

[112] Wallace,K; Burt,AD; Wright,MC. Liver fibrosis. *Biochem J,* 2008 *411*, 1-18.

[113] Poli,G. Pathogenesis of liver fibrosis: role of oxidative stress. *Mol Aspects Med,* 2000 *21*, 49-98.

[114] Atzori,L; Poli,G; Perra,A. Hepatic stellate cell: a star cell in the liver. *Int J Biochem Cell Biol,* 2009 *41*, 1639-1642.

[115] Plentz,RR; Caselitz,M; Bleck,JS; Gebel,M; Flemming,P; Kubicka,S; Manns,MP; Rudolph,KL. Hepatocellular telomere shortening correlates with chromosomal instability and the development of human hepatoma. *Hepatology,* 2004 *40*, 80-86.

[116] Farazi,PA; Glickman,J; Jiang,S; Yu,A; Rudolph,KL; DePinho,RA. Differential impact of telomere dysfunction on initiation and progression of hepatocellular carcinoma. *Cancer Res,* 2003 *63*, 5021-5027.

[117] Knight,B; Yeoh,GC; Husk,KL; Ly,T; Abraham,LJ; Yu,C; Rhim,JA; Fausto,N. Impaired preneoplastic changes and liver tumor formation in tumor necrosis factor receptor type 1 knockout mice. *J Exp Med,* 2000 *192*, 1809-1818.

[118] Pikarsky,E; Porat,RM; Stein,I; Abramovitch,R; Amit,S; Kasem,S; Gutkovich-Pyest,E; Urieli-Shoval,S; Galun,E; Ben Neriah,Y. NF-kappaB functions as a tumour promoter in inflammation-associated cancer. *Nature,* 2004 *431*, 461-466.

[119] Maeda,S; Kamata,H; Luo,JL; Leffert,H; Karin,M. IKKbeta couples hepatocyte death to cytokine-driven compensatory proliferation that promotes chemical hepatocarcino-genesis. *Cell,* 2005 *121*, 977-990.

[120] Luedde,T; Beraza,N; Kotsikoris,V; van Loo,G; Nenci,A; De Vos,R; Roskams,T; Trautwein,C; Pasparakis,M. Deletion of NEMO/IKKgamma in liver parenchymal cells causes steatohepatitis and hepatocellular carcinoma. *Cancer Cell,* 2007 *11*, 119-132.

[121] Sakurai,T; He,G; Matsuzawa,A; Yu,GY; Maeda,S; Hardiman,G; Karin,M. Hepatocyte necrosis induced by oxidative stress and IL-1 alpha release mediate carcinogen-induced compensatory proliferation and liver tumorigenesis. *Cancer Cell,* 2008 *14*, 156-165.

[122] Naugler,WE; Sakurai,T; Kim,S; Maeda,S; Kim,K; Elsharkawy,AM; Karin,M. Gender disparity in liver cancer due to sex differences in MyD88-dependent IL-6 production. *Science,* 2007 *317*, 121-124.

[123] Naugler,WE; Karin,M. The wolf in sheep's clothing: the role of interleukin-6 in immunity, inflammation and cancer. *Trends Mol Med,* 2008 *14*, 109-119.

[124] Taub,R. Liver regeneration: from myth to mechanism. *Nat Rev Mol Cell Biol,* 2004 *5*, 836-847.

[125] Calvisi,DF; Ladu,S; Gorden,A; Farina,M; Conner,EA; Lee,JS; Factor,VM; Thorgeirsson,SS. Ubiquitous activation of Ras and Jak/Stat pathways in human HCC. *Gastroenterology,* 2006 *130*, 1117-1128.

[126] Ogata,H; Kobayashi,T; Chinen,T; Takaki,H; Sanada,T; Minoda,Y; Koga,K; Takaesu,G; Maehara,Y; Iida,M; Yoshimura,A. Deletion of the SOCS3 gene in liver parenchymal cells promotes hepatitis-induced hepatocarcinogenesis. *Gastroenterology,* 2006 *131*, 179-193.

[127] Niwa,Y; Kanda,H; Shikauchi,Y; Saiura,A; Matsubara,K; Kitagawa,T; Yamamoto,J; Kubo,T; Yoshikawa,H. Methylation silencing of SOCS-3 promotes cell growth and migration by enhancing JAK/STAT and FAK signalings in human hepatocellular carcinoma. *Oncogene,* 2005 *24*, 6406-6417.

[128] Tanaka,Y; Furuta,T; Suzuki,S; Orito,E; Yeo,AE; Hirashima,N; Sugauchi,F; Ueda,R; Mizokami,M. Impact of interleukin-1beta genetic polymorphisms on the development of hepatitis C virus-related hepatocellular carcinoma in Japan. *J Infect.Dis,* 2003 *187*, 1822-1825.

[129] Hirankarn,N; Kimkong,I; Kummee,P; Tangkijvanich,P; Poovorawan,Y. Interleukin-1beta gene polymorphism associated with hepatocellular carcinoma in hepatitis B virus infection. *World J Gastroenterol,* 2006 *12*, 776-779.

[130] Gonzalez,FJ. Role of HNF4alpha in the superinduction of the IL-1beta-activated iNOS gene by oxidative stress. *Biochem J,* 2006 *394*, e3-e5.

[131] Calvisi,DF; Pinna,F; Ladu,S; Pellegrino,R; Muroni,MR; Simile,MM; Frau,M; Tomasi,ML; De Miglio,MR; Seddaiu,MA; Daino,L; Sanna,V; Feo,F; Pascale,RM. Aberrant iNOS signaling is under genetic control in rodent liver cancer and potentially prognostic for the human disease. *Carcinogenesis,* 2008 *29*, 1639-1647.

[132] Breuhahn,K; Longerich,T; Schirmacher,P. Dysregulation of growth factor signaling in human hepatocellular carcinoma. *Oncogene,* 2006 *25*, 3787-3800.

[133] De Souza,AT; Hankins,GR; Washington,MK; Orton,TC; Jirtle,RL. M6P/IGF2R gene is mutated in human hepatocellular carcinomas with loss of heterozygosity. *Nat Genet,* 1995 *11*, 447-449.

[134] Sue,SR; Chari,RS; Kong,FM; Mills,JJ; Fine,RL; Jirtle,RL; Meyers,WC. Transforming growth factor-beta receptors and mannose 6-phosphate/insulin-like growth factor-II receptor expression in human hepatocellular carcinoma. *Ann Surg,* 1995 *222*, 171-178.

[135] Gong,Y; Cui,L; Minuk,GY. The expression of insulin-like growth factor binding proteins in human hepatocellular carcinoma. *Mol Cell Biochem,* 2000 *207*, 101-104.

[136] Pennacchietti,S; Michieli,P; Galluzzo,M; Mazzone,M; Giordano,S; Comoglio,PM. Hypoxia promotes invasive growth by transcriptional activation of the met protooncogene. *Cancer Cell,* 2003 *3*, 347-361.

[137] Seol,DW; Chen,Q; Zarnegar,R. Transcriptional activation of the hepatocyte growth factor receptor (c-met) gene by its ligand (hepatocyte growth factor) is mediated through AP-1. *Oncogene,* 2000 *19*, 1132-1137.

[138] Ishizaki,Y; Ikeda,S; Fujimori,M; Shimizu,Y; Kurihara,T; Itamoto,T; Kikuchi,A; Okajima,M; Asahara,T. Immunohistochemical analysis and mutational analyses of beta-catenin, Axin family and APC genes in hepatocellular carcinomas. *Int J Oncol,* 2004 *24*, 1077-1083.

[139] Pang,R; Yuen,J; Yuen,MF; Lai,CL; Lee,TK; Man,K; Poon,RT; Fan,ST; Wong,CM; Ng,IO; Kwong,YL; Tse,E. PIN1 overexpression and beta-catenin gene mutations are distinct oncogenic events in human hepatocellular carcinoma. *Oncogene,* 2004 *23,* 4182-4186.

[140] Ding,Z; Qian,YB; Zhu,LX; Xiong,QR. Promoter methylation and mRNA expression of DKK-3 and WIF-1 in hepatocellular carcinoma. *World J Gastroenterol,* 2009 *15,* 2595-2601.

[141] Merle,P; de la,MS; Kim,M; Herrmann,M; Tanaka,S; Von Dem,BA; Kew,MC; Trepo,C; Wands,JR. Functional consequences of frizzled-7 receptor overexpression in human hepatocellular carcinoma. *Gastroenterology,* 2004 *127,* 1110-1122.

[142] Yau,TO; Chan,CY; Chan,KL; Lee,MF; Wong,CM; Fan,ST; Ng,IO. HDPR1, a novel inhibitor of the WNT/beta-catenin signaling, is frequently downregulated in hepatocellular carcinoma: involvement of methylation-mediated gene silencing. *Oncogene,* 2005 *24,* 1607-1614.

[143] Musch,A; Rabe,C; Paik,MD; Berna,MJ; Schmitz,V; Hoffmann,P; Nischalke,HD; Sauerbruch,T; Caselmann,WH. Altered expression of TGF-beta receptors in hepatocellular carcinoma--effects of a constitutively active TGF-beta type I receptor mutant. *Digestion,* 2005 *71,* 78-91.

[144] Gotzmann,J; Huber,H; Thallinger,C; Wolschek,M; Jansen,B; Schulte-Hermann,R; Beug,H; Mikulits,W. Hepatocytes convert to a fibroblastoid phenotype through the cooperation of TGF-beta1 and Ha-Ras: steps towards invasiveness. *J Cell Sci,* 2002 *115,* 1189-1202.

[145] Park,YN; Chae,KJ; Oh,BK; Choi,J; Choi,KS; Park,C. Expression of Smad7 in hepatocellular carcinoma and dysplastic nodules: resistance mechanism to transforming growth factor-beta. *Hepatogastroenterology,* 2004 *51,* 396-400.

[146] Kira,S; Nakanishi,T; Suemori,S; Kitamoto,M; Watanabe,Y; Kajiyama,G. Expression of transforming growth factor alpha and epidermal growth factor receptor in human hepatocellular carcinoma. *Liver,* 1997 *17,* 177-182.

[147] Yeh,YC; Tsai,JF; Chuang,LY; Yeh,HW; Tsai,JH; Florine,DL; Tam,JP. Elevation of transforming growth factor alpha and its relationship to the epidermal growth factor and alpha-fetoprotein levels in patients with hepatocellular carcinoma. *Cancer Res,* 1987 *47,* 896-901.

[148] Berasain,C; Castillo,J; Prieto,J; Avila,MA. New molecular targets for hepatocellular carcinoma: the ErbB1 signaling system. *Liver Int,* 2007 *27,* 174-185.

[149] Prange,W; Schirmacher,P. Absence of therapeutically relevant c-erbB-2 expression in human hepatocellular carcinomas. *Oncol Rep,* 2001 *8,* 727-730.

[150] Natarajan,A; Wagner,B; Sibilia,M. The EGF receptor is required for efficient liver regeneration. *Proc Natl Acad Sci U.S A,* 2007 *104,* 17081-17086.

[151] Avila,MA; Berasain,C; Sangro,B; Prieto,J. New therapies for hepatocellular carcinoma. *Oncogene,* 2006 *25,* 3866-3884.

[152] Choudhury,S; Pan,J; Amin,S; Chung,FL; Roy,R. Repair kinetics of trans-4-hydroxynonenal-induced cyclic 1,N2-propanodeoxyguanine DNA adducts by human cell nuclear extracts. *Biochemistry,* 2004 *43,* 7514-7521.

[153] Roy,R; Biswas,T; Hazra,TK; Roy,G; Grabowski,DT; Izumi,T; Srinivasan,G; Mitra,S. Specific interaction of wild-type and truncated mouse N-methylpurine-DNA glycosylase with ethenoadenine-containing DNA. *Biochemistry,* 1998 *37,* 580-589.

[154] Barash,H; Gross,R; Edrei,Y; Ella,E; Israel,A; Cohen,I; Corchia,N; Ben Moshe,T; Pappo,O; Pikarsky,E; Goldenberg,D; Shiloh,Y; Galun,E; Abramovitch,R. Accelerated carcinogenesis following liver regeneration is associated with chronic inflammation-induced double-strand DNA breaks. *Proc Natl Acad Sci U.S A,* 2010 *107,* 2207-2212.

[155] Meira,LB; Bugni,JM; Green,SL; Lee,CW; Pang,B; Borenshtein,D; Rickman,BH; Rogers,AB; Moroski-Erkul,CA; McFaline,JL; Schauer,DB; Dedon,PC; Fox,JG; Samson,LD. DNA damage induced by chronic inflammation contributes to colon carcinogenesis in mice. *J Clin Invest,* 2008 *118,* 2516-2525.

[156] Choudhury,S; Zhang,R; Frenkel,K; Kawamori,T; Chung,FL; Roy,R. Evidence of alterations in base excision repair of oxidative DNA damage during spontaneous hepatocarcinogenesis in Long Evans Cinnamon rats. *Cancer Res,* 2003 *63,* 7704-7707.

[157] Jia,G; Tohyama,C; Sone,H. DNA damage triggers imbalance of proliferation and apoptosis during development of preneoplastic foci in the liver of Long-Evans Cinnamon rats. *Int J Oncol,* 2002 *21,* 755-761.

[158] Laurent-Puig,P; Zucman-Rossi,J. Genetics of hepatocellular tumors. *Oncogene,* 2006 *25,* 3778-3786.

[159] Imbeaud,S; Ladeiro,Y; Zucman-Rossi,J. Identification of novel oncogenes and tumor suppressors in hepatocellular carcinoma. *Semin Liver Dis,* 2010 *30,* 75-86.

[160] Miyoshi,Y; Iwao,K; Nagasawa,Y; Aihara,T; Sasaki,Y; Imaoka,S; Murata,M; Shimano,T; Nakamura,Y. Activation of the beta-catenin gene in primary hepatocellular carcinomas by somatic alterations involving exon 3. *Cancer Res,* 1998 *58,* 2524-2527.

[161] Hsu,HC; Jeng,YM; Mao,TL; Chu,JS; Lai,PL; Peng,SY. Beta-catenin mutations are associated with a subset of low-stage hepatocellular carcinoma negative for hepatitis B virus and with favorable prognosis. *Am J Pathol.,* 2000 *157,* 763-770.

[162] Legoix,P; Bluteau,O; Bayer,J; Perret,C; Balabaud,C; Belghiti,J; Franco,D; Thomas,G; Laurent-Puig,P; Zucman-Rossi,J. Beta-catenin mutations in hepatocellular carcinoma correlate with a low rate of loss of heterozygosity. *Oncogene,* 1999 *18,* 4044-4046.

[163] Cieply,B; Zeng,G; Proverbs-Singh,T; Geller,DA; Monga,SP. Unique phenotype of hepatocellular cancers with exon-3 mutations in beta-catenin gene. *Hepatology,* 2009 *49,* 821-831.

[164] Fujito,T; Sasaki,Y; Iwao,K; Miyoshi,Y; Yamada,T; Ohigashi,H; Ishikawa,O; Imaoka,S. Prognostic significance of beta-catenin nuclear expression in hepatocellular carcinoma. *Hepatogastroenterology,* 2004 *51,* 921-924.

[165] Taniguchi,K; Roberts,LR; Aderca,IN; Dong,X; Qian,C; Murphy,LM; Nagorney,DM; Burgart,LJ; Roche,PC; Smith,DI; Ross,JA; Liu,W. Mutational spectrum of beta-catenin, AXIN1, and AXIN2 in hepatocellular carcinomas and hepatoblastomas. *Oncogene,* 2002 *21,* 4863-4871.

[166] Zucman-Rossi,J; Benhamouche,S; Godard,C; Boyault,S; Grimber,G; Balabaud,C; Cunha,AS; Bioulac-Sage,P; Perret,C. Differential effects of inactivated Axin1 and activated beta-catenin mutations in human hepatocellular carcinomas. *Oncogene,* 2007 *26,* 774-780.

[167] Laurent-Puig,P; Legoix,P; Bluteau,O; Belghiti,J; Franco,D; Binot,F; Monges,G; Thomas,G; Bioulac-Sage,P; Zucman-Rossi,J. Genetic alterations associated with hepatocellular carcinomas define distinct pathways of hepatocarcinogenesis. *Gastroenterology,* 2001 *120*, 1763-1773.

[168] Hsu,IC; Metcalf,RA; Sun,T; Welsh,JA; Wang,NJ; Harris,CC. Mutational hotspot in the p53 gene in human hepatocellular carcinomas. *Nature,* 1991 *350*, 427-428.

[169] Vautier,G; Bomford,AB; Portmann,BC; Metivier,E; Williams,R; Ryder,SD. p53 mutations in british patients with hepatocellular carcinoma: clustering in genetic hemochromatosis. *Gastroenterology,* 1999 *117*, 154-160.

[170] Hayashi,H; Sugio,K; Matsumata,T; Adachi,E; Takenaka,K; Sugimachi,K. The clinical significance of p53 gene mutation in hepatocellular carcinomas from Japan. *Hepatology,* 1995 *22*, 1702-1707.

[171] Honda,K; Sbisa,E; Tullo,A; Papeo,PA; Saccone,C; Poole,S; Pignatelli,M; Mitry,RR; Ding,S; Isla,A; Davies,A; Habib,NA. p53 mutation is a poor prognostic indicator for survival in patients with hepatocellular carcinoma undergoing surgical tumour ablation. *Br J Cancer,* 1998 *77*, 776-782.

[172] Bluteau,O; Jeannot,E; Bioulac-Sage,P; Marques,JM; Blanc,JF; Bui,H; Beaudoin,JC; Franco,D; Balabaud,C; Laurent-Puig,P; Zucman-Rossi,J. Bi-allelic inactivation of TCF1 in hepatic adenomas. *Nat Genet,* 2002 *32*, 312-315.

[173] Rebouissou,S; Amessou,M; Couchy,G; Poussin,K; Imbeaud,S; Pilati,C; Izard,T; Balabaud,C; Bioulac-Sage,P; Zucman-Rossi,J. Frequent in-frame somatic deletions activate gp130 in inflammatory hepatocellular tumours. *Nature,* 2009 *457*, 200-204.

[174] Boyault,S; Rickman,DS; de Reynies,A; Balabaud,C; Rebouissou,S; Jeannot,E; Herault,A; Saric,J; Belghiti,J; Franco,D; Bioulac-Sage,P; Laurent-Puig,P; Zucman-Rossi,J. Transcriptome classification of HCC is related to gene alterations and to new therapeutic targets. *Hepatology,* 2007 *45*, 42-52.

[175] Lee,JW; Soung,YH; Kim,SY; Lee,HW; Park,WS; Nam,SW; Kim,SH; Lee,JY; Yoo,NJ; Lee,SH. PIK3CA gene is frequently mutated in breast carcinomas and hepatocellular carcinomas. *Oncogene,* 2005 *24*, 1477-1480.

[176] Zhang,X; Xu,HJ; Murakami,Y; Sachse,R; Yashima,K; Hirohashi,S; Hu,SX; Benedict,WF; Sekiya,T. Deletions of chromosome 13q, mutations in Retinoblastoma 1, and retinoblastoma protein state in human hepatocellular carcinoma. *Cancer Res,* 1994 *54*, 4177-4182.

[177] Bae,JJ; Rho,JW; Lee,TJ; Yun,SS; Kim,HJ; Choi,JH; Jeong,D; Jang,BC; Lee,TY. Loss of heterozygosity on chromosome 10q23 and mutation of the phosphatase and tensin homolog deleted from chromosome 10 tumor suppressor gene in Korean hepatocellular carcinoma patients. *Oncol Rep,* 2007 *18*, 1007-1013.

[178] De Souza,AT; Hankins,GR; Washington,MK; Orton,TC; Jirtle,RL. M6P/IGF2R gene is mutated in human hepatocellular carcinomas with loss of heterozygosity. *Nat Genet,* 1995 *11*, 447-449.

[179] Oka,Y; Waterland,RA; Killian,JK; Nolan,CM; Jang,HS; Tohara,K; Sakaguchi,S; Yao,T; Iwashita,A; Yata,Y; Takahara,T; Sato,S; Suzuki,K; Masuda,T; Jirtle,RL. M6P/IGF2R tumor suppressor gene mutated in hepatocellular carcinomas in Japan. *Hepatology,* 2002 *35*, 1153-1163.

[180] Yamada,T; De Souza,AT; Finkelstein,S; Jirtle,RL. Loss of the gene encoding mannose 6-phosphate/insulin-like growth factor II receptor is an early event in liver carcinogenesis. *Proc Natl Acad Sci U.S A,* 1997 *94,* 10351-10355.

[181] Yao,YJ; Ping,XL; Zhang,H; Chen,FF; Lee,PK; Ahsan,H; Chen,CJ; Lee,PH; Peacocke,M; Santella,RM; Tsou,HC. PTEN/MMAC1 mutations in hepatocellular carcinomas. *Oncogene,* 1999 *18,* 3181-3185.

[182] Chen,TC; Hsieh,LL; Kuo,TT; Ng,KF; Wu Chou,YH; Jeng,LB; Chen,MF. p16INK4 gene mutation and allelic loss of chromosome 9p21-22 in Taiwanese hepatocellular carcinoma. *Anticancer Res,* 2000 *20,* 1621-1626.

[183] Kita,R; Nishida,N; Fukuda,Y; Azechi,H; Matsuoka,Y; Komeda,T; Sando,T; Nakao,K; Ishizaki,K. Infrequent alterations of the p16INK4A gene in liver cancer. *Int J Cancer,* 1996 *67,* 176-180.

[184] Boige,V; Laurent-Puig,P; Fouchet,P; Flejou,JF; Monges,G; Bedossa,P; Bioulac-Sage,P; Capron,F; Schmitz,A; Olschwang,S; Thomas,G. Concerted nonsyntenic allelic losses in hyperploid hepatocellular carcinoma as determined by a high-resolution allelotype. *Cancer Res,* 1997 *57,* 1986-1990.

[185] Lin,Y; Shi,CY; Li,B; Soo,BH; Mohammed-Ali,S; Wee,A; Oon,CJ; Mack,PO; Chan,SH. Tumour suppressor p53 and Rb genes in human hepatocellular carcinoma. *Ann Acad Med Singapore,* 1996 *25,* 22-30.

[186] Park,HJ; Yu,E; Shim,YH. DNA methyltransferase expression and DNA hypermethylation in human hepatocellular carcinoma. *Cancer Lett,* 2006 *233,* 271-278.

[187] Kaneto,H; Sasaki,S; Yamamoto,H; Itoh,F; Toyota,M; Suzuki,H; Ozeki,I; Iwata,N; Ohmura,T; Satoh,T; Karino,Y; Satoh,T; Toyota,J; Satoh,M; Endo,T; Omata,M; Imai,K. Detection of hypermethylation of the p16(INK4A) gene promoter in chronic hepatitis and cirrhosis associated with hepatitis B or C virus. *Gut,* 2001 *48,* 372-377.

[188] Tannapfel,A; Wittekind,C. Genes involved in hepatocellular carcinoma: deregulation in cell cycling and apoptosis. *Virchows Arch,* 2002 *440,* 345-352.

[189] Yu,J; Ni,M; Xu,J; Zhang,H; Gao,B; Gu,J; Chen,J; Zhang,L; Wu,M; Zhen,S; Zhu,J. Methylation profiling of twenty promoter-CpG islands of genes which may contribute to hepatocellular carcinogenesis. *BMC Cancer,* 2002 *2,* 29.

[190] Kubo,T; Yamamoto,J; Shikauchi,Y; Niwa,Y; Matsubara,K; Yoshikawa,H. Apoptotic speck protein-like, a highly homologous protein to apoptotic speck protein in the pyrin domain, is silenced by DNA methylation and induces apoptosis in human hepatocellular carcinoma. *Cancer Res,* 2004 *64,* 5172-5177.

[191] McConnell,BB; Vertino,PM. TMS1/ASC: the cancer connection. *Apoptosis,* 2004 *9,* 5-18.

[192] Kanai,Y; Ushijima,S; Hui,AM; Ochiai,A; Tsuda,H; Sakamoto,M; Hirohashi,S. The E-cadherin gene is silenced by CpG methylation in human hepatocellular carcinomas. *Int J Cancer,* 1997 *71,* 355-359.

[193] Kwon,GY; Yoo,BC; Koh,KC; Cho,JW; Park,WS; Park,CK. Promoter methylation of E-cadherin in hepatocellular carcinomas and dysplastic nodules. *J Korean Med Sci,* 2005 *20,* 242-247.

[194] Yamada,S; Nomoto,S; Fujii,T; Takeda,S; Kanazumi,N; Sugimoto,H; Nakao,A. Frequent promoter methylation of M-cadherin in hepatocellular carcinoma is associated with poor prognosis. *Anticancer Res,* 2007 *27*, 2269-2274.

[195] Bian,J; Wang,Y; Smith,MR; Kim,H; Jacobs,C; Jackman,J; Kung,HF; Colburn,NH; Sun,Y. Suppression of in vivo tumor growth and induction of suspension cell death by tissue inhibitor of metalloproteinases (TIMP)-3. *Carcinogenesis,* 1996 *17*, 1805-1811.

[196] Lu,GL; Wen,JM; Xu,JM; Zhang,M; Xu,RB; Tian,BL. [Relationship between TIMP-3 expression and promoter methylation of TIMP-3 gene in hepatocellular carcinoma]. *Zhonghua Bing.Li Xue.Za Zhi.,* 2003 *32*, 230-233.

[197] Wong,CM; Ng,YL; Lee,JM; Wong,CC; Cheung,OF; Chan,CY; Tung,EK; Ching,YP; Ng,IO. Tissue factor pathway inhibitor-2 as a frequently silenced tumor suppressor gene in hepatocellular carcinoma. *Hepatology,* 2007 *45*, 1129-1138.

[198] Tischoff,I; Tannapfe,A. DNA methylation in hepatocellular carcinoma. *World J Gastroenterol,* 2008 *14*, 1741-1748.

[199] Matsukura,S; Soejima,H; Nakagawachi,T; Yakushiji,H; Ogawa,A; Fukuhara,M; Miyazaki,K; Nakabeppu,Y; Sekiguchi,M; Mukai,T. CpG methylation of MGMT and hMLH1 promoter in hepatocellular carcinoma associated with hepatitis viral infection. *Br J Cancer,* 2003 *88*, 521-529.

[200] Zhang,YJ; Chen,Y; Ahsan,H; Lunn,RM; Lee,PH; Chen,CJ; Santella,RM. Inactivation of the DNA repair gene O6-methylguanine-DNA methyltransferase by promoter hypermethylation and its relationship to aflatoxin B1-DNA adducts and p53 mutation in hepatocellular carcinoma. *Int J Cancer,* 2003 *103*, 440-444.

[201] Su,PF; Lee,TC; Lin,PJ; Lee,PH; Jeng,YM; Chen,CH; Liang,JD; Chiou,LL; Huang,GT; Lee,HS. Differential DNA methylation associated with hepatitis B virus infection in hepatocellular carcinoma. *Int J Cancer,* 2007 *121*, 1257-1264.

[202] Zhang,YJ; Chen,Y; Ahsan,H; Lunn,RM; Chen,SY; Lee,PH; Chen,CJ; Santella,RM. Silencing of glutathione S-transferase P1 by promoter hypermethylation and its relationship to environmental chemical carcinogens in hepatocellular carcinoma. *Cancer Lett,* 2005 *221*, 135-143.

[203] Zhong,S; Tang,MW; Yeo,W; Liu,C; Lo,YM; Johnson,PJ. Silencing of GSTP1 gene by CpG island DNA hypermethylation in HBV-associated hepatocellular carcinomas. *Clin Cancer Res,* 2002 *8*, 1087-1092.

[204] Wang,J; Qin,Y; Li,B; Sun,Z; Yang,B. Detection of aberrant promoter methylation of GSTP1 in the tumor and serum of Chinese human primary hepatocellular carcinoma patients. *Clin Biochem,* 2006 *39*, 344-348.

[205] Okochi,O; Hibi,K; Sakai,M; Inoue,S; Takeda,S; Kaneko,T; Nakao,A. Methylation-mediated silencing of SOCS-1 gene in hepatocellular carcinoma derived from cirrhosis. *Clin Cancer Res,* 2003 *9*, 5295-5298.

[206] Yoshida,T; Ogata,H; Kamio,M; Joo,A; Shiraishi,H; Tokunaga,Y; Sata,M; Nagai,H; Yoshimura,A. SOCS1 is a suppressor of liver fibrosis and hepatitis-induced carcinogenesis. *J Exp Med,* 2004 *199*, 1701-1707.

[207] Tischoff,I; Markwarth,A; Witzigmann,H; Uhlmann,D; Hauss,J; Mirmohammad-sadegh,A; Wittekind,C; Hengge,UR; Tannapfel,A. Allele loss and epigenetic inactivation of 3p21.3 in malignant liver tumors. *Int J Cancer,* 2005 *115*, 684-689.

[208] Aravalli,RN; Steer,CJ; Cressman,EN. Molecular mechanisms of hepatocellular carcinoma. *Hepatology,* 2008 *48*, 2047-2063.

[209] Kutay,H; Bai,S; Datta,J; Motiwala,T; Pogribny,I; Frankel,W; Jacob,ST; Ghoshal,K. Downregulation of miR-122 in the rodent and human hepatocellular carcinomas. *J Cell Biochem,* 2006 *99*, 671-678.

[210] Gramantieri,L; Ferracin,M; Fornari,F; Veronese,A; Sabbioni,S; Liu,CG; Calin,GA; Giovannini,C; Ferrazzi,E; Grazi,GL; Croce,CM; Bolondi,L; Negrini,M. Cyclin G1 is a target of miR-122a, a microRNA frequently down-regulated in human hepatocellular carcinoma. *Cancer Res,* 2007 *67*, 6092-6099.

[211] Meng,F; Henson,R; Wehbe-Janek,H; Ghoshal,K; Jacob,ST; Patel,T. MicroRNA-21 regulates expression of the PTEN tumor suppressor gene in human hepatocellular cancer. *Gastroenterology,* 2007 *133*, 647-658.

[212] Marquardt,JU; Thorgeirsson,SS. Stem cells in hepatocarcinogenesis: evidence from genomic data. *Semin Liver Dis,* 2010 *30*, 26-34.

[213] Hsia,CC; Evarts,RP; Nakatsukasa,H; Marsden,ER; Thorgeirsson,SS. Occurrence of oval-type cells in hepatitis B virus-associated human hepatocarcinogenesis. *Hepatology,* 1992 *16*, 1327-1333.

[214] Roskams,T; Desmet,V. Ductular reaction and its diagnostic significance. *Semin Diagn.Pathol.,* 1998 *15*, 259-269.

[215] Libbrecht,L; Desmet,V; Van Damme,B; Roskams,T. Deep intralobular extension of human hepatic 'progenitor cells' correlates with parenchymal inflammation in chronic viral hepatitis: can 'progenitor cells' migrate? *J Pathol.,* 2000 *192*, 373-378.

[216] Lowes,KN; Brennan,BA; Yeoh,GC; Olynyk,JK. Oval cell numbers in human chronic liver diseases are directly related to disease severity. *Am J Pathol.,* 1999 *154*, 537-541.

[217] Durnez,A; Verslype,C; Nevens,F; Fevery,J; Aerts,R; Pirenne,J; Lesaffre,E; Libbrecht,L; Desmet,V; Roskams,T. The clinicopathological and prognostic relevance of cytokeratin 7 and 19 expression in hepatocellular carcinoma. A possible progenitor cell origin. *Histopathology,* 2006 *49*, 138-151.

[218] Roskams,T. Liver stem cells and their implication in hepatocellular and cholangiocarcinoma. *Oncogene,* 2006 *25*, 3818-3822.

[219] Tang,Y; Kitisin,K; Jogunoori,W; Li,C; Deng,CX; Mueller,SC; Ressom,HW; Rashid,A; He,AR; Mendelson,JS; Jessup,JM; Shetty,K; Zasloff,M; Mishra,B; Reddy,EP; Johnson,L; Mishra,L. Progenitor/stem cells give rise to liver cancer due to aberrant TGF-beta and IL-6 signaling. *Proc Natl Acad Sci U.S A,* 2008 *105*, 2445-2450.

[220] Knight,B; Tirnitz-Parker,JE; Olynyk,JK. C-kit inhibition by imatinib mesylate attenuates progenitor cell expansion and inhibits liver tumor formation in mice. *Gastroenterology,* 2008 *135*, 969-79, 979.

In: Liver Cancer: Causes, Diagnosis and Treatment
Editor: Benjamin J. Valverde

ISBN: 978-1-61209-115-0
© 2011 Nova Science Publishers, Inc.

*Chapter III*

# Liver Cancer Prevention and Treatment with Resveratrol

## *Anupam Bishayee*[*]

Cancer Therapeutics and Chemoprevention Group,
Department of Pharmaceutical Sciences,
Northeastern Ohio Universities Colleges of Medicine and Pharmacy,
Rootstown, OH, USA

## Abstract

Primary liver cancer, the majority of which represents hepatocellular carcinoma (HCC), is one of the most lethal cancers in the world with an annual incidence of over 700,000 cases. HCC most commonly develops in patients with chronic liver disease, the etiology of which includes viral infections (hepatitis B and C), alcoholic liver damage and ingestion of dietary carcinogens, such as aflatoxins and nitrosamines. Although, surgical resection and liver transplantation are currently available treatment options, only 10% of HCC patients qualify for these modalities. In view of the limited therapeutic alternatives and poor prognosis of liver cancer, chemoprevention and novel therapeutic approaches could be extremely valuable in lowering the present prevalence of the disease. Oxidative stress and inflammation are intimately connected to each other in the multistage hepatocarcinogenesis and these have been proposed as potential targets for the prevention and therapy of inflammation-associated HCC. A variety of bioactive food components, obtained from various fruits, vegetables, nuts and spices, have been shown to modify molecular targets involved with oxidative stress and chronic inflammation with resultant attenuation of carcinogenesis. Resveratrol, a naturally occurring antioxidant and antiinflammatory agent found in grapes and red wine, has emerged as a promising molecule that inhibits carcinogenesis with a pleiotropic mode of action. Although anticancer activities of resveratrol have been studied extensively in various cancer

---

[*] For correspondence: Anupam Bishayee, M. Pharm., Ph.D., Department of Pharmaceutical Sciences, Northeastern Ohio Universities Colleges of Medicine and Pharmacy, 4209, State Route 44, Rootstown, OH 44272, USA, Tel: 330-325-6449, Fax: 330-325-5936, Email: abishayee@neoucom.edu.

models, the preventive and therapeutic potential of resveratrol in liver cancer is only beginning to be unraveled. This chapter reviews the current cutting-edge discoveries on the potent cytotoxic effects of resveratrol against various liver cancer cells *in vitro* as well as the chemopreventive and therapeutic potential of this dietary agent *in vivo*. Available toxicity and pharmacokinetic data are also presented for clinical relevance. The current limitations, potential challenges, innovative approaches as well as the future directions of resveratrol research to explore its full potential in the prevention and therapy of liver cancer are also critically examined.

# Abbreviations

CAV1 = caveolin-1
COX-2 = cyclooxygenase-2
DENA = diethylnitrosamine
5-FU = 5-fluorouracil
$GST_P$ = placental glutathione S-transferase
HCC = hepatocellular carcinoma
IL = interleukin
iNOS = inducible nitric oxide synthase
i.p. = intraperitoneal
MAPK = mitogen-activated protein kinase
MMP = matrix metalloproteinase
MR-3 = 3,5,4′-trimethoxystilbene
NF-κB = nuclear factor-kappa B
Nrf2 = nuclear factor-E2 related factor 2
NO = nitric oxide
PB = phenobarbital
ROS = reactive oxygen species
TIMP = tissue inhibitor of metalloproteinase
TNF-α = tumor necrosis factor-α

# The Disease

Liver cancer is the fifth most common cancer in men and the eight frequent malignancy in women [American Cancer Society, 2007]. Clearly, a male predominance of this disease has been established with a male to female ratio of 2-4:1. More than 700,000 new cases of primary liver cancer are diagnosed worldwide every year and hepatocellular carcinoma (HCC) accounts for about 85-90% of these cancers [El-Serag *et al.*, 2007]. Liver cancer has a poor prognosis with a life expectancy of approximately 6 months from the time of the diagnosis. It represents the third leading cause of cancer death worldwide with an estimated 680,000 deaths in 2007. More than 80% of new cases are detected primarily in developing countries with 55% occurring in China alone [Thun *et al.*, 2010]. The incidence of HCC has been rising in several regions around the world, including east and southeast Asia, sub-

Saharan Africa, southern Europe and North America. In the United States, a 70% increase has been registered during the last 25 years [El-Serag, 2004]. More than 22,000 new cases and about 18,000 deaths are estimated to occur in 2009 alone in the United States primarily due to liver cancer [American Cancer Society, 2009]. The majority of liver cancer cases are attributable to underlying infections caused by the hepatitis B virus and the hepatitis C virus; however, several other risk factors, such as excessive alcohol consumption, non-alcoholic steatohepatitis, obesity, iron overload as well as dietary carcinogens (e.g., aflatoxins and nitrosamines) are also involved in its etiology [Bartsch and Montesano, 1984; Bosch et al., 2004; Kensler et al., 2004; Pang et al., 2006; Schütte et al., 2009].

# The Treatment

Although surgical resection is considered the optimal treatment approach, only 10-20% of HCC patients qualify for this option. In addition, for those undergoing resection, the recurrence rates can be 50% within several years of surgery [Llovet et al., 2003]. While liver transplantation has been successful for the treatment of limited-stage liver cancer patients, regrettably only a small number of patients are candidates for transplantation. The potential of this option is also limited due to organ shortage and the rapid and frequent recurrence of HCC in the transplanted liver. At present, there is no proven effective systemic chemotherapy for HCC. Although sorafenib is currently the only drug approved by the United States Food and Drug Administration for the treatment of unresectable HCC, recent studies indicate severe unfavorable side effects including a significant risk of bleeding [Je et al., 2009]. Alternate treatment modalities including transcatheter arterial chemoembolization, targeted intra-arterial delivery of Yttrium-90 microspheres, percutaneous intratumor ethanol injection and radiofrequency ablation are primarily for palliation and are applicable only to patients with localized liver tumors. Moreover, the implementation of these new modalities has also increased the complexity of HCC management [Senthil et al., 2010]. In the absence of a proven effective systemic therapy for liver cancer, novel chemopreventive approaches as well as therapeutic regimens are urgently needed to lower the current morbidity and mortality associated with this lethal malignancy.

# Inflammation, Oxidative Stress and Liver Cancer

Compelling evidence over the past few years strongly suggests the role of inflammation in the initiation, promotion and progression of HCC [Prieto, 2008]. Despite intrinsic differences among etiological factors for HCC, a common denominator of the genesis of malignancy is the perpetuation of a wound-healing response and the subsequent inflammatory reaction [Mantovani et al., 2008; Berasain et al., 2009]. Though numerous studies have shown the significant alterations in several cytokines and their signaling pathways in liver cirrhosis and HCC, the critical components linking inflammation and liver cancer are only beginning to be unraveled [Naugler et al., 2007; Rogers et al., 2007]. Cyclooxygenase-2 (COX-2), an enzyme with a critical role in the production of inflammatory mediators including prostaglandins, is chronically overexpressed in chronic liver inflammation and cirrhosis as well as experimental and human HCC. Consequently, blocking COX-2 may prove effective in the chemoprevention of HCC [Wu, 2006; Giannitrapani et al., 2009]. Another enzyme with a pivotal influence in mediating inflammation is inducible nitric oxide synthase (iNOS), which plays a significant role in experimental as well as human HCC [Ahn et al., 1999; Rahman et al., 2001; Calvisi et al., 2008]. Accordingly, inhibitors of elevated iNOS expression may be potential candidates for liver cancer chemoprevention and treatment. The nuclear factor-kappa B (NF-κB) is one of the most ubiquitous eukaryotic transcription factors that regulate expression of genes involved in the regulation of cell proliferation, survival, inflammation, invasion, angiogenesis and metastasis, which are involved in the promotion as well as the progression of cancers [Karin and Greten, 2005; Sethi et al., 2008]. The genes that are known to be regulated by NF-κB include both COX-2 and iNOS. Recently, a connection between inflammation and cancer through the NF-κB pathway has been established [Karin, 2008]. It has been demonstrated that almost 90% of HCC cases possess a natural history of unresolved inflammation and fibrosis or cirrhosis [Muriel, 2009]. Accordingly, the molecular regulator of HCC has been termed the *"inflammation-fibrosis-cancer axis"* [Elsharkawy and Mann, 2007] and NF-κB has been proposed as a potential *"master orchestrator"* of this axis [Muriel, 2009]. Emerging evidence suggests that suppression of the proinflammatory pathways regulated by NF-κB could lead to prevention and treatment of malignancies linked to chronic inflammatory conditions [Aggarwal et al., 2009; Paur et al., 2010].

Oxidative stress, through generation of reactive oxygen species (ROS), functions as a predisposing factor to hepatocellular carcinogenesis and is a common and major driving force of HCC in chronic liver ailments [Cortez-Pinto, 2001; Lai, 2002; Kawanishi et al., 2006]. Environmental insults due to chemical toxicants, such as nitrosamines, acts as tumor initiators and/or promoters by inducing a steady-state increase in the generation of ROS [Gius and Spitz, 2006]. Oxidative stress has been implicated in the propagation of inflammatory responses involved in carcinogenesis [Bartsch and Nair, 2005; Kawanishi et al., 2006]. Induction of several antioxidant and drug metabolizing enzymes is believed to be an important means of protecting against carcinogenesis and considered to be of advantage for cancer prevention. A promising means for upregulating levels of these cytoprotective enzymes in the human population is the consumption of plant-based foods and other natural products. The increased levels of cytoprotective enzymes induced by these phytochemicals over the course of a human lifetime could lead to reduced rate of carcinogenesis. Induction of such enzymes by various dietary phytochemicals has been recognized as one of the highly effective strategies for preventing cancer in human population [Talalay, 2000; Kwak et al., 2001a; Eggler et al., 2008; Jana and Mandlekar, 2009; Bishayee and Darvesh, 2010]. The nuclear factor-E2 related factor 2 (Nrf2) is a transcription factor of the basic leucine-zipper family and plays an essential role in the antioxidant-response element-mediated expression of many antioxidant and phase 2 detoxifying enzymes [Itoh et al., 1997; Kwak et al., 2001b]. Nrf2 is known to play an important role in the regulation of inflammation as well as expression of several antioxidant and detoxifying enzymes in response to oxidative and electrophilic stress [Osburn and Kensler, 2008; Li et al., 2008]. Nrf2 is an important modulator of susceptibility to develop carcinogen-induced tumors in various organs, including liver [Kitamura et al., 2007; Nishimura et al., 2008; Khor et al., 2008]. All these studies strongly suggest that Nrf2 could be a viable target in the inhibition of hepatocellular carcinogenesis.

# Resveratrol and Cancer

Natural dietary components, obtained from several fruits, vegetables, nuts and spices, have drawn significant attention due to their demonstrated ability to suppress carcinogenesis in experimental animal models with some of these substances able to partially prevent or delay cancer formation in several high-risk populations [WCRF/AICR, 2007]. A large number of bioactive food components have been shown to modify molecular targets involved with inflammation and redox signaling resulting in suppression of carcinogenesis [Rahman *et al.*, 2005; Kim *et al.*, 2009]. The plant polyphenol resveratrol (3,4′,5-trihydroxy-*trans*-stilbene, Figure 1) is one such agent, which has been shown to possess many biological activities relevant to human diseases [Baur and Sinclair, 2006; Shankar *et al.*, 2007; Shakibaei *et al.*, 2009]. It has been detected in more than 70 plant species, including grapes, berries, peanuts, plums and pine as well as in red wine. With epidemiological evidence indicating an inverse correlation between red wine consumption and the incidence of cardiovascular disease (*"French paradox"*), it has been suggested that the resveratrol in red wine may be responsible for this phenomenon [Kopp, 1998]. Subsequent studies have shown that resveratrol can prevent or slow the progression of a wide variety of inflammation-related illnesses, including cancer, neurodegenerative diseases, cardiovascular ailments, ischemic injury and viral infections [Baur and Sinclair, 2006; Das and Das, 2007; Saiko *et al.*, 2008].

Jang *et al.* [1997] demonstrated, for the first time, the chemopreventive effects of resveratrol in inhibiting multi-stage carcinogenesis, including initiation, promotion and progression. Subsequently, resveratrol has been shown to exhibit antiproliferative effects against a wide variety of human tumor cells *in vitro* [reviewed by Aggarwal *et al.*, 2004; Kundu and Surh, 2008], which have led to numerous preclinical animal studies to evaluate the cancer chemopreventive and chemotherapeutic potential of resveratrol. Resveratrol has been shown to prevent chemically-induced carcinogenesis in multiple organs and inhibit the growth of xenografted tumors in animals [reviewed by Bishayee, 2009]. An epidemiological study has shown a 50% or greater reduction in breast cancer risk in woman with resveratrol consumption from grapes [Levi *et al.*, 2005]. Several clinical trials, including one sponsored by the National Cancer Institute, are currently underway for oral resveratrol as a pure compound or resveratrol-rich products, for prevention and treatment of colon cancer [reviewed by Bishayee, 2009]. Interestingly, the liver is one of the principal target organs of resveratrol [Bertelli *et al.*, 1998; Vitrac *et al.*, 2003]. Resveratrol has also been shown to inhibit hepatic carcinogen activating enzymes and induce hepatic phase 2 conjugating enzymes *in vitro* as well as *in vivo* [Ciolino *et al.*, 1998; Hebbar *et al.*, 2005; Canistro *et al.*, 2009]. Resveratrol is known to protect rat liver cells against oxidative stress possibly by modulating antioxidant enzymes [Rubiolo and Vega, 2008; Rubiolo *et al.*, 2008]. Despite its great promise, the chemopreventive and therapeutic potential of resveratrol in liver cancer has not been investigated until recently [reviewed by Mann *et al.*, 2009; Bishayee *et al.*, 2010a].

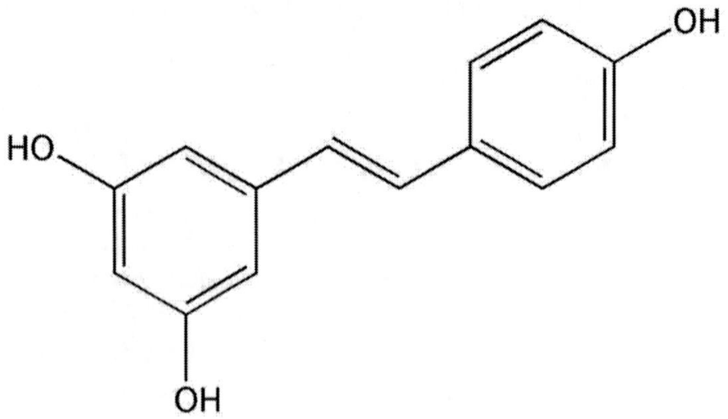

Figure 1. Chemical structure of resveratrol.

# Resveratrol and Liver Cancer

## Studies Using Cell Culture Models

As summarized in Table 1, several *in vitro* studies have examined the antitumor effects of resveratrol against various liver cancer cells. The cytotoxic potential of resveratrol against hepatic cancer cells was first reported by Delmas and coworkers [2000]. According to this study, resveratrol inhibited the proliferation of rat hepatoma Fao and human hepatoblastoma HepG$_2$ cells in both concentration- and time-dependent fashion. Accompanying studies have shown the ability of resveratrol in preventing or delaying the cells from entering mitosis and in increasing the number of cells arrested in the S as well as G$_2$/M phase. Resveratrol was found to attenuate hepatic growth factor-induced scattering and invasion of HepG$_2$ cells as well as cell proliferation possibly due to a post-receptor mechanism rather than apoptosis induction [DeLèdinghen *et al.*, 2001]. Kozuki and colleagues [2001] showed that resveratrol suppressed both the proliferation and invasion of AH109A rat ascites hepatoma cells at higher concentrations but inhibited only the invasion at lower concentrations. Resveratrol-loaded rat serum restrained only the invasion. Results of this study propose that the antiinvasive effect of resveratrol is independent of its antiproliferative activity and rather related to its antioxidant property. Additional studies from the same laboratory confirmed the involvement of the antioxidant property of resveratrol as sera from rats orally administered resveratrol were found to repress ROS-induced invasion of AH109A cells [Miura *et al.*, 2004]. Resveratrol, isolated from the seeds of *Paeonia lactiflora*, a plant used widely in Chinese traditional medicine, has been shown to exert cytotoxic effects on HepG$_2$ cells [Kim *et al.*, 2002]. Kuo *et al.* [2002] investigated the antiproliferative effects of resveratrol in two human liver cancer cell lines, such as HepG$_2$ and Hep3B and reported that resveratrol inhibited cell proliferation in p53-positive HepG$_2$ cells only. Mechanistic studies revealed that resveratrol-treated cells were arrested in the G$_1$ phase and underwent apoptotic death via the p53-dependent pathway with an increase in p21 and Bax expression. Resveratrol was found to

**Table 1. Effects of resveratrol on various liver cancer cells and underlying mechanisms**

| Cell lines | Effects | Mechanisms | Conc. (µM) | References |
|---|---|---|---|---|
| Fao; HepG$_2$ | ↓proliferation | cell cycle regulation | 1–150 | Delmas *et al.*, 2000 |
| HepG$_2$ | ↓proliferation; ↓invasion | receptor-related mechanism | 2.5–50 | De Lèdinghen *et al.*, 2001 |
| AH109A | ↓proliferation; ↓invasion | ↓oxidative stress | 25–200 | Kozuki *et al.*, 2001; Miura *et al.*, 2004 |
| HepG$_2$ | ↓proliferation |  | 5.2x10-5 (IC$_{50}$) | Kim *et al.*, 2002 |
| HepG$_2$ | ↓proliferation | G$_1$ phase; ↑apoptosis; ↑p53; ↑p21; ↑Bax | 4.4x10$^{-6}$–9x10$^{-5}$ | Kuo *et al.*, 2002 |
| H22 | ↓proliferation | ↑apoptosis | 5.5–88 | Sun *et al.*, 2002 |
| HepG$_2$ | ↓invasion | ↓HIF-1α; ↓VEGF | 5–100 | Zhang *et al.*, 2005 |
| HepG$_2$ | no cytotoxicity | ↑apoptosis; cell cycle regulation | 1–100 | Kocsis *et al.*, 2005 |
| H4IIE | ↓proliferation | ↑apoptosis; ↑caspase 2, 3, 8/10; ↑DNA fragmentation | 5–350 | Michels *et al.*, 2006 |
| HepG$_2$ | ↓proliferation |  | 5–100 (µg/mL) | Jo *et al.*, 2006 |
| HepG$_2$ | ↓proliferation | ↑apoptosis; cell cycle regulation | 2.5–320 | Stervbo *et al.*, 2006 |
| HepG$_2$ | ↓proliferation | ↑apoptosis; cell cycle arrest in G$_1$ and G$_2$/M phase; ↓ROS; ↑iNOS; ↑eNOS; ↑NO | 10$^{-6}$–1 | Notas *et al.*, 2006 |
| HepG$_2$ | ↓invasion | ↓MMP-9; ↓NF-κB | 50, 100 | Yu *et al.*, 2008 |
| HepG2 | ↓proliferation | ↑NADPH; ↑detoxifying enzymes | 1–100 | Colin *et al.*, 2008 |
| HepG$_2$; PLC/PRF-5 | ↓invasion |  | 1–100 | Braconi *et al.*, 2009 |
| HepG$_2$ | ↓proliferation | ↑apoptosis; cell cycle regulation; ↑Bax; ↑Bim; ↑Puma; ↑caspase; ↓ERK | 12.5–100 | Zhou *et al.*, 2009 |

Table 1. (Continued)

| HepG$_2$ ; CAV1 | ↓proliferation | ↑apoptosis; cell cycle regulation; ↑p38 MAPK activity; ↑caspase-3 | 20–300 | Yang *et al.*, 2009 |
|---|---|---|---|---|
| SK-HEP-1 | ↓proliferation | ↑ROS; ↑Rab 37; ↓annexin A8; ↓thymidine kinase; ↓maspin; ↓peroxiredoxin-2; ↓G protein | | Choi *et al.*, 2009 |
| HepG$_2$ | ↓proliferation | ↓cyclin D1; ↓P38 MAPK; ↓Akt; ↓Pak1 | 10–300 | Parekh *et al.*, 2010 |
| HepG$_2$; Hep3B | ↓proliferation; ↓invasion | ↓MMP-2/9; ↑TIMP-1/2 | 10–100 | Weng *et al.*, 2010 |
| SK-CHA-1 | ↓proliferation | ↑G$_1$/S phase cells; ↑LDH; ↑ALP; ↑TG | 8–64 | Roncoroni *et al.*, 2008 |

Abbreviations: ALP, alkaline phosphatase; ERK, extracellular signal-regulated kinase; IC$_{50}$, half maximal inhibitory concentration; CAV1, caveolin-1; Conc., concentration; eNOS, endothelial nitric oxide synthase; G protein, guanine nucleotide-binding protein; HIF-1α, hypoxia-inducible factor-1α; iNOS, inducible nitric oxide synthase; LDH, lactate dehydrogenase; MAPK, mitogen-activated protein kinase; MMP-2/9, matrix metalloproteinase-2/9; NADPH, nicotinamide adenine dinucleotide phosphate; NF-κB, nuclear factor-κB; NO, nitric oxide; Rab 37, Ras-related protein; ROS, reactive oxygen species; TG, transglutaminase; TIMP-1/2, tissue inhibitor of metalloproteinase-1/2; VEGF, vascular endothelial growth factor.

inhibit the growth of H22 hepatoma cells in a concentration- and time-dependent manner [Sun et al., 2002]. Another interesting observation of this study was a synergistic antitumor effect of resveratrol and the anticancer drug 5-fluorouracil (5-FU). A direct evidence of apoptosis was considered as the underlying mechanism of antihepatocarcinogenic activity of resveratrol. Zhang et al. [2005] showed that resveratrol inhibited the hypoxia-stimulated invasiveness of HepG$_2$ cells through its potent inhibitory effect on hypoxia-inducible factor-1$\alpha$ and its downstream target gene, vascular endothelial growth factor. In contrast to previous studies, Kocsis and colleagues [2005] did not find any cytotoxicity of resveratrol at the concentration range of 1-100 μM. Cell cycle analysis revealed an increase of S phase cells at low concentrations of resveratrol (10-50 μM) and a decrease at high concentrations (100-200 μM). The ratio of apoptotic cells was found to increase following resveratrol treatment at or above 50 μM typically after 48 h. Michels et al. [2006] observed resveratrol-mediated killing of metabolically active H4IIE rat hepatoma cells due to induction of apoptosis via activation of caspases 2, 3 and 8/10. In another study (Jo et al., 2006), the cytotoxicity of resveratrol on HepG$_2$ cells was found to be superior to two procyanidin-rich fractions derived from grapes though the related mechanisms were not studied. Stervbo and coworkers [2006] confirmed the inhibitory effects of resveratrol on the proliferation of HepG$_2$ cells. In line with previous studies, the investigators observed apoptotic as well as cell cycle effects with regards to mitotic interference; however this study provided evidence that HepG$_2$ cells treated with resveratrol for just 2 h exhibited evidence for hindrance of DNA synthesis. Notas et al. [2006] observed apoptosis through cell cycle arrest as the central mechanism by which resveratrol interferes with HepG$_2$ cell proliferation. This study also showed that resveratrol exerted antioxidant effects and altered the nitric oxide (NO)/nitric oxide synthase (NOS) system by increasing expressions and activities of iNOS and endothelial NOS enzymes as well as NO production. All these effects were achieved at nanomolar or picomolar levels, compatible with the concentrations of free resveratrol in biological fluids following consumption of resveratrol-rich foods and beverages. It has been shown that resveratrol inhibited tumor necrosis factor-$\alpha$ (TNF-$\alpha$)-mediated invasion and matrix metalloproteinase-9 (MMN-9) expression in HepG$_2$ cells. These effects were associated with the downregulation of NF-$\kappa$B signaling pathway [Yu et al., 2008]. Colin et al. [2008] compared the antiproliferative effects of trans-resveratrol, trans-ε-viniferin and their respective acetate derivatives as well as a polyphenolic mixture extracted from grapevine shoots, known as vineatrol. Resveratrol triacetate showed a slightly better antiproliferative activity than resveratrol. Vineatrol was found to be the most potent compound indicating a possible synergistic effect of both resveratrol and ε-viniferin. By utilyzing the in situ autofluorescence technique, the researchers also observed that resveratrol and related compounds induced cellular NADPH and green fluorescent cytoplasmic granular structures which may indicate a mechanism involving induction of xenobiotic detoxifying enzymes. A computational bioinformatics analysis of phenotype-associated gene expression has identified resveratrol as one of the leading therapeutic agents for HCC. Ancillary studies have confirmed that noncytotoxic concentration (10 μM) of resveratrol reduced the invasion of HepG$_2$ and PLC/RPF-5 [Braconi et al., 2009]. Resveratrol at a lower concentration induced a substantial but reversible S phase delay and mild DNA synthesis inhibition in HepG$_2$ cells without causing apoptotic cell death. At higher concentration, resveratrol triggered apoptosis mediated primarily by the mitochondrial pathway. Mechanistically, MEK inhibition has been implicated as an important early signaling event for resveratrol-mediated apoptosis [Zhou *et al.*, 2009]. The possible role of caveolin-1 (CAV1), a member of the caveolin family with function as a tumor suppressor that is poorly expressed in HCC, in the cytotoxic and pro-apoptotic actions of resveratrol has been investigated in HepG$_2$ cells transfected with various CAV mutants. The results have clearly demonstrated that resveratrol can induce a concentration- and time-dependent death of HepG$_2$ cells and the over-expression of CAV1 can enhance the cytotoxic and proapoptotic effects of resveratrol. Another interesting observation of this study is that overexpression of CAV1 improves the transport of resveratrol into HepG$_2$ cells via its cholesterol shuttle domain rather than the scaffolding domain, inhibiting cell proliferation and inducing apoptosis mediated through the p38 mitogen-activated protein kinase (MAPK) pathway and caspase-3 expression [Yang *et al.*, 2009]. Resveratrol inhibited cell proliferation, generated ROS, and caused DNA single-strand breaks in SK-HEP-1 cells. It also upregulated Ras-related protein and downregulated annexin A8, thymidine kinase, maspin, peroxiredoxin-2, and guanine nucleotide-binding protein [Choi *et al.*, 2009]. In a recent study, resveratrol has been shown to downregulate cyclin D1 as well as p38 MAPK, Akt and Pak1 expression and activity in HepG$_2$ cells, suggesting that the growth inhibitory response of resveratrol is associated with the downregulation of cell proliferation and survival pathways [Parekh *et al.*, 2011]. Resveratrol and its methoxy analog 3,5,4'-trimethoxystilbene (MR-3) have also been reported to possess antiproliferative and antiinvasive activities in HepG$_2$ and Hep3B cells; however MR-3 has been found to be more potent than resveratrol. The antiinvasive mechanisms of these two compounds could be mediated through the inhibition of MMP-2 and MMP-9 as well as induction of tissue inhibitor of metalloproteinase-1 (TIMP-1) and TIMP-2 [Weng *et al.*, 2010].

Cholangiocarcinoma, a malignancy originating from the epithelial cells of the biliary tree, represents approximately 3% of all the gastrointestinal neoplasia with an increasing incidence of the intrahepatic form [Khan *et al.*, 2005]. Recently, Roncoroni and colleagues [2008] investigated the effects of resveratrol on SK-ChA-1 human cholangiocarcinoma cells, cultured in the classical two-dimensional setting as well as in the three-dimensional spheroids. Resveratrol treatment suppressed SK-ChA-1 cell growth in both cell culture systems with a simultaneous cell cycle perturbation characterized by an accumulation of cells in the G$_1$/S phase. Further studies have shown that resveratrol elevated lactate dehydrogenase and alkaline phosphatase activities in the culture medium as well as promoted transglutaminase activity in the cell lysates. This study underscores potential of resveratrol in treating unresectable human cholangiocarcinoma.

## Studies Using Animal Models

Unlike *in vitro* studies, there are relatively fewer studies that have investigated the antitumor potential of resveratrol in various *in vivo* preclinical models of liver cancer (Table 2). Carbó *et al.* [1999] reported the first study on the chemotherapeutic potential of resveratrol in rodents. In this study, resveratrol administration to rats inoculated with fast growing Yoshida AH-130 hepatoma cells was found to demonstrate a significant reduction in the tumor cell count with an increase in the number of cells in the G$_2$/M phase of cell cycle and apoptosis of tumor cell population. Resveratrol-supplemented food suppressed the growth and metastasis of AH109A ascites hepatoma cells implanted into Donryu rats. Dietary resveratrol was also found to lower the serum lipid peroxide level and suppress the serum triglyceride as well as lipoprotein levels [Miura et al., 2003]. Parenteral administration of resveratrol inhibited the growth of H22 tumor cells transplanted into mice perhaps due to its effects on nonspecific host immunomodulatory activity [Liu et al., 2003]. In another study, the investigators first developed external tumors by injecting H22 cells into the groin of BALB/c mice and subsequently transplanted the tumor tissue into the liver. Resveratrol treatment was found to abrogate hepatic tumor growth through reduced expression of cell cycle proteins, namely cyclin B1 and p34cdc2 [Yu et al., 2003]. The efficacy of resveratrol in combination with 5-FU was also tested against the H22 transplanted murine tumor model. Akin to the *in vitro* study mentioned earlier, 5-FU's ability to reverse tumor growth was again increased when resveratrol was administered concomitantly. The same study also showed decreased 5-FU toxicity in mice concurrently given resveratrol, and a substantial increase in the number of cells arrested in mitosis [Wu et al., 2004]. Resveratrol's ability to augment the therapeutic effect of 5-FU could be beneficial in the treatment of HCC. The activity of CAV1 mutants on the growth of HepG$_2$ cells in nude mice receiving resveratrol treatment has been evaluated. Wild type HepG$_2$ cells or HepG$_2$ cells expressing various CAV1 mutants were implanted in mice that received resveratrol treatment on every alternate day for 21 days, starting the treatment 10 days following tumor cell injection. Although resveratrol significantly inhibited the growth of various types of HepG$_2$ cells, a maximum tumor regression was achieved against xenografts of HepG$_2$ cells expressing CAV1 [Yang et al., 2009]. The involvement of CAV1 in the antitumor and proapoptotic actions of resveratrol through modulation of cellular sensitivity may represent a novel approach in overcoming multi-drug resistance in the therapy of human HCC.

The chemopreventive potential of resveratrol or resveratrol-rich products against chemically-induced hepatocarcinogenesis in rodents has also been investigated (Table 2). Experimental liver cancer in rodents induced by diethylnitrosamine (DENA), a potent environmental and dietary hepatocarcinogen [Hecht, 1997; Brown, 1999; Loeppky, 1999], has been considered as one of the best characterized experimental models of HCC, allowing the screening of potential anticancer compounds on various phases of neoplastic transformation and development [Chatterjee and Bishayee, 1998; Chakraborty et al., 2007]. DENA-induced preneoplastic foci, neoplastic and HCC nodule formation in rodents closely mimics HCC development in humans [Peto et al., 1991; Verna et al., 1996]. Recently, a cross-species comparison of gene expression patterns has established that DENA-induced liver tumors in rodents closely resemble a subclass of human HCC [Lee et al., 2004]. Kweon and colleagues [2003] studied the effects of dietary grape extract (known to contain resveratrol) on the development of placental glutathione S-transferase (GST$_P$)-positive preneoplastic hepatic foci induced in rats by intraperitoneal (i.p.) injection of potent hepatocarcinogen DENA followed by partial hepatectomy. The results of this study provided evidence of an inhibitory effect of chronic grape diet on the occurrence of GST$_P$-positive foci. The grape diet also suppressed the extent of hepatic lipid peroxidation and fatty acid synthase activity, which could provide mechanistic basis of the observed chemopreventive action. Tharappel et al. [2008] used another experimental hepatocarcinogenesis model utilizing DENA as the initiating carcinogen and 3,3',4',4-tetrachlorobiphenyl (a polychlorinated biphenyl) as the promoting agent and noticed that dietary resveratrol did not modify the number and volume of GST$_P$-positive foci in rat liver. The presence of extremely low amount

**Table 2. Effects of resveratrol on development and growth of liver cancer in various animal model systems**

| Animal Models | Effects | Mechanisms | Dose/duration | Route | References |
|---|---|---|---|---|---|
| *Resveratrol in xenografted liver cancer* | | | | | |
| Wistar rats implanted with AH-130 hepatoma cells | Arrested tumor growth | ↑cells at G2/M; ↑apoptosis | 1 mg/kg; 7 days | i.p. | Carbó *et al.*, 1999 |
| Donryu rats implanted with AH109A hepatoma cells | Suppressed tumor growth and metastasis | ↓TBARS; ↓serum triglycerides; ↓VLDL; ↓LDL | 10-50 ppm; 20 days | diet | Miura *et al.*, 2003 |
| BALB/c mice implanted with H22 hepatoma cells | Inhibited tumor weights | immunomodulatory activity | 500-1500 mg/kg; 10 days | abd | Liu *et al.*, 2003 |
| BALB/c mice implanted with H22 hepatoma cells | Reduced tumor volumes | ↓cyclin B1; ↓p34cdc2; | 5-15 mg/kg; 10 days | abd | Yu *et al.*, 2003 |
| BALB/c mice transplanted with H22 cancer cells | Worked synergistically with 5-FU for cancer treatment | ⊥ S-phase | 5-15 mg/kg; 10 days | abd | Wu *et al.*, 2004 |
| CAV1-expressing HepG2 cells transplanted in BALB/c mice | Inhibited tumor growth | ↓cell proliferation; ↑apoptosis; ↑caspase-3 | 15 mg/kg; every alternate day for 21 days | i.p. | Yang *et al.*, 2009 |
| *Resveratrol in chemically-induced hepatocarcinogenesis* | | | | | |
| DENA-initiated hepatocarcinogenesis in Sprague-Dawley rats | Reduced GSTP-positive hepatic preneoplastic foci | ↓lipid peroxidation; ↓FAS | 15% [w/w] grape extract in diet; 11 weeks | diet | Kweon *et al.*, 2003 |
| DENA-initiated and PCB-77-promoted hepatocarcinogenesis in Spargue-Dawley rats | Did not modify hepatocarcinogenesis | | 0.005% in diet; ~10 weeks | diet | Tharappel *et al.*, 2008 |

**Table 2. (Continued)**

| DENA-initiated and PB-promoted hepatocarcinogenesis in Spargue-Dawley rats | Suppressed incidence, number and multiplicity of hepatic nodule formation | ↓cell proliferation; ↑Bax; ↓Bcl-2↑apoptosis; ↓HSP70; ↓COX-2; ↓iNOS; ↓3-NT; ↓TBARS; ↓PC; ↓NF-κB; ↑Nrf2 | 50-300 mg/kg; 20 weeks | diet | Bishayee & Dhir, 2009; Bishayee *et al.*, 2010b,c |

Abbreviations: abd, abdominal injection; CAV1, caveolin-1; COX-2, cyclooxygenase-2; DENA, diethylnitrosamine; FAS, fatty acid synthase; 5-FU, 5-fluorouracil; $GST_P$, placental glutathione S-transferase; HSP70, heat shock protein70; iNOS, inducible nitric oxide synthase; i.p., intraperitoneal; LDL, low-density lipoprotein; NF-κB, nuclear factor-κB; Nrf2, nuclear factor E2 related factor; 3-NT, 3-nitrotyrosine; PB, phenobarbital; PCB-77, polychlorinated biphenyl-77; PC, protein carbonyl; TBARS, thiobarbituric acid reactive substances; VLDL, very low-density lipoprotein.

of resveratrol in the diet (0.005% w/w) resulting in an extremely low dose (compared to the other *in vivo* studies presented here) could explain the lack of antihepatocarcinogenic effect of resveratrol in this experimental model.

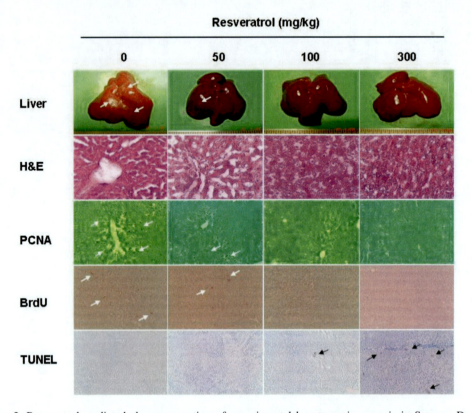

Figure 2. Resveratrol-mediated chemoprevention of experimental hepatocarcinogenesis in Sprague-Dawley rats as evidenced from inhibition of hepatocyte nodule formation, improved histopathological appearance, suppression of cell proliferation and induction of apoptosis. Initiation of hepatocarcinogenesis was performed by DENA (200 mg/kg, i.p.) followed by promotion with PB (0.05% in drinking water). The rats had free access to food supplemented with resveratrol equivalent to 0, 50, 100 or 300 mg/kg/day 4 weeks prior to the initiation and continued for total 20 weeks. Visible hepatic nodules were counted at the end of the study. Hepatic histopathology was studied by hematoxylin and eosin (H&E) staining and immunohistochemistry was performed to detect proliferating cell nuclear antigen (PCNA)- and 5-bromo-2'-deoxyuridine (BrdU)-positive cells. Terminal deoxynucleotidyl transferase dUTP nick end labeling (TUNEL) assay was performed to monitor apoptotic cells [adapted from Bishayee and Dhir, 2009, with permission].

In order to delineate the role of resveratrol on chemoprevention of hepatocellular carcinogenesis, our laboratory has initiated a series of experiments employing a well-characterized and clinically relevant two-stage rat liver tumorigenesis model initiated with DENA and promoted by phenobarbital (PB) [Bishayee and Chatterjee, 1995; Bishayee *et al.*, 1999, 2000]. In our recently published study [Bishayee and Dhir, 2009], the rats had free access to food supplemented with resveratrol equivalent to 0, 50, 100 or 300 mg/kg body weight/day. Resveratrol treatment was started 4 weeks prior to the initiation and continued for 20 weeks. Resveratrol dose-dependently reduced the incidence, total number and average number/liver (multiplicity) of visible hepatocyte nodules (Figure 2), the precursors of HCC [Farber and Sarma, 1987]. Histopathological examination of hematoxylin and eosin-stained liver tissue confirmed the antihepatocarcinogenic effect of resveratrol (Figure 2).

Immunohistochemical detection of cell proliferation and apoptosis indicated a decrease in cell proliferation and an increase of apoptotic cells in the livers of resveratrol-supplemented rats, respectively (Figure 2). The resveratrol-induced apoptogenic signal during DENA-initiated hepatocarcinogenesis was associated with the downregulation of Bcl-2 and upregulation of Bax expression [Bishayee and Dhir, 2009]. We have observed the involvement of inflammatory insult and oxidative stress in DENA-induced hepatocarcinogenesis in rats [Bishayee et al., 2010b,c] which is in agreement with prior studies [Maeda *et al.*, 2005; Ueno *et al.*, 2005; Naugler *et al.*, 2007; Zhao *et al.*, 2008]. Resveratrol also dose-dependently suppressed DENA-induced elevated expressions of hepatic preneoplastic and inflammatory markers, namely heat shock protein 70, COX-2 and NF-κB p65 and attenuated the translocation of NF-κB p65 to the nucleus by stabilizing the inhibitor of κB (Figure 3) [Bishayee *et al.*, 2010b]. DENA-induced hepatic lipid peroxidation, protein oxidation (protein carbonyl formation) as well as iNOS and 3-nitrotyrosine expression were also inhibited by resveratrol treatment, whereas resveratrol elevated hepatic protein and mRNA expression of Nrf2 in DENA-initiated animals (Figure 4) [Bishayee *et al.*, 2010c]. We have also observed that resveratrol treatment reversed the DENA-induced alteration of the level and expression of hepatic TNF-α, interleukin-1β (IL-1β) as well as IL-6 [Mbimba *et al.*, 2011]. All these results provide convincing evidence that resveratrol exerts chemoprevention of experimental hepatocarcinogenesis possibly by suppressing the inflammatory cascades and combating oxidative stress through modulation of NF-κB and Nrf2 signaling pathways respectively. Since both oxidative stress and inflammation play extremely crucial roles in the development and progression of human liver cancer, our findings underscore the potential of targeting these events as a strategy for achieving liver cancer chemoprevention and intervention by dietary agent resveratrol. Accumulating evidence suggests that not all of the antiinflammatory agents (COX-2 inhibitors) are ideal candidates for chemoprevention due to the risk of adverse cardiovascular events [Yona and Arber, 2004; Cervello and Montalto, 2006; Fujimura *et al.*, 2007]. Accordingly, we have evaluated the effects of chemopreventive doses of resveratrol on cardiac performance using transthoracic echocardiography (a non-invasive technique) during experimental hepatocarcinogenesis initiated with DENA and promoted by PB. Our results clearly indicate that resveratrol does not exhibit any cardiotoxicity but rather improves the cardiac function in a dose-responsive fashion in a chemopreventive setting [Luther *et al.*, 2011].

# Mechanisms of Action of Resveratrol in Liver Cancer

The numerous studies presented here indicate that the liver cancer chemopreventive and therapeutic effects of resveratrol are due to its unique ability to influence multiple cellular pathways rather than it having effects on a single target. A large number of studies suggest that the anti-liver cancer effects of resveratrol are mostly due to inhibition of cell proliferation and induction of apoptosis through cell cycle regulation. It is also possible that resveratrol could affect the progression of HCC by its inhibitory effects on invasion, angiogenesis and metastasis. Resveratrol is a potent antiinflammatory agent [Das and Das, 2007] and one of the

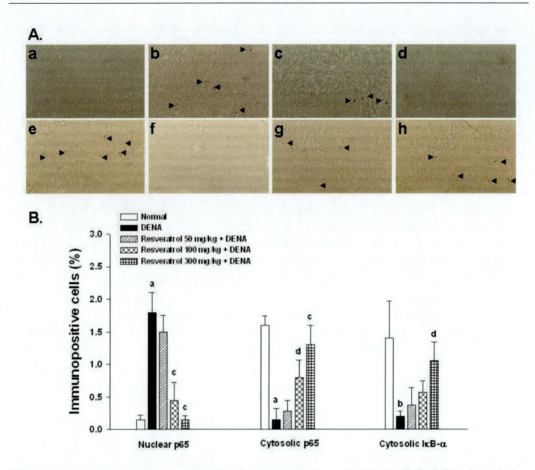

Figure 3. Effects of resveratrol on hepatic NF-κB p65 translocation and inhibitor of κB (IκB-α) degradation during DENA-evoked hepatic neoplasia in Sprague-Dawley rats. (A) Representative immunohistochemical localization of NF-κB p65 in nucleus (a-d) and IκB-α in cytosol (e-h) (magnification: 100x). Rats were sacrificed 20 weeks following the commencement of the study and immunohistochemistry was performed to detect NF-κB p65 as well as IκB-α. Arrows indicate immunohistochemical staining. Different experimental groups are: (a) and (e) normal control; (b) and (f) DENA control; (c) and (g) resveratrol 100 mg/kg + DENA and (d) and (h) resveratrol 300 mg/kg + DENA. (B) Quantification of NF-κB p65- and IκB-α-immunopositive cells in rat livers of several experimental groups. One thousand hepatocytes were counted per animal and the results were based on 4 animals per group. Each bar represents the mean±SD (n = 4). [a]$P<0.001$ and [b]$P<0.01$ as compared to normal group; [c]$P<0.001$ and [d]$P<0.01$ as compared to DENA control [adapted from Bishayee et al., 2010b, with permission].

possible mechanisms of its observed liver cancer preventive action could involve down regulation of the inflammatory responses. Prior studies [Kim et al., 2006; Cichocki et al., 2008; Yang et al., 2008; Chávez et al., 2008] have indicated that resveratrol could counteract NF-κB-mediated early inflammatory events. Our recent studies [Bishayee et al., 2010b] have also indentified NF-κB as one of the targets of resveratrol in the chemoprevention of experimental hepatocarcinogenesis. We have also shown that Nrf2 could be another important target of resveratrol in the inhibition of rat liver carcinogenesis [Bishayee et al., 2010c]. A large body of evidence indicates that targeted activation of the Nrf2 signaling accounts for the

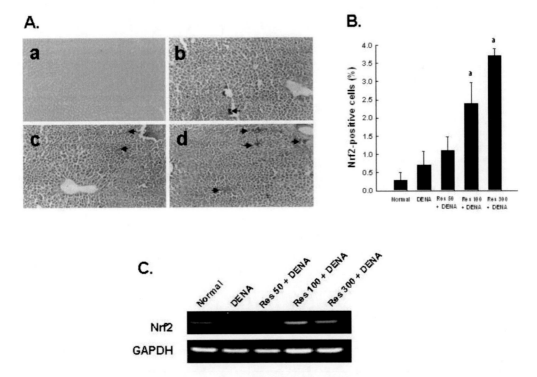

Figure 4. Effects of resveratrol on Nrf2 expression during DENA hepatocarcinogenesis in rats at 20 weeks. (A) Representative observation of hepatic Nrf2 immunoreactivity in different groups: (a) very limited expression in normal liver, (b) marginal elevated expression in DENA control, (c) resveratrol-mediated induction in 100 mg/kg and (d) 300 mg/kg group. (B) Immunochemical estimation of Nrf2 in livers of various groups. One thousand hepatocytes were counted per animal and the results were based on 4 animals per group. Each bar represents the mean±SD (n = 4). $^a P<0.05$ compared to DENA control. (C) Resveratrol-mediated induction of *Nrf2* gene expression. Total hepatic RNA was isolated, subjected to reverse transcription and resulting cDNA was subjected to reverse transcriptase-polymerase chain reaction using specific primer sequence [adapted from Bishayee et al., 2010c, with permission].

chemopreventive effects of several phytochemicals capable of suppressing oxidative and inflammatory stress [reviewed by Eggler et al., 2008; Khor et al., 2008; Surh et al., 2008; Kensler and Wakabayashi, 2010]. Induction of cytoprotective enzymes by dietary chemopreventive agents through the Nrf2 pathway is currently considered to be an important and viable part of preventing cancer in the human population. Considering all, prevention of oxidative stress-associated hepatocarcinogenesis through activation of Nrf2 signaling by dietary antioxidant resveratrol seems to be a promising strategy in the prevention of human liver cancer.

# Preclinical Toxicity and Pharmacokinetic Studies

During the last decade, several laboratories have evaluated the potential preclinical *in vivo* toxicity of resveratrol primarily in rodents (Table 3). Juan *et al.* [2002] did not observe

**Table 3. Preclinical toxicity studies of resveratrol**

| Species | Observations | Route | Dose | Duration | References |
|---|---|---|---|---|---|
| Sprague Dawley rats | Did not exhibit any hematologic, histopathologic as well as biochemical changes | p.o. | 20 mg/kg/day | 28 days | Juan *et al.*, 2002 |
| CD rats | 300 mg /kg/day:  did not produce any adverse effects in both male and female rats<br><br>1000 mg/kg/day:  produced a slight increase in WBC and lymphocyte count in male rats; it also produced body weight changes as well as slight decrease in adrenal weights in female rats<br><br>3000 mg/kg/day:  produced decrease in body weights, nephropathy, increase in kidney weights, renal lesions, it also elevated several clinical markers of liver metabolism, however no changes in liver histology were observed | p.o. | 300, 1000, 3000 mg/kg/day | 28 days | Crowell *et al.*, 2004 |
| CD rats | 300 and 1000 mg/kg/day: suppressed genes for phase 1 DME and enzyme expression in rat liver<br><br>All doses: dose-dependent increase was observed in gene and enzyme induction of several phase 2 detoxifying liver enzymes | p.o. | 300, 1000, 3000 mg/kg/day | 28 days | Hebber *et al.*, 2005 |
| C57BL/6 p53 knockout mice | All the doses administered did not produce any malignant or benign neoplasm | p.o. | 1000, 2000, 4000 mg/kg/day | 28 days | Horn *et al.*, 2007 |
| F2 hybrid four- way cross mice | Chronic administration produced nephrotoxocity as evidenced by increase in markers of lipid and protein oxidation | d.w. | 14.09 mg/L | 12 months | Wong *et al.*, 2009 |
| New Zealand white rabbits | Did not produce any dermal or ophthalmic irritation | Skin patch, ophthalmic application | 500 mg (dermal), 100 mg (ophthalmic) | 28 days | Williams *et al.*, 2009 |
| Sprague Dawley rats | Neither produced any increase in micronucleated immature erythrocytes nor any genotoxicity | p.o. | 500, 1000, 2000 mg/kg/day | 2 days | |

Table 3.(Continued)

| Wistar rats | Did not produce any systemic toxicity at all the administered doses | diet | 50, 150, 500 mg/kg/day | 28 days | |
| Wistar rats | Did not produce any reproductive organ as well as embryo-fetal toxicity in both male and female rats | diet | 120, 300, 750 mg/kg/day | 90 days | |

Abbreviations: DME, drug metabolizing enzymes; d.w., drinking water; p.o., *per os*; WBC, white blood corpuscles.

## Table 4. Clinical pharmacokinetic and safety studies of pure resveratrol and resveratrol containing beverages

| Objectives | Subjects* | Study results | Route | Dose | References |
|---|---|---|---|---|---|
| Bioavailability | Healthy males (2) | Pure compound appeared in whole blood and serum in 30 min | p.o. | 25 mg/person | Soleas *et al.*, 2001a |
| Bioavailability | Healthy humans (10) | Plasma free and conjugates peaked in 30 min; nearly 25% recovered in urine over 24 h | p.o. | 25 mg/person | Soleas *et al.*, 2001b |
| Bioavailability | Healthy males (12) | Peak glucuronide and sulfate conjugates appeared in serum in 30 min; urinary 24 h excretion was 16-17% of the dose | p.o. | 25 mg/70 kg | Goldberg *et al.*, 2003 |
| Bioavailability | Healthy males (3); Healthy females (3) | Absorption was 70% with plasma half-life of 9.2 h; mostly excreted in urine | p.o., i.v. | 25 mg/person | Walle *et al.*, 2004 |
| Bioavailability | Healthy humans (7) | Two glucuronide conjugates observed in serum | p.o. | 1 g/person | Wang *et al.*, 2004 |
| Bioavailability | Healthy humans (4) | Six major conjugate metabolites were detected and separated from serum and urine | p.o. | 1 g/person | Boocock *et al.*, 2007a |
| Bioavailability | Healthy males (3) | Pure resveratrol and its derivatives were detectable in plasma and urine; 25-50% resveratrol was recovered in urine during 24 h | p.o. | 0.03, 0.5, 1 mg/kg | Meng *et al.*, 2004 |
| Bioavailability | Healthy males (11) | Pure resveratrol and its glucuronide conjugates detected in plasma LDL samples | p.o. | 5.4 mg/person | Urpi-Sardà *et al.*, 2005 |

**Table 4.(Continued)**

| Bioavailability | Healthy males (11) | Pure resveratrol and glucuronide and sulfate conjugates detected in plasma LDL and urine samples | p.o. | 5.4 mg/person | Urpi-Sardà et al., 2007 |
|---|---|---|---|---|---|
| Urinary excretion | Healthy males (10); Healthy females (10) | Showed increase in total metabolites which may be utilized as biomarkers for clinical studies | p.o. | 0.36, 0.4, 2.6 mg/person | Zamora-Ros et al., 2006 |
| Urinary excretion | High-cardiovascular risk volunteers (1000) | Glucuronide and sulfate metabolites detected in urine, utilized as biomarker for wine consumption | p.o. | NQ | Zamora-Ros et al., 2009 |
| Bioavailability | Healthy males (14); Healthy females (11) | Pure or glucuronide conjugate was found in serum; meals did not affect bioavailability | p.o. | 3,4, 7.5, 33 μg/kg | Vitaglione et al., 2005 |
| Pharmacokinetics | Healthy humans (24) | Presence of food significantly delayed, but did not affect the extent of absorption | p.o. | 400 mg/person | Vaz-da-Silva et al., 2008 |
| Bioavailability | Healthy males (9) | Sulfate and glucuronide conjugated metabolites present in plasma and urine; 50% metabolites are bound to plasma proteins | p.o. | 85.5 mg/70 kg | Burkon & Somoza, 2008 |
| Phase I study | Healthy humans (40) | Did not exhibit adverse effects, peak plasma levels occurred in 1.5 h; 77% of all urinary species excreted in 24 h | p.o. | 0.5, 1, 2.5, 5 g/person | Boocock et al., 2007b |
| Pharmacokinetics | Healthy males (20); Healthy females (20) | Peak plasma concentrations at 1.5 h, only mild adverse effects were observed | p.o. | 25, 50, 100, 150 mg, 6 times/day | Almeida et al., 2009 |

*The number of human subjects is indicated in the parenthesis.
 Abbreviations:  i.v., intravenous; LDL, low density lipoprotein; NQ, not quantified, p.o., per os.

any evidence of systemic toxicity as well as hematologic and histopathologic alterations in rats administered 20 mg/kg/day for 28 days. Crowell *et al.* [2004] investigated the potential toxicity of three incremental doses of resveratrol in both male and female rats for 28 days. Enteral administration of a high dose of (3000 mg/kg/day) produced nephropathy and renal toxicity. This dose resulted in an increase in several clinical markers of liver metabolism including elevated blood urea nitrogen and creatinine levels without producing any hepatotoxicity. Interestingly, a low dose (300 mg) did not produce any adverse effects. Hebbar *et al.* [2005] used a similar dosing regimen to study the effect of resveratrol on rodent liver phase 1 and 2 gene and enzyme expression. Lower doses of resveratrol suppressed the phase 1 gene and enzyme expression. Dose-dependent increases in several phase 2 enzymes as well as their genes were observed with a significant increase being observed at the highest resveratrol dose of 3000 mg/kg/day. Parenteral administration of resveratrol (1000, 2000 or 4000 mg/kg/day) in p53 knockout mice did not induce malignant or benign neoplasm, demonstrating the absence of any carcinogenic potential of resveratrol even at high doses [Horn *et al.*, 2007]. Chronic supplementation of resveratrol in drinking water produced hepatotoxicity as evidenced by increased markers of oxidative stress [Wong *et al.*, 2009]. Resveratrol did not manifest any dermal or ophthalmic irritation in rabbits. Resveratrol administration was found to be devoid of any genotoxicity in rats. Additionally, both subchronic and chronic administration of resveratrol showed an absence of systemic as well as reproductive organ toxicity in rats [Williams *et al.*, 2009]. Based upon these studies, it can be concluded that a high (3000 mg/kg/day) dose of resveratrol produces renal toxicity in rodents. Resveratrol exhibits a complete absence of genotoxicity, oncogenicity as well as systemic and reproductive toxicity. All these studies highlight the relative safety profiles of resveratrol in doses that are found to be effective in the prevention and therapy of liver cancer as described earlier.

The pharmacokinetic profile of resveratrol, namely its absorption, distribution, metabolism and elimination has been extensively studied in rodents. We have recently reviewed the preclinical pharmacokinetic studies on resveratrol in detail [Bishayee *et al.*, 2010d].

# Clinical Toxicity and Pharmacokinetic Studies

Besides preclinical rodent studies, several investigators have studied the bioavailability, metabolism and safety of resveratrol in human subjects. Resveratrol, either as a pure compound or available from red wine or other beverages was examined in the clinical studies outlined in Table 4. It has been shown that resveratrol is rapidly absorbed after oral administration and undergoes extensive phase 2 metabolism primarily forming glucuronide and sulfate conjugates which are excreted in urine. Soleas *et al.* [2001a,b] in their pioneering work demonstrated that resveratrol was well absorbed in healthy males with the compound appearing in blood and serum in 30 min and in the urine at 24 h. Similar results were obtained in studies carried out by Goldberg *et al.* [2003]. Resveratrol administered mixed with a beverage (red wine, grape juice or vegetable juice) showed peak plasma levels 30 min after administration. This study also showed the presence of both glucuronide and sulfate conjugates of resveratrol in serum demonstrating the extensive metabolism of resveratrol.

This result was further supported by the observation that only 17% of resveratrol was excreted unmetabolized in the urine. Walle and co-workers [2004] studied the pharmacokinetics of [14]C-resveratrol after both oral and intravenous administration. Nearly 70% of the compound was absorbed and showed a plasma half-life of 9.2 h. An extremely interesting observation in this study was that only a small amount of resveratrol was found unmetabolized in the serum implying that the intestinal and hepatic conjugation of resveratrol was rapid as well as the rate limiting step. Two distinct glucuronide conjugates and six major conjugate metabolites have been identified after oral administration of 1 g of resveratrol [Wang et al., 2004; Boocock et al., 2007a]. Another study highlighted the effect of dose on metabolism of resveratrol. Administration of a low oral dose of resveratrol (0.03 mg/kg) resulted in the recovery of more than half of resveratrol in unmetabolized form in the urine, however a higher oral dose (1 mg/kg) resulted in only 25% of resveratrol being excreted unmetabolized in the urine [Meng et al., 2004].

Red wine is an extremely important dietary source of resveratrol in several regions of the world. Urpí-Sardà and fellow workers [2005, 2007] studied the uptake of resveratrol following moderate consumption of red wine. Using instrumental analytical methods of liquid chromatography and mass spectrometry the researchers determined the presence of free as well as glucuronide conjugates of resveratrol in human low density lipoprotein. Resveratrol, along with its glucuronide and sulfate conjugates were also found in urine samples in healthy males after moderate consumption of red wine. Zamora-Ros et al. [2006, 2009] evaluated the potential use of resveratrol metabolites as biomarkers of wine consumption. Results from their studies suggested the usefulness of both glucuronide and sulfate conjugates of resveratrol found in urine as useful biomarkers for wine consumption. These results would be extremely useful in ensuring compliance during clinical studies as well for epidemiological evaluation.

Several studies have evaluated the effect of food consumption on the bioavailability of resveratrol. In one study the effect of fasting, standard meal and meal with high lipid content were examined. The bioavailability of resveratrol as well as its glucuronide conjugates was found to be independent of food consumption or lipid content of the meal [Vitaglione et al., 2005]. Results from another study suggested that although the presence of food delayed the rate of absorption, the extent to which resveratrol was absorbed was not significantly affected [Vaz-da-Silva et al., 2008]. The pharmacokinetic profile of *trans*-resveratrol-3-*O*-β-D-glycoside, which is also known as piceid and is a major dietary form of resveratrol, was studied by Burkon and Somoza [2008]. Both sulfate and glucuronide conjugates were found to be present in both plasma and urine. Nearly 50% of resveratrol was found to be plasma protein bound. It was also found that about 35% of piceid was excreted unmetabolized in the urine.

Two studies evaluated the safety of resveratrol in humans [Boocock et al., 2007b; Almeida et al., 2009]. Resveratrol showed peak plasma levels 1.5 h after oral administration in both studies. While the former group of researchers reported an absence of any adverse effects after oral consumption of resveratrol, the latter reported a few mild adverse effects.

It is certainly clear from the clinical studies highlighted in this section that resveratrol is well absorbed following oral administration. However, the complete pharmacokinetic profile of resveratrol has not yet been completely elucidated. A major lacuna in this area remains the influence of genetic and ethnic polymorphism of metabolizing enzymes. This is an extremely important area of research considering the fact that resveratrol undergoes rapid and major phase 2 metabolism forming sulfate and glucuronide conjugates. Another caveat is that the clinical studies reviewed in this section have been conducted with a limited number of human subjects. Although these studies offer some information regarding the clinical pharmacokinetics of resveratrol, there exists a critical need for future studies evaluating the safety, bioavailability and metabolic profile in resveratrol in a large number of human subjects.

## Conclusions and Future Directions

Due to limited treatment options as well as a severely grave prognosis, liver cancer is an ideal candidate for chemoprevention. Although the primary prevention of HCC through hepatitis B and C vaccination and reduction of environmental carcinogens are likely to yield significant benefits, these approaches are not without their accompanying challenges. It is still necessary to target therapy towards those patients at a high risk of developing human HCC. Secondary prevention would include slowing down or halting tumor growth and preventing disease recurrence after surgery. However, efficient secondary preventions of HCC are not currently available. Using naturally occurring dietary compounds endowed with potent antioxidant and antiinflammatory actions as preventing and therapeutic agents for inflammation-associated cancers has become a fascinating strategy. One distinct example of inflammation-related cancer is HCC as it arises most frequently in the setting of chronic liver inflammation due to viral infection, metabolic injury as well as toxic insults. Resveratrol, a naturally occurring antioxidant and antiinflammatory agent, has emerged as a promising molecule that inhibits carcinogenesis with a pleiotropic mode of action. Based on our studies as well as those carried out in other laboratories, it is possible that the antioxidant and antiinflammatory effects of resveratrol could prevent the development of HCC. All these findings clearly reinforce its potential for liver cancer chemoprevention and therapy. Accordingly, continued efforts are needed, especially mechanism-based pre-clinical studies, to establish resveratrol as an effective chemopreventive agent against HCC. Prophylactic interventions with resveratrol as well as supplementation of foods rich in resveratrol may represent a practical approach to prevent the development of HCC. The complex molecular mechanisms of HCC coupled with cross-talks among several disrupted signaling pathways have made it almost impossible to block HCC development by interfering with a single pathway. Future studies utilizing various preclinical liver cancer models relevant to human HCC would expand the scope of the positive, coordinated regulation of a wide variety of mediators of inflammatory pathways and antioxidant defense mechanisms, and underscore the potential of targeting these events as a strategy for achieving liver cancer chemoprevention and treatment. Moreover, understanding of the downstream molecular targets of resveratrol would provide a wealth of information on which future clinical trials of resveratrol in high-risk populations could be designed effectively. These studies are expected to benefit the development of resveratrol as a clinically effective drug for the treatment of human HCC.

A large number of recent studies clearly indicate that combinations of two or more compounds could impart greater therapeutic benefit possibly by lowering their doses and consequently reducing the undesirable toxic manifestations. Prior studies have shown that resveratrol has the ability to potentiate the effects of standard anticancer drugs and ionizing radiation. Several preclinical animal studies as well as clinical observations as highlighted in this chapter provide evidence that this natural product is well tolerated and pharmacologically safe. In the light of these favorable attributes, resveratrol may be used in combination with other chemotherapeutic agents to achieve better therapeutic outcome in liver cancer patients.

From this chapter, it becomes clear to the reader that resveratrol shows efficacy as liver cancer preventive and therapeutic agent in spite of its low bioavailability. It has been hypothesized that resveratrol metabolites could be responsible, at least in part, for the observed beneficial effects of the parent molecule. More studies are needed to clearly delineate the effects of resveratrol metabolites and conjugates against liver cancer cells as well as relevant animal models to confirm this possibility. Novel drug formulation and delivery systems including liposomal-, neosomal- and nanoparticle-based approaches could enhance the targeted delivery of resveratrol in liver resulting in better efficacy. Furthermore, new direction of resveratrol research should aim at designing and synthesizing novel resveratrol analogs with better antitumor activity with accompanying improved pharmacokinetic properties.

In conclusion, existing data on the effects of resveratrol on cultured hepatocellular cancer cells as well as preclinical animal models of hepatic carcinoma coupled with its excellent safety profile unequivocally suggest a great potential of this natural antioxidant and antiinflammatory agent in the prevention and treatment of inflammation-driven liver cancer. Nevertheless, a considerable amount of work remains to be performed before the full potential of this *"miracle molecule"* in the prevention and intervention of liver cancer is realized.

# Acknowledgments

The author sincerely thanks Cornelis J. Van der Schyf, D.Sc., DTE, for his constant support and encouragement and Altaf S. Darvesh, Ph.D., and Roslin J. Thoppil, B.S., for carefully reading the manuscript and providing constructive suggestions. Our research on resveratrol and liver cancer chemoprevention is partly supported by a Research Incentive Grant from the Ohio Board of Regents, State of Ohio, USA.

# References

Aggarwal, BB; Bhardwaj, A; Aggarwal, RS; Seeram, NP; Shishodia, S; Takada, Y. Role of resveratrol in prevention and therapy of cancer: preclinical and clinical studies. *Anticancer Res*, 2004, 24, 2783-2840.

Aggarwal, BB; Vijayalekshmi, RV; Sung B. Targeting inflammatory pathways for prevention and therapy of cancer: short-term friend, long-term foe. *Clin Cancer Res*, 2009, 15, 425-430.

Ahn, B; Han, BS; Kim, DJ; Ohshima, H. Immunohistochemical localization of inducible nitric oxide synthase and 3-nitrotyrosine in rat liver tumors induced by N-nitrosodiethylamine. *Carcinogenesis*, 1999, 20, 1337-1344.

Almeida, L; Vaz-da-Silva, M; Falcão, A; Soares, E; Costa, R; Loureiro, AI; *et al.* Pharmacokinetic and safety profile of trans-resveratrol in a rising multiple-dose study in healthy volunteers. *Mol Nutr Food Res*, 2009, 53, S7-S15.

American Cancer Society. Global Cancer Facts and Figures 2007. Atlanta: American Cancer Society, 2007.

American Cancer Society. Cancer Facts and Figures 2009. Atlanta: American Cancer Society, 2009.

Bartsch, H; Montesano, R. Relevance of nitrosamines to human cancer. *Carcinogenesis*, 1984, 5, 1381-1393.

Bartsch, H; Nair, J. Accumulation of lipid peroxidation-derived DNA lesions: potential lead markers for chemoprevention of inflammation-driven malignancies. *Mutat Res*, 2005, 591, 34-44.

Baur, JA; Sinclair, DA. Therapeutic potential of resveratrol: the in vivo evidence. *Nat Rev Drug Discov*, 2006, 5, 493-506.

Berasain, C; Casillo, J; Perugorria, MJ; Latasa, MU; Prieto, J; Avila, MA. Inflammation and liver cancer: new molecular links. *Ann NY Acad Sci*, 2009, 1155, 206-221.

Bertelli, AA; Giovanni, L; Stradi, R; Urisen, S; Tillement, JP; Bertelli A. Evaluation of kinetic parameters of natural phytoalexin in resveratrol orally administered in wine to rats. *Drug Expt Clin Res*, 1998, 24, 51-55.

Bishayee A. Cancer prevention and treatment with resveratrol: from rodent studies to clinical trials. *Cancer Prev Res*, 2009, 2, 409-418.

Bishayee, A; Chatterjee, M. Inhibitory effect of vanadium on rat liver carcinogenesis initiated with diethylnitrosamine and promoted by phenobarbital. *Br J Cancer*, 1995, 71, 1214-1220.

Bishayee, A; Dhir, N. Resveratrol-mediated chemoprevention of diethylnitrosamine-initiated hepatocarcinogenesis: inhibition of cell proliferation and induction of apoptosis. *Chem-Biol Interact*, 2009, 179, 131-144.

Bishayee, A; Darvesh, A. Oxidative stress in cancer and neurodegenerative diseases: prevention and treatment by dietary antioxidants, Handbook of Free Radicals: Formation, Types and Effects, Kozyrev, D; Slutsky, V (Eds.) Nova Science Publishers, Inc., New York, 2010, 1-55.

Bishayee, A; Roy, S; Chatterjee, M. Characterization of selective induction and alteration of xenobiotic biotransforming enzymes by vanadium during diethylnitrosamine-induced chemical rat liver carcinogenesis. *Oncol Res*, 1999, 11, 41-53.

Bishayee, A; Sarkar, A; Chatterjee, M. Further evidence for chemopreventive potential of β-carotene against experimental hepatocarcinogenesis: diethylnitrosamine-initiated and phenobarbital promoted hepatocarcinogenesis is prevented more effectively by β-carotene than by retinoic acid. *Nutr Cancer*, 2000, 37, 89-98.

Bishayee, A; Politis, T; Darvesh, AS. Resveratrol in the chemoprevention and treatment of hepatocellular carcinoma. *Cancer Treat Rev*, 2010a, 36, 43-53.

Bishayee, A; Waghray, A; Barnes, KF; Mbimba, T; Bhatia, D; Chatterjee, M; *et al.* Suppression of the inflammatory cascade is implicated in resveratrol chemoprevention of experimental hepatocarcinogenesis. *Pharm Res*, 2010b, 27, 1080-1091.

Bishayee, A; Barnes, KF; Bhatia, D; Darvesh, AS; Carroll, RT. Resveratrol suppresses oxidative stress and inflammatory response in diethylnitrosamine-initiated rat hepatocarcinogenesis. *Cancer Prev Res*, 2010c, 3, 753-763.

Bishayee, A; Darvesh, AS; Politis, T; McGory, R. Resveratrol and liver disease: from bench to bedside and community. *Liver Int*, 2010d, 30, 1103-1114.

Boocock, DJ; Patel, KR; Faust, GE; Normolle, DP, Marczlo, TH; Crowell, JA; *et al.* Quantitation of *trans*-resveratrol and detection of its metabolites in human plasma and urine by high performance liquid chromatography. *J Chromatogr B Analyt Technol Biomed Life Sci*, 2007a, 848, 182-187.

Boocock DJ, Faust GE, Patel KR, Schinas, AM; Brown, VA; Ducharme, MP; *et al.* Phase I dose escalation pharmacokinetic study in healthy volunteers of resveratrol, a potential cancer chemopreventive agent. *Cancer Epidemiol Biomarkers Prev*, 2007b, 16, 1246-1252.

Bosch, FX; Ribes, J; Diaz, M; Cleries, R. Primary liver cancer: worldwide incidence and trends. *Gastroenterology*, 2004, 127, S5-S16.

Braconi, C; Meng, F; Swenson, E; Khrapenko, L; Huang, N; Patel, T. Candidate therapeutic agents for hepatocellular cancer can be identified from phenotype-associated gene expression signatures. *Cancer*, 2009, 115, 3738-3748.

Brown JL. N-Nitrosamines. *Occup Med*, 1999, 14, 839-848.

Burkon, A; Somoza, V. Quantification of free and protein-bound *trans*-resveratrol metabolites and identification of *trans*-resveratrol-C/O-conjugated diglucuronides – two resveratrol metabolites in human plasma. *Mol Nutr Food Res*, 2008, 52, 549-557.

Calvisi, DF; Pinna, F; Ladu, S; Pellegrino, R; Muroni, MR; Simile, MM; *et al.* Aberrant iNOS signaling is under genetic control in rodent liver cancer and potentially prognostic for the human disease. *Carcinogenesis*, 2008, 29, 1639-1647.

Canistro, D; Bonamassa, B; Pozzetti, L; Sapone, A; Abdel-Rahman, SZ; Biagi, GL; *et al.* Alteration of xenobiotic metabolizing enzymes by resveratrol in liver and lung of CD1 mice. *Food Chem Toxicol*, 2009, 47, 454-461.

Carbó, N; Costelli, P; Baccino, FM; López-Soriano, FJ; Argilés, JM. Resveratrol, a natural product present in wine, decreases tumour growth in a rat tumour model. *Biochem Biophys Res Commun*, 1999, 254, 739-743.

Cervello, M; Montalto, G. Cyclooxygenase in hepatocellular carcinoma. *World J Gastroenterol*, 2006, 12, 5113-5121.

Chakraborty, T; Chatterjee, A; Rana, A; Dhachinamoorthi, D; Kumar, PA; Chatterjee, M. Carcinogen-induced early molecular events and its implication in the initiation of chemical hepatocarcinogenesis in rats: chemopreventive role of vanadium on this process. *Biochim Biophys Acta*, 2007, 1772, 48-59.

Chatterjee, M; Bishayee A. Vanadium - a new tool for cancer prevention, Vanadium in the Environment, Part 2: Health Effects, Nriagu, JO (Ed.), John Wiley and Sons, Inc., New York, 1998, 347-390.

Chávez, E; Reyes-Gordillo, K; Segovia, J; Shibayama, M; Tsutsumi, V; Vergara, P; *et al.* Resveratrol prevents fibrosis, NF-κB activation and TGF-β increases by chronic CCl$_4$ treatment in rats. *J Appl Toxicol*, 2008, 28, 35-43.

Choi, HY; Chong, SA; Nam, MJ. Resveratrol induces apoptosis in human SK-HEP-1 hepatic cancer cells. *Cancer Genomics Proteomics*, 2009, 6, 263-268.

Cichocki, M; Paluszczak, J; Szaefer, H; Piechowiak, A; Rimando, AM; Baer-Dubowska, W. Pterostilbene is equally potent as resveratrol in inhibiting 12-*O*-tetradecanoylphorbol-

13-acetate activated NFκB, AP-1, COX-2, and iNOS in mouse epidermis. *Mol Nutr Food Res*, 2008, 52, S62-S70.

Ciolino, HP; Daschner, PJ; Yeh, GC. Resveratrol inhibits transcription of CYP1A1 in vitro by preventing activation of the aryl hydrocarbon receptor. *Cancer Res*, 1998, 58, 5707-5712.

Colin, D; Lancon, A; Delmas, D; Lizard, G; Abrossinow, J; Kahn, E; *et al*. Antiproliferative activities of resveratrol and related compounds in human hepatocyte derived HepG2 cells are associated with biochemical cell disturbance revealed by fluorescence analyses. *Biochimie*, 2008, 90, 1674-1684.

Cortez-Pinto H. Oxidative stress in alcoholic and nonalcoholic liver disease. Falk symposium 121. Steatohepatitis (NASH and ASH), Leuscher U; Dancygier M (Ed.), Kluwer Academic Publishers, Dordrecht, 2001, 54-61.

Crowell, JA; Korytko, PJ; Morrissey, RL, Booth, TD; Levine, BS. Resveratrol-associated renal toxicity. *Toxicol Sci*, 2004, 82, 614-619.

Das S; Das DK. Anti-inflammatory responses of resveratrol. *Inflammation Allergy Drug Target*, 2007, 6, 168-173.

DeLėdinghen, V; Monovoisin, A; Neaud, V; Krisa, S; Payrastre, B; *et al*. *Trans*-resveratrol, a grapevine-derived polyphenol, blocks hepatocyte growth factor-induced invasion of hepatocellular carcinoma cells. *Int J Oncol*, 2001, 19, 83-88.

Delmas, D; Jannin, B; Malki, MC; Latruffe, N. Inhibitory effect of resveratrol on the proliferation of human and rat hepatic derived cell lines. *Oncol Rep*, 2000, 7, 847-852.

Eggler, A; Gay, KA; Mesecar, AD. Molecular mechanisms of natural products in chemoprevention: induction of cytoprotective enzymes by Nrf2. *Mol Nutr Food Res*, 2008, 52, S84-S94.

El-Serag, HB. Hepatocellular carcinoma: recent trends in the United States. *Gastroenterology*, 2004, 127, S27-S34.

El-Serag, HB; Rudolph, KL. Hepatocellular carcinoma: epidemiology and molecular carcinogenesis. *Gastroenterology*, 2007, 132, 2557-2576.

Elsharkawy, AM; Mann, DA. Nuclear factor-κB and the hepatic inflammation-fibrosis-cancer axis. *Hepatology*, 2007, 46, 590-597.

Farber, E; Sarma, DS. Hepatocarcinogenesis: a dynamic cellular perspective. *Lab Invest*, 1987, 56, 4-22.

Fujimura, T; Ohta, T; Oyama, K; Miyashita, T; Miwa, K. Cycloxygenase-2 (COX-2) in carcinogenesis and selective COX-2 inhibitors for chemoprevention in gastrointestinal cancers. *J Gastrointest Cancer*, 2007, 38, 78-82.

Giannitrapani, L; Ingrao, S; Soresi, M; Maria Florena, A; La Spada, E; Sandonato, L; *et al*. Cyclooxygenase-2 expression in chronic liver diseases and hepatocellular carcinoma. *Ann NY Acad Sci*, 2009, 1155, 293-299.

Gius, D; Spitz DR. Redox signaling in cancer biology. *Antioxid Redox Signal*, 2006, 8, 1249-1252.

Goldberg, DM; Yan, J; Soleas, GJ. Absorption of three wine-related polyphenols in three different matrices by healthy subjects. *Clin Biochem*, 2003, 36, 79-87.

Hebbar, V; Shen, G; Hu, R; Kim, B-R; Chen, C; Korytko, PJ; *et al*. Toxicogenomics of resveratrol in rat liver. *Life Sci*, 2005, 76, 2299-2314.

Hecht, SS. Approaches to cancer prevention based on an understanding of N-nitrosamine carcinogenesis. *Proc Soc Exp Biol Med*, 1997, 216, 181-191.

Horn, TL; Cwik, MJ; Morrissey, RL; Kapetanovic, I; Crowell, JA; Booth, TD; *et al.* Oncogenicity evaluation of resveratrol in p53 (+/-) (p53 knockout) mice. *Food Chem Toxicol*, 2007, 45, 55-63.

Itoh, K; Chiba, T; Takahashi, S; Ishii, T; Igarashi, K; Katoh, Y; *et al.* An Nrf2/small Maf heterodimer mediates the induction of phase II detoxifying enzyme genes through antioxidant response elements. *Biochem Biophys Res Commun*, 1997, 236, 313-322.

Jana, S; Mandlekar, S. Role of phase II drug metabolizing enzymes in cancer chemoprevention. *Curr Drug Metab*, 2009, 10, 595-616.

Jang, M; Cai, L; Udeani, GO; Slowing, KV; Thomas, CF; Beecher, CWW; *et al.* Cancer chemopreventive activity of resveratrol, a natural product derived from grapes. *Science*, 1997, 275, 218-220.

Je, Y; Schutz, FAB; Choueiri, TK. Risk of bleeding with vascular endothelial growth factor receptor tyrosine-kinase inhibitors sunitinib and sorafenib: a systematic review and mata-analysis of clinical trials. *Lancet Oncol*, 2009, 10, 967-974.

Jo, JY; de Mejia, EG; Lila, MA. Cytotoxicity of bioactive polymeric fractions from grape cell culture on human hepatocellular carcinoma, murine leukemia and non-cancerous PK15 kidney cells. *Food Chem Toxicol*, 2006, 44, 1758-1767.

Juan, ME; Vinardell, MP; Planas, JM. The daily oral administration of high doses of *trans*-resveratrol to rats for 28 days is not harmful. *J Nutr*, 2002, 132, 257-260.

Karin, M. The IκB kinase – a bridge between inflammation and cancer. *Cell Res*, 2008, 18, 334-432.

Karin, M; Greten, FR. NF-κB: linking inflammation and immunity to cancer development and progression. *Nat Rev Immunol*, 2005, 5, 749-759.

Kawanishi, S; Hiraku, Y; Pinlaor, S; Ma, N. Oxidative stress and nitrative DNA damage in animals and patients with inflammatory diseases in relation to inflammation-related carcinogenesis. *Biol Chem*, 2006, 387, 365-372.

Kensler, TW; Wakabayashi N. Nrf2: friend or foe for chemoprevention. *Carcinogenesis*, 2010, 31, 90-99.

Kensler, TW; Egner, PA; Wang, J-B; Zhu, Y-R; Zhang, B-C; Lu, P-X; *et al.* Chemoprevention of hepatocellular carcinoma in aflatoxin endemic areas. *Gastroenterology*, 2004, 127, S310-S318.

Khan, SA; Thomas, CH; Davidson, BR; Taylor-Robinson, SD. Cholangiocarcinoma. *Lancet*, 2005, 366, 1303-1314.

Khor, TO; Yu, S; Kong, A-N. Dietary cancer chemopreventive agents – targeting inflammation and Nrf2 signaling pathway. *Planta Med*, 2008, 74, 1540-1547.

Kim, HJ; Chang, EJ; Bae, SJ; Shim, SM; Park, HD; Rhee, CH; *et al.* Cytotoxic and antimutagenic stilbenes from seeds of *Paeonia lactiflora*. *Arch Pharm Res*, 2002, 3, 293-299.

Kim, YA; Lim, S-Y; Rhee, S-H; Park, KY; Kim, C-H; Choi, BT; *et al.* Resveratrol inhibits inducible nitric oxide synthase and cyclooxygenase-2 expression in β-amyloid-treated C6 glioma cells. *Int J Mol Med*, 2006, 17, 1069-1075.

Kim, YS; Young, MR; Bobe, G; Colbum, NH; Milner, JA. Bioactive food components, inflammatory targets, and cancer prevention. *Cancer Prev Res*, 2009, 2, 200-208.

Kitamura, Y; Umemura, T; Kanki, K; Kodama, Y; Kitamoto, S; Saito, K; *et al*. Increased susceptibility to hepatocarcinogenicity of Nrf2-deficient mice exposed to 2-amino-3-methylimidazo[4,5-*f*]quinoline. *Cancer Sci*, 2007, 98, 19-24.

Kocsis, Z; Marcsek, ZL; Jakab, MG; Szende, B; Tompa, A. Chemopreventive properties of *trans*-resveratrol against the cytotoxicity of chloroacetanilide herbicides in vitro. *Int J Hyg Environ-Health*, 2005, 208, 211-218.

Kopp P. Resveratrol, a phytoestrogen found in red wine. A possible explanation for the conundrum of the 'French paradox'? *Eur J Endocrinol*, 1998, 138, 619-620.

Kozuki, Y; Miura, Y; Yagasaki, K. Resveratrol suppresses hepatoma cell invasion independently of its anti-proliferative action. *Cancer Lett*, 2001, 167, 151-156.

Kundu, JK; Surh, Y-J. Cancer chemopreventive and therapeutic potential of resveratrol: mechanistic perspectives. *Cancer Lett*, 2008, 269, 243-261.

Kuo, P; Chiang, L; Lin, C. Resveratrol-induced apoptosis is mediated by p53-dependent pathway in Hep G2 cells. *Life Sci*, 2002, 72, 23-34.

Kwak, MK; Egner, A; Dolan, P; Ramos-Gomez, M; Groopman, JD; Itoh, K; *et al*. Role of phase 2 enzyme induction in chemoprotection by dithiolethiones. *Mutat Res*, 2001a, 480-481, 305-315.

Kwak, MK; Itoh, K; Yamamoto, M; Suttwer, TR; Kensler TW. Role of transcription factor Nrf2 in the induction of hepatic phase 2 and antioxidative enzymes in vivo by the cancer chemopreventive agent, 3H-1,2-dimethiole-3-thione. *Mol Med*, 2001b, 7, 135-145.

Kweon, S; Kim, Y; Choi, H. Grape extracts suppress the formation of preneoplastic foci and activity of fatty acid synthase in rat liver. *Exp Mol Med*, 2003, 35, 371-378.

Lai, MM. Hepatitis C virus proteins: direct link to hepatic oxidative stress, steatosis, carcinogenesis and more. *Gastroenterology*, 2002, 122, 568-571.

Lee, JS; Chu, IS; Mikaelyan, A; Calvisi, DF; Heo, J; Reddy, JK; *et al*. Application of comparative functional genomics to identify best-fit mouse models to study human cancer. *Nat. Genetics*, 2004, 36, 1306-1311.

Levi, F; Pasche, C; Lucchini, F; Ghidoni, R; Ferraroni, M; La Vecchia, C. Resveratrol and breast cancer risk. *Eur J Cancer Prev*, 2005, 14, 139-142.

Li, W; Khor, TO; Xu, C; Shen, G; Jenog, W-S; Yu, S; *et al*. Activation of Nfr2-antioxidant signaling attenuates NF-κB-inflammatory response and elicits apoptosis. *Biochem Pharmacol*, 2008, 76, 1485-1489.

Liu, H-S; Pan, C-E; Yang, W; Liu, X-M. Antitumor and immunomodulatory activity of resveratrol on experimentally implanted tumor of H22 in Balb/c mice. *World J Gastroenterol*, 2003, 9, 1474-1476.

Llovet, JM; Burroughs, A; Bruix, J. Hepatocellular carcinoma. *Lancet*, 2003, 362, 1907-1917.

Loeppky RN. The mechanism of bioactivation of N-nitrosodiethanolamine. *Drug Metab Rev*, 1999, 31, 175-193.

Luther, DJ; Ohanyan, V; Shamhart, PE; Hodnichak, CM; Sisakian, H; Booth, TD; *et al*. Chemopreventive doses of resveratrol do not produce cardiotoxicity in a rodent model of hepatocellular carcinoma. *Invest New Drugs*, 2011, 29, 380-391.

Maeda, S; Kamata, H; Luo, JL; Leffert, H; Karin, M. IKKβ couples hepatocyte death to cytokine-driven compensatory proliferation that promotes chemical hepatocarcinogenesis. *Cell*, 2005, 121, 977-990.

Mann, CD; Neal, CP; Garcea, G; Manson, MM; Dennison, AR; Berry, DP. Phytochemicals as potential chemopreventive and chemotherapeutic agents in hepatocarcinogenesis. *Eur J Cancer Prev*, 2009, 18, 13-25.

Mantovani, A; Allavena, P; Sica, A; Balkwill, F. Cancer-related inflammation. *Nature*, 2008, 454, 436-444.

Mbimba, T; Awale, P; Bhatia, D; Geldenhuys, WJ; Darvesh, AS; Carroll, RT; *et al.* Alteration of hepatic proinflammatory cytokines is involved in the resveratrol-mediated chemoprevention of chemically-induced hepatocarcinogenesis. *Curr Pharm Biotechnol*, 2011, in press.

Meng, X; Maliaki, P; Lu, H; Lee, M-J; Yang, CS. Urinary and plasma levels of resveratrol and quercetin in humans, mice, and rats after ingestion of pure compounds and grape juice. *J Agric Food Chem*, 2004, 52, 935-942.

Michels, G; Wätjen, W; Weber, N; Niering, P; Chovolou, Y; Kampkötter, A; *et al.* Resveratrol induces apoptotic cell death in rat H4IIE hepatoma cells but necrosis in C6 glioma cells. *Toxicology*, 2006, 225, 173-182.

Miura, D; Miura, Y; Yagasaki, K. Hypolipidemic action of dietary resveratrol, a phytoalexin in grapes and red wine, in hepatoma-bearing rats. *Life Sci*, 2003, 73, 1393-1400.

Miura, D; Miura, Y; Yagasaki K. Resveratrol inhibits hepatoma cell invasion by suppressing gene expression on hepatocyte growth factor via its reactive oxygen species-scavenging property. *Clin Exp Metas*, 2004, 25, 445-451.

Muriel, P. NF-κB in liver diseases: a target for drug therapy. *J Appl Toxicol*, 2009, 29, 91-100.

Naugler, WE; Sakurai, T; Kim, S; Maeda, S; Kim, KH; Elsharkawy, AM; *et al.* Gender disparity in liver cancer due to sex differences in MyD88-dependent IL-6 production. *Science*, 2007, 317, 121-124.

Nishimura, J; Dewa, Y; Okamura, T; Jin, M; Saegusa, Y; Kawai, M; *et al.* Role of Nrf2 and oxidative stress on fenofibrate-induced hepatocarcinogenesis in rats. *Toxicol Sci*, 2008, 106, 339-349.

Notas, G; Figli, A; Kampa, M; Vercauteren, J; Kouroumalis, E; Castanas, E. Resveratrol exerts its antiproliferative effect on HepG2 hepatocellular carcinoma cells, by inducing cell cycle arrest, and NOS activation. *Biochim Biophys Acta*, 2006, 1760, 1657-1666.

Osburn, WO; Kensler TW. Nrf2 signaling: an adaptive response pathway for protection against environmental toxic insults. *Mutat Res*, 2008, 659, 31-39.

Pang, R; Tse, E; Poon, TP. Molecular pathways in hepatocellular carcinoma. *Cancer Lett*, 2006, 240, 157-169.

Parekh, P; Motiwale, L; Naik, N; Rao, KVK. Downregulation of cyclin D1 is associated with decreased levels of p38 MAP kinases, Akt/PKB and Pak1 during chemopreventive effects of resveratrol in liver cancer cells. *Exp Toxicol Pathol*, 2011, 63, 167-173.

Paur, I; Balstad, TR; Kolberg, M; Pedersen, MK; Austenaa, LM; Jacobs, DR Jr; *et al.* Extract of oregano, coffee, thyme, clove, and walnuts inhibits NF-κB in monocytes and in transgenic reporter mice. *Cancer Prev Res*, 2010, 3, 653-663.

Peto, R; Gary, R; Brantom, P; Grasso, P. Dose and time relationships for tumor induction in the liver and esophagus of 4080 inbred rats by chronic ingestion of N-nitrosodiethylamine or N-nitrosodimethylamine. *Cancer Res*, 1991, 51, 6452-6469.

Prieto J. Inflammation, HCC and sex: IL-6 in the centre of the triangle. *J Hepatol*, 2008, 48, 380-381.

Rahman, MA; Dhar, DK; Yamaguchi, E; Maruyama, S; Sato, T; Hayashi, H; *et al.* Coexpression of inducible nitric oxide synthase and COX-2 in hepatocellular carcinoma and surrounding liver: possible involvement of COX-2 in the angiogenesis of hepatitis C virus-positive cases. *Clin Cancer Res*, 2001, 7, 1325-1332.

Rahman, I; Biswas, SK; Kirkham, PA. Regulation of inflammation and redox signaling by dietary polyphenols. *Biochem Pharmacol*, 2005, 72, 1439-1452.

Rogers, AB; Theve, EJ; Feng, Y; Fry, RC; Taghizadeh, K; Clapp, KM; *et al.* Hepatocellular carcinoma associated with liver-gender disruption in male mice. *Cancer Res*, 2007, 67, 11536-11546.

Roncoroni, L; Elli, L; Dolfini, E; Erba, E; Dogliotti, E; Terrani, C; *et al.* Resveratrol inhibits cell growth in a human cholangiocarcinoma cell line. *Liver Int*, 2008, 28, 1426-1436.

Rubiolo, JA; Vega, FV. Resveratrol protects primary rat hepatocytes against necrosis induced by reactive oxygen species. *Biomed Pharmacother*, 2008, 62, 606-612.

Rubiolo, JA; Mithieux, G; Vega, FV. Resveratrol protects primary rat hepatocytes against oxidative stress damage: activation of the Nrf2 transcription factor and augmented activities of antioxidant enzymes. *Eur J Pharmacol*, 2008, 591, 66-72.

Saiko, P; Szakmary, A; Jaeger, W; Szekeres, T. Resveratrol and its analogs: defense against cancer, coronary disease and neurodegenerative maladies or just a fad? *Mutat Res*, 2008, 658, 68-94.

Schütte, K; Bornschein, J; Malfertheiner, P. Hepatocellular carcinoma – epidemiological trends and risk factors. *Dig Dis*, 2009, 27, 80-92.

Senthil, M; Mailey, B; Leong, L; Chung, V; Yen, Y; Chen, YJ; *et al.* Liver-directed regional therapy in the multi-disciplinary management of hepatocellular cancer. *Curr Cancer Ther Rev*, 2010, 6, 19-25.

Sethi, G; Sung, S; Aggarwal, BB. Nuclear factor-κB activation: from bench to bedside. *Exp Biol Med*, 2008, 233, 21-31.

Shakibaei, M; Harikumar, KB; Aggarwal BB. Resveratrol addiction: to die or not to die. *Mol Nutr Food Res*, 2009, 53, 115-128.

Shankar, S; Singh, G; Srivastava, RK. Chemoprevention by resveratrol: molecular mechanisms and therapeutic potential. *Front Biosci*, 2007, 12, 4839-4854.

Soleas, GJ; Yan, J; Goldberg, DM. Ultrasensitivity assay for the three polyphenols (catechins, quercetin and resveratrol) and their conjugates in biological fluids utilizing gas chromatography with mass selective detection. *J Chromatogr B*, 2001a, 757, 161-172.

Soleas, GJ; Yan, J; Goldberg, DM. Measurement of *trans*-resveratrol, (+)-catechin and quercetin in rat and human blood and urine by gas chromatography with mass selective detection. *Methods Enzymol*, 2001b, 335, 130-145.

Stervbo, U; Vang, O; Bonnesen, C. Time- and concentration-dependent effects of resveratrol in HL-60 and HepG2 cells. *Cell Prolif*, 2006, 39, 479-493.

Sun, Z; Pan, C; Liu, H; Wang, G. Anti-hepatoma activity of resveratrol in vitro. *World J Gastroenterol*, 2002, 8, 79-81.

Surh, Y-J; Kundu, JK; Na, HK. Nrf2 as a master redox switch in turning on the cellular signaling involved in the induction of cytoprotective genes by some chemopreventive phytochemicals. *Planta Med*, 2008, 74, 1526-1539.

Talalay P. Chemoprotection against cancer by induction of phase 2 enzymes. *Biofactors*, 2000, 12, 5-11.

Tharappel, JC; Lehmler, H-J; Srinivasan, C; Robertson, LW; Spear, BT; Glauert, HP. Effect of antioxidant phytochemicals on the hepatic tumor promoting activity of 3,3',4,4'-tetrachlorobiphenyl [PCB-77]. *Food Chem Toxicol*, 2008, 46, 3467-3474.

Thun, MJ; DeLancey, JO; Center, MM; Jemal, A; Ward, EM. The global burden of cancer: priorities for prevention. *Carcinogenesis*, 2010, 31, 100-110.

Ueno, S; Aoki, D; Kubo, F; Hiwatashi, K; Matsushita, K; Oyama, T; *et al*. Roxithromyc inhibits constitutive activation of nuclear factor κB by diminishing oxidative stress in a rat model of hepatocellular carcinoma. *Clin Cancer Res*, 2005, 11, 5645-5650.

Urpí-Sardà, M; Jáuregui, O; Lamuela-Raventós, RM; Jaeger, W; Miksits, M; Covas, M-I; *et al*. Uptake of diet resveratrol into the human low-density lipoprotein: identification and quantification of resveratrol metabolites by liquid chromatography coupled with tanden mass spectrometry. *Anal Chem*, 2005, 77, 3149-3155.

Urpí-Sardà, M; Zamora-Ros, R; Raventos-Lamuela, R; Cherubini, A; Jauregui, O; de la Torre, R; *et al*. HPLC-tandem mass spectrometric method to characterize resveratrol metabolism in humans. *Clin Chem*, 2007, 53, 292-299.

Vaz-da-Silva, M; Loureiro, AI; Falcao, A; Nunes, T; Rocha, J-F; Fernandez-Lopes, C; *et al*. Effect of food on the pharmacokinetic profile of trans-resveratrol. *Int J Clin Pharmacol Ther*, 2008, 46, 564-570.

Verna, L; Whysner, J; Williams, GM. N-nitrosodiethylamine mechanistic data and risk assessment: bioactivation, DNA-adduct formation, mutagenicity, and tumor initiation. *Pharmacol Ther*, 1996, 71, 57-81.

Vitaglione, P; Sforza, S; Galaverna, G; Ghidini, C; Caporaso, N; Vescovi, PP; *et al*. Bioavailability of trans-resveratrol from red wine in humans. *Mol Nutr Food Res*, 2005, 49, 495-504.

Vitrac, X; Desmoulière, A; Brouillaud, B; Krisa, S; Deffieux, G; Barthe, N; *et al*. Distribution of $[^{14}C]$-trans-resveratrol, a cancer chemopreventive polyphenol, in mouse tissues after oral administration. *Life Sci*, 2003, 72, 2219-2233.

Walle, T; Hsieh, F; DeLegge, MH; Oatis, JE; Walle, UK. High absorption but very how bioavailability of oral resveratrol in humans. *Drug Metab Disp*, 2004, 32, 1377-1382.

Wang, LX; Heredia, A; Song, H; Zhang, Z; Yu, B; Davis, C; *et al*. Resveratrol glucuronides as the metabolites of resveratrol in humans: characterization, synthesis and anti-HIV activity. *J Pharm Sci*, 2004, 93, 2448-2457.

Weng, CJ; Wu, CF; Huang, HW; Wu, CH; Ho, CT; Yen, GC. Evaluation of anti-invasion effect of resveratrol and related methoxy analogues on human hepatocarcinoma cells. *J Agric Food Chem*, 2010, 58, 2866-2894.

Williams, LD; Burdock, GA; Edwards, JA; Beck, M; Bausch, J. Safety studies conducted on high-purity *trans*-resveratrol in experimental animals. *Food Chem Toxicol*, 2009, 47, 2170-2182.

Wong, YT; Gruber, J; Jenner, AM; Ng, MPE; Ruan, R; Tay, FEH. Elevation of oxidative-damage biomarkers during aging in F2 hybrid mice: protection by chronic oral intake of resveratrol. *Free Radic Biol Med*, 2009, 46, 799-809.

World Cancer Research Fund/American Institute for Cancer Research. Food, Nutrition, Physical Activity, and the Prevention of Cancer: a Global Perspective. Washington, DC: AICR, 2007.

Wu T. Cyclooxygenase-2 in hepatocellular carcinoma. *Cancer Treat Rev*, 2006, 32, 28-44.

Wu, S-L; Sun, Z-J; Yu, L; Meng, K-W; Qin, X-L; Pan, C. Effect of resveratrol and in combination with 5-FU on murine liver cancer. *World J Gastroenterol*, 2004, 10, 3048-3052.

Yang, Z; Yang, S; Misner, BJ; Chiu, R; Liu, F; Meyskens, FL. Nitric oxide initiates progression of human melanoma via a feedback loop mediated by apurinic/apyrimidinic endonuclease-1/redox factor-1, which is inhibited by resveratrol. *Mol Cancer Ther*, 2008, 7, 3751-3760.

Yang, H-l; Chen, W-Q; Cao, X; Worschech, A; Du, L-F; Fang, W-Y; *et al.* Caveolin-I enhances resveratrol-mediated cytotoxicity and transport in a hepatocellular carcinoma model. *J Transl Med*, 2009, 7, 22.

Yona, D; Arber, N. Coxibs and cancer prevention. *J Cardiovasc Pharmacol*, 2004, 47, S76-S81.

Yu, L; Sun, Z-J; Wu, SL; Pan, C-E. Effect of resveratrol on cell cycle proteins in murine transplantable liver cancer. *World J Gastroenterol*, 2003, 9, 2341-2343.

Yu, H; Pan, C; Zhao, S; Wang, Z; Zhang, H; Wu, W. Resveratrol inhibits tumor necrosis factor-$\alpha$-mediated matrix metalloproteinase-9 expression and invasion of human hepatocellular carcinoma cells. *Biomed Pharmacother*, 2008, 62, 366-372.

Zamora-Ros, R; Urpí-Sardà, M; Lamuela-Raventós, RM; Estruch, R; Vázquez-Agell, M; Serrano-Martinez, M; *et al.* Diagnostic performance of urinary resveratrol metabolites as a biomarker of moderate wine consumption. *Clin Chem*, 2006, 52, 1373-1380.

Zamora-Ros, R; Urpí-Sardà, M; Lamuela-Raventós, RM; Estruch, R; Martinez-González, MA; Bulló, M; *et al.* Resveratrol metabolites in urine as a biomarker of wine intake in free-living subjects: the PREDIMED study. *Free Rad Biol Med*, 2009, 46, 1562-1566.

Zhang, Q; Tang, X; Oing, YL; Zhang, ZF; Brown, J; Le, AD. Resveratrol inhibits hypoxia-induced accumulation of hypoxia-inducible factor-1$\alpha$ and VEGF expression in human tongue squamous cell carcinoma and hepatoma cells. *Mol Cancer Ther*, 2005, 10, 1465-1474.

Zhao, X; Zhang, J-J; Wang, X; Bu, X-Y; Lou, Y-Q; Zhang, G-L. Effect of berbarine on hepatocyte proliferation, inducible nitric oxide synthase expression, cytochrome P450 2E1 and 1A2 activities in diethylnitrosamine- and phenobarbital-treated rats. *Biomed Pharmacother*, 2008, 62, 567-572.

Zhou, R; Fukui, M; Choi, HJ; Zhu, BT. Induction of a reversible, non-cytotoxic S-phase delay by resveratrol: implications for a mechanism of lifespan prolongation and cancer protection. *Br J Pharmacol*, 2009, 158, 462-474.

In: Liver Cancer: Causes, Diagnosis and Treatment
Editor: Benjamin J. Valverde

ISBN: 978-1-61209-115-0
© 2011 Nova Science Publishers, Inc.

*Chapter IV*

# Signaling Pathways in Hepatocellular Carcinoma

## *Edith Y. T. Tse and Judy W. P. Yam* [*]
Department of Pathology, Li Ka Shing Faculty of Medicine,
The University of Hong Kong, Hong Kong

## Abstract

Hepatocellular carcinoma (HCC) is a prevalent malignancy worldwide. It is often diagnosed at the advanced stage and the overall prognosis is unsatisfactory due to high rates of postoperative recurrence and metastasis. High incidence and severe casualty have led to the attention of the public health problem caused by HCC. HCC is developed from a multistep process which emerged through chronic hepatitis/cirrhosis and dysplastic nodules from normal liver. The genomic alterations and dysregulations of multiple intracellular signaling pathways reveal the heterogeneity and complexity of HCC. Profound evidence has demonstrated that cross-talks between different signaling pathways have made the pathogenesis of HCC even more intriguing. In this review, we provide a comprehensive overview on the salient signaling pathways in HCC, including growth factors regulated pathways and Rho-ROCK signaling cascad, zero in on the molecules along these pathways which are the key players in the initiation and progression of HCC. A better understanding of the molecular mechanisms of HCC would facilitate and advance the identification of prognostic markers, the improvement of therapeutic management and the development of novel therapies.

---

[*] Corresponding Author: Judy W.P. Yam, Department of Pathology, The University of Hong Kong, University Pathology Building, Queen Mary Hospital, Hong Kong. Tel: (852) 2255-4864; Fax: (852) 2218-5212; E-mail: judyyam@pathology.hku.hk.

# Introduction

HCC is the fifth most common cancer in the world and the third most common cause of cancer mortality. High incidence and severe casualty have led to the attention of major public health problem. HCC displayed interesting epidemiologic features including apparent variations among geographic regions, races, sex and presence of well documented environmental risk factors. Patients with associated cirrhosis caused by chronic hepatitis infection and long-term heavy alcohol consumption are at the greatest risk of developing HCC. Late presentation and high recurrence rate of HCC due to metastasis has led to poor prognosis of HCC. Surgical resection remains the main solution for resectable cases. However, most patients with advanced HCC are inoperable and chemotherapy has not been proven to be effective. Molecular targeted therapy may be envisioned as a potential treatment for liver malignancy. Therefore, intense research on elucidating the molecular complexity of HCC warrants further efforts to identify valid targets for more effective clinical management and development of new therapies for this highly aggressive disease.

# Growth factors/Receptors Regulated Pathways

## Granulin-epithelial Precursor (GEP)

GEP is an autocrine growth factor which evokes multifaceted biological processes and has been implicated in early embryogenesis (Qin *et al.*, 2005), tissue remodeling (He *et al.*, 2003), inflammation (Guo *et al.*, 2010), tumorigenesis (Ong and Bateman, 2003) and neurodegenerative diseases (Baker *et al.*, 2006). It is also named as progranulin, proepithelin, acrogranin and PC-derived growth factor. Although GEP is a secretory factor, it is also localized inside the cells. These intracellular GEP were suggested to act as transcriptional repressor that regulates functions of viral and cellular transcription factors (Hoque *et al.*, 2010; Hoque *et al.*, 2005).

Genome-wide expression profiling comparing mRNA expressions of paired HCCs and adjacent nontumorous liver tissues revealed GEP as one of the significantly upregulated genes in tumor tissues (Cheung *et al.*, 2004). In over hundred of tissues examined, GEP was upregulated in 72% of cases. The clinical relevance of GEP overexpression was further reflected by its significant association with large tumor size, venous infiltration and early recurrence after surgery. GEP expression was also correlated with the expression and mutation status of p53 in human cancers. In both HCC and breast cancers, statistical analysis revealed significant overall positive association between GEP and p53 expressions (Cheung *et al.*, 2006; Serrero and Ioffe, 2003). This tight association was only found in HCCs with wildtype p53 but not in HCCs with p53 mutations. Modulation of p53 expression by GEP was further demonstrated in HepG2 hepatoma cell line. Overexpression of GEP resulted in the enhancement of p53 protein level whereas suppression of GEP reduced p53 expression in cells (Cheung *et al.*, 2006). Apart from clinical analysis, functional assays showed that silencing of GEP in HCC cells reduced cell proliferation, invasion, anchorage-independent growth and *in vivo* tumorigenicity (Cheung *et al.*, 2004). These compelling studies suggest that GEP is a promising therapeutic target for HCC. More importantly, GEP is a secretory factor which makes it a good tumor marker for screening patient and monitoring treatment response. GEP monoclonal antibody (mAb) was generated and tested for its efficacy as a therapeutic agent (Ho *et al.*, 2008). It was shown that GEP mAb did not exert adverse effect on normal liver cells but inhibited hepatoma cells in culture. In an animal model implanted with human HCC, GEP mAb effectively decreased serum GEP level and hindered tumor development. GEP mAb was also shown to impede cell growth by suppressing p44/p42 MAPK and Akt pathways and inhibit tumor angiogenesis via the reduction of vascular endothelial growth factor (VEGF) level (Ho *et al.*, 2008). Other than p44/p42 MAPK and Akt pathways, GEP has been shown to induce chondrogenesis via ERK1/2 signaling (Feng *et al.*, 2010). In ovarian cancer cells, silencing of GEP reduced proliferation and invasion through downregulation of cyclin D and CDK4 and inactivation of matrix metalloproteinase (MMP)-2 (Liu *et al.*, 2007).

Involvement of GEP in chemoresistance has been revealed in ovarian cancer and HCC (Cheung *et al.*, In press; Pizarro *et al.*, 2007). Overexpression of GEP was associated with the chemoresistant phenotype of ovarian cancer cell lines. Ovarian cancer cell line with higher GEP expression showed higher resistance to cisplatin treatment (Pizarro *et al.*, 2007). Furthermore, in nude mice model with cisplatin chemotherapy, tumors derived from GEP transfectants progressively increased in size, whereas tumors derived from control transfectants stopped growing in response to cisplatin. Recent study showed that expressions of GEP and ATP-dependent binding cassette (ABC)B5 were tightly correlated, suggesting a role of GEP in chemoresistance (Cheung *et al.*, In press). Chemoresistant cells expressing GEP had higher level of ABCB5, while knockdown of ABCB5 resulted in enhanced doxorubicin uptake and increased apoptosis in cells. Cancer stem cells are naturally resistant to chemotherapeutic agents. CD133 positive HCC cancer stem cells confer chemoresistance via the activation of Akt survival pathway has been reported (Ma *et al.*, 2008). Indeed, analysis of GEP and ABCB5 coexpressing cells revealed expression of hepatic cancer stem cell markers such as CD133 and EpCAM (Cheung *et al.*, In press). In the physiological context, a significant correlation between GEP and ABCB5 expression levels were found in human HCC samples.

## Hepatocyte Growth Factor (HGF)/MET signaling

HGF (hepatocyte growth factor) is a well-recognized potent mitogen for hepatocytes (Lee et al., 1998; Nakamura et al., 1984). HGF binds to its specific cell surface tyrosine kinase receptor Met, which is encoded by the proto-oncogene c-met (Bottaro et al., 1991) (Figure 1). Upon HGF stimulation, Met undergoes autophoshorylation of tyrosine(Tyr) residues, $Tyr^{1234}$ and $Tyr^{1235}$, that resided in the tyrosine kinase domain of the receptor, followed by paraphosphorylation of adaptor proteins Gab-1 and Grb2, which generate phosphotyrosine docking sites for a variety of downstream effectors, such as PI3K, PLCγ, Crk adaptor protein, SHP-2 and Pak (Lai et al., 2009). The binding of HGF to Met elicits a series of cellular biological responses by triggering a spectrum of signal transduction pathways, including the Grb2-Ras-MAPK (mitogen-activated Protein kinase) cascade (Fournier et al., 1996), the PI3K pathway (Royal and Park, 1995)and the STAT (signal transducer and activator of transcription) pathway (Boccaccio et al., 1998). Under normal conditions, the HGF-Met axis contributes indispensably with other cytokines and growth factors to coordinate optimal cell proliferation, survival, morphogenesis and angiogenesis during embryonic development and wound healing. However, as in transformed cells, the signaling pathways kindled by HGF-Met orchestrate to switch on the invasive growth program, thereby promoting angiogenesis and metastasis in many cancers (Lesko and Majka, 2008; Ma et al., 2003). Extensive studies in various human cancers have characterized the roles of HGF-Met signaling in cancer cell invasion and metastasis as reviewed by Birchmeier *et al.* (Birchmeier et al., 2003).

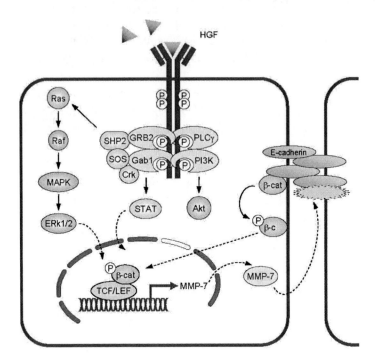

Figure 1. HGF/Met pathway in HCC. Upon HGF stimulation, Met undergoes autophoshorylation of tyrosineresidues in the kinase domain leading to the formation of docking sites for various downstream effectors. Activation of Met initiates a spectrum of signal transduction pathways, including the Grb2-Ras-MAPK, the PI3K/Akt and STAT pathways. Activated Met also stimulates phosphorylation of β-catenin. Phosphorylated β-catenin dissociates from E-cadherin and translocates into the nucleus where it binds with TCF/LEF transcription factor and activates the transcription of MMP-7. Secreted MMP-7 then cleaves E-cadherin and induces cell scattering.

In HCC, HGF and its receptor Met cooperate in a paracrine fashion; HGF is produced by stellate cells and myofibroblasts (Guirouilh et al., 2000; Guirouilh et al., 2001; Neaud et al., 1997), as well as Kupffer cells and sinusoidal endothelial cells (Matsumoto and Nakamura, 1992), while Met is expressed by hepatocytes. Higher HGF serum level in HCC patients was correlated with greater tumor size (Yamagamim et al., 2002), poorer survival (Vejchapipat et al., 2004) and more invasive, intrahepatic metastasis-positive tumors (Osada et al., 2008). The involvement of HGF in HCC angiogenesis has been demonstrated. HGF treatment upregulates VEGF expression in HCC cells via upregulation of the transcription factor Egr-1, which binds to VEGF promoter and initiate transcription of the gene (Lee and Kim, 2009). Ding *et al.* found that a population of HCC cells that have undergone epithelial-mesenchymal transition (EMT) was capable of HGF secretion, and these mesenchymal cells exhibited higher proliferative rate and a more motile and invasive phenotype as compared to their epithelial counterparts (Ding et al., 2010b). This compelling evidence suggested that HGF secreted by mesenchymal tumor cells might promote the proliferation and invasiveness of the epithelial tumor in a feed-forward mechanism. In general, Met is expressed in most HCC tissues (Kiss et al., 1997; Suzuki et al., 1994). Overexpression of Met in tumorous liver is associated with intrahepatic metastasis, vascular invasion and disease survival (Kaposi-Novak et al., 2006; Ueki et al., 1997), and is predominantly detected in tumors of poor differentiation (Daveau et al., 2003). Somatic mutations have been reported in childhood HCC (Park et al., 1999). Animal model showed that transgenic mice with Met overexpressing hepatocytes developed HCC readily (Wang *et al.*, 2001). Mechanistically, Met promotes hepatocytes survival by binding directly with the death receptor Fas, preventing Fas from ligand binding and self-aggregation, thus inhibiting its apoptotic effect (Wang et al., 2002). Recently, Pan *et al.* suggested the involvement of HGF/Met/β-catenin/MMP-7/E-cadherin signaling pathway in HCC metastasis. Activation of the HGF/Met axis in HCC cell initiated Wnt/β-catenin signaling, which subsequently downregulated E-cadherin and increased the production and secretion of MMP-7. The secreted MMP-7 then cleaved the ectodomain of E-cadherin, resulted in cell scattering, a morphological indication of the acquisition of motile phenotype and the initial step of metastasis (Pan et al., 2010)

## Insulin-like Growth Factor/IGF-1 Receptor (IGF/IGF-1R) Signaling

The IGF-1R signaling cascade is initiated upon the binding of IGF-1 and -2 to IGF-1R (Alexia et al., 2004). IGF-1R then undergoes autophosphorylation, which in turn phosphorylates insulin receptor substrate(IRS) 1-4, leading to the activation of downstream signaling pathways including the MAPK and the PI3K/Akt pathways (Figure 2). IGF-1R signaling modulates cell survival by controlling cell proliferation and apoptosis, its regulatory effects on cell motility and anchorage-independent growth have also been reported (Pollak et al., 2004). In HCC, the effect of IGF-2 transcends that of IGF-1 in deregulating the IGF-1R signaling. Dramatic upregulation of IGF-2 expression was found in cirrhotic liver, HCC tissues and cell lines as compared to non-tumorous liver (Cariani et al., 1988; Park et al., 1995; Sedlaczek et al., 2003; Su et al., 1994). Increased transcriptional activity of IGF-2 via preferential activation and hypomethylation of the P3 promoter was attributed to IGF-2 overexpression (Eriksson et al., 2001; Sohda et al., 1996). Excess bioavailability of IGF-2 enhanced the mitogenic effect of the IGF-R signaling. Suppression of IGF-2 production in HCC cells substantially inhibited cell growth and increased apoptosis (Lin et al., 1997; Lund et al., 2004). The positive regulatory effect of IGF-2 in *in vivo* hepatocarcinogenesis via an autocrine mechanism has also been demonstrated (Schirmacher et al., 1992). Under normal conditions, the expression of IGF-1R is tightly controlled by the gene products of tumor suppressor gene or negative growth regulators to be maintained at a very low level (Werner and Roberts, 2003). In HCC cells and tissues, upregulation of IGF-1R was observed (Scharf et al., 1998; Stefano et al., 2006). Increased IGF-1R transcriptional activity was found to be potentiated by p53mt249 (third base mutant of codon 249 in p53 gene) (Lee *et al.*, 2003) and HBx (Kim et al., 1996). Conversely, blockade of IGF-1R activity in HCC cells suppressed proliferation and induced apoptosis (Hopfner et al., 2006; Zhang et al., 2006). In HCC animal models, the pivotal role of the IGF-2/IGF-1R axis in HCC cell motility and invasiveness has been clearly demonstrated (Nussbaum et al., 2008), inhibition of either IGF-2 or IGF-1R suppressed *in vivo* metastasis but had no effect on tumor growth (Chen et al., 2009).

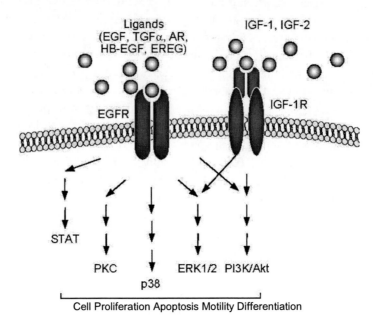

Figure 2. Growth factors regulated pathways in HCC.The IGF-1R signaling cascade is initiated upon the binding of IGF-1 and -2 to IGF-1R leading to the activation of the MAPK and the PI3K/Akt pathways.Binding of ligands (EGF, TGFα, AR, HB-EGF and EREG) to EGFR elicits a number of pathways including MAPK, p38, PKC, PI3K/Akt ans STAT pathways. These pathways are involved in cell survival, differentiation, motility and apoptosis.

## Epidermal Growth Factor Receptor (EGFR) Signaling

EGFR is a family of tyrosine kinases comprised of four members, EGFR (ErbB1), Her2 (ErbB2), ErbB3 and ErbB4. EGFRs and their ligands cooperate in an autocrine fashion. Upon ligand binding, numerous signaling pathways are initiated, including the MAPK cascade, the p38-MAPK cascade, the protein kinase C (PKC) pathway, the PI3K/Akt pathway and the STAT pathway. These pathways then activate transcriptions of a battery of genes that regulate cell-cycle progression, cell survival, differentiation and motility (Fabregat et al., 2007; Jorissen et al., 2003). Among the EGFR family, EGFR (ErbB1) has been most extensively evaluated. Ligands of EGFR include EGF, transforming growth factor α (TGFα), amphiregulin (AR), heparin-binding EGF (HB-EGF) and epiregulin (EREG). These ligands are tethered in the membrane and proteolytic cleavage induced by the a disintegrin and metalloprotase (ADAM) family is necessary for the activation of ligands(Ohtsu et al., 2006). The EGFR signaling is tightly coordinated and essential in liver regeneration after injury (Berasain et al., 2005; Kiso et al., 1995; Michalopoulos and DeFrances, 1997; Toyoda et al., 1995; Webber et al., 1993). EGFR and its ligands are expressed in normal hepatocytes, yet prolonged activation of the EGFR signaling pathway in liver with persistent damage and chronic inflammation is believed to equip the premalignant cells with growth advantage

(Drucker et al., 2006). In accordance with this idea, expressions of EGFR ligands were found upregulated in chronically injured and cirrhotic liver tissues (Berasain et al., 2005; Chung et al., 2000; Kiso et al., 1999). In HCC, overexpression of EGFR was correlated with higher proliferation rate, intrahepatic metastasis and tumor de-differentiation (Ito et al., 2001). EGFR ligands and ADAM17 expressions were as well elevated in HCC (Castillo et al., 2006; Chung et al., 2000; Ding et al., 2004; Inui et al., 1994; Moon et al., 2006). Upregulation of EGFR was observed in HCC cell lines, cell proliferation was enhanced upon treatment of the EGFR ligands (Castillo et al., 2006; Hisaka et al., 1999). Conversely, suppression of AR expression with RNAi inhibited cell proliferation and reduced the resistance to TGFβ and doxorubicin-induced apoptosis (Castillo et al., 2006). Perturbation of the signaling pathway using specific EGFR inhibitors suppressed cell growth, induced cell-cycle arrest and apoptosis (Ortiz et al., 2008). The involvement of EGFR signaling in *in vivo* hepatocarcinogenesis was demonstrated by the readiness of TGFα or EGF transgenic mice to develop HCC (Borlak et al., 2005; Webber et al., 1994). EGFR also mediates signal induced by the secretory protein epidermal growth factor-like domain 7 (Egfl7), which overexpression was observed in HCC and correlated with poor prognosis. A positive association of Egfl7 expression and metastatic potential was observed in HCC cell lines. Knockdown of Egfl7 impeded HCC cell motility and suppressed intrahepatic and pulmonary metastases. Egfl7 promoted cell migration via focal adhesion kinase(FAK) phosphorylation and this activation is EGFR-dependent (Wu et al., 2009). Mutations of EGFR have also been reported in various malignancies. EGFR variant type III, a ligand-independent and constitutively active mutant of EGFR which is expressed exclusively in cancerous but not normal tissues, was found overexpressed in HCC cases and correlated with disease progression and recurrence (Ou et al., 2005). Expression of this mutant in HCC promoted *in vitro* and *in vivo* cell growth, *in vitro* cell motility and the chemoresistance towards 5-fluorouracil treatment (Wang et al., 2009).

## Crosstalk between Different Growth Factor Signaling Pathways

The common downstream signaling molecules shared by different growth factor signaling pathways allow them to crosstalk and interact. It has been shown in various cancers that IGF-1R activation induced the secretion of EGFR ligands such as AR, TGFα and HB-EGF (Adams et al., 2004). Indeed in HCC cells, the mitogenic effect induced by IGF-2 involved the autocrine or paracrine activation of EGFR by AR (Desbois-Mouthon et al., 2006). Interestingly, Desbois-Mouthon *et al.* further demonstrated the combinatorial effect of IGF-1R and EGFR signaling on HCC cell proliferation. Treatment of anti-IGF-1R antibody, AVE1642, in combination with Gefitinib, an EGFR inhibitor, imposed dramatic additive growth inhibitory effect on HCC cells as compared to AVE1642 treatment alone. The augmented growth suppression was attributed to the inhibition of Akt phosphorylation. They further showed that treatment of AVE1642 alone upregulated the expression and activity of HER3, binding partner of EGFR, which explained the moderate growth inhibitory effect induced by AVE1642 alone. Co-treatment of Gefitinib suppressed the HER3 activation and therefore imposing a synergistic effect on growth suppression (Desbois-Mouthon et al., 2009). Crosstalk between HGF and EGFR modulates the mitogenic signal imposed on hepatocytes. On one hand, HGF induced TGFα production and imposed a secondary effect in augmenting the EGFR signaling. On the other hand, EGF and TGFα triggered Met phosphorylation by activating EGFR. Interestingly, suppression of EGFR activation by TGFα antibodies or antisense oligonucleotide substantially inhibited HGF-mediated proliferation, suggesting that EGFR signaling transcends that of Met (Scheving et al., 2002).

# Rho/ROCK Signaling Cascade

## Rho GTPases

Rho (*Ras homology*) family GTPases, belonging to the Ras superfamily, modulate various cellular events, including cell polarity, motility, differentiation, proliferation and apoptosis, which play critical role in tumor initiation and progression (Figure 3). Three Rho family members, Rho, Rac and Cdc42, have been well characterized and widely studied in human cancers. Rho GTPases cycle between the inactive GDP-bound and active GTP-bound states, this cycle is tightly regulated by guanine nucleotide exchange factors(GEFs), GTPases activating proteins(GAPs) and guanine nucleotide hydrolysis dissociation inhibitors(GDIs). GEFs catalyze the exchange of GDP to GTP thus activating the GTPase, while GAPs inactivate the GTPase by catalyzing the hydrolysis of GTP. GDIs maintain the GTPase inactive by restraining the dissociation of GTPase from GDP, as well as controlling the shuttle of GTPase between cytoplasm and plasma membrane. Active GTPases activate a wide variety of downstream effectors including protein kinases, phospholipases and scaffold proteins, which mediate the upstream GTPases activity to a diversity of signaling pathways(Heasman and Ridley, 2008). In the context of HCC, aberrant expressions and activations of the Rho GTPases, as well as the deregulations of their upstream regulators, GEFs, GAPS and GDIs, and downstream effectors such as ROCK and PAK1 have been extensively reported. We will highlight the alterations of these critical components and their subsequent functional implications in HCC.

### Rho Subfamily

Rho subfamily members, RhoA, RhoB and RhoC have entirely different cellular functions even though there is 85% homology in their amino acid sequences. RhoA regulates the actomyosin contractility and the formation of stress fiber; RhoB plays a role in membrane trafficking whereas RhoC is involved in cell adhesion and invasion. RhoA and RhoC are located in the cytoplasm and plasma membrane, while RhoB localizes on endosomes (Wheeler and Ridley, 2004). Elevated mRNA and protein expressions of RhoA (Fukui *et al.*, 2006; Iizuka *et al.*, 2006; Li *et al.*, 2006; Wang *et al.*, 2007) and RhoC (Chen et al., 2002; Wang et al., 2004) in HCC tissues as compared to the non-tumorous liver have been frequently reported and were associated with metastasis and poor prognosis. RhoA induces cell motility through its downstream effector ROCK (Riento and Ridley, 2003). Overexpression of RhoA was found to promote the *in vitro* and *in vivo* tumorigenesis and invasiveness of hepatoma (Itoh et al., 1999; Yoshioka et al., 1999) and HCC cells (Xue et al., 2008b), playing a central role in tumor initiation and progression. Activation of RhoA by EIF5A2 (eukaryotic initiation factor 5A2) has recently been shown (Tang et al., 2010), resulting in rearrangement of cytoskeleton and induction of EMT, a critical event in invasion and metastasis. RhoC, on the other hand, has been shown in mammary adenocarcinoma to be involved in metastasis but not required for tumor initiation (Hakem et al., 2005). RhoC regulates HCC invasiveness and metastasis by modulating the expression of MMP-2 and MMP-9 (Xue et al., 2008a). In contrary to the other Rho family members, RhoB was found to function as a tumor suppressor (Liu et al., 2001) and its expression is often downregulated in HCC (Chen et al., 2002; Delpuech et al., 2002). A recent study showed that upon expression of microRNA(miR)-21, which directly targeted the 3'UTR of RhoB and suppressed its expression, the motility and invasiveness of HCC cells were enhanced, clearly demonstrating the negative regulatory role of RhoB in HCC aggressiveness (Connolly et al., 2010).

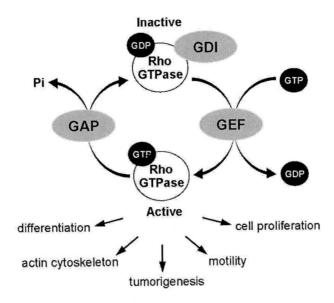

Figure 3. Regulation of Rho GTPases. Rho GTPases exist as inactive GDP-bound and active GTP-bound states. The molecular switches of Rho GTPases are tightly regulated by guanine nucleotide exchange factor (GEF), GTPases activating protein (GAP) and guanine nucleotide hydrolysis dissociation inhibitor (GDI). GEFs catalyze the exchange of GDP to GTP thus activating the GTPase, while GAPs inactivate the GTPase by catalyzing the hydrolysis of GTP. GDIs maintain the GTPase inactive by restraining the dissociation of GTPase from GDP, as well as controlling the shuttle of GTPase between cytoplasm and plasma membrane. Active GTPases regulate a diversity of signaling pathways.

## *Rac Subfamily*

Rac subfamily members Rac1, Rac2, Rac3 and RhoG, play important role in cell migration via the formation of lamellipodia and focal adhesion complexes. Rac1 has been most frequently studied in HCC; its expression was found to be upregulated and correlated with poor prognosis (Liu et al., 2008; Yang et al., 2010). Higher Rac1 expression and activity were found in metastatic HCC cells as compared to the non-metastatic cells (Lee *et al.*, 2005; Liu *et al.*, 2008). The positive regulatory role of Rac1 on HCC cell motility and metastasis has been demonstrated in *in vitro* and *in vivo* models (Liu et al., 2008). Like RhoA, Rac1 was activated by EIF5A2 and promoted EMT process (Tang et al., 2010). Interestingly, Rac1 can also be activated by the hepatitis B virus(HBV) viral protein HBx. HBx interacted directly with the Rac1 nucleotide exchange factor by binding to the SH3 motif (Tan et al., 2008). Furthermore, nuclear localization of Rac1 was correlated with the expression of VEGF and associated with an increase of metastatic potential in HCC. Notably, expression of constitutively active Rac1 upregulated hypoxia-inducible factor-1α and provoked the secretion of VEGF, which further suggested the potential role of Rac1 in promoting HCC angiogenesis under hypoxia (Lee *et al.*, 2006).

### Cdc42 Subfamily

Cdc42 subfamily is consisted of Cdc42, RhoJ, RhoQ, RhoU and RhoV. Cdc42 regulates cell polarity and migration through the formation of filopodia. In Cdc42-deficient mice, hepatomegaly and signs of liver transformation were developed after birth; HCC was eventually developed followed by lung metastases (van Hengel et al., 2008). These results implied Cdc42 as a suppressor to hepatocarcinogenesis. Yet the expression of Cdc42 in human liver tissues suggested otherwise. Overexpression of Cdc42 was observed in HBV- (Chang et al., 2007) and HCV- (Cooper et al., 2007) related HCC. Moreover, recent study showed that activation of Cdc42 encouraged HCC cell motility, invasiveness and metastasis by inducing filopodia formation and EMT (Chen et al., 2010). Cdc42 appears to be a complex player in HCC as compared to the other GTPases in the Rho and Rac subfamilies, further investigations are required to elucidate the functional role of Cdc42.

## Regulators of Rho GTPases

### Guanine Nucleotide Exchange Factors(GEFs)

GEFs catalyze the exchange of GDP to GTP, leading to the activation of GTPases. Despite its significant role in GTPases activation, studies concerning the functional involvement of GEFs in HCC are scarce. Chen *et al.* recently found a dramatic overexpression of ARHGEF9, which encodes a GEF for Cdc42, in metastatic HCC tissues. ARHGEF9, regulated by chromodomain helicase/ATPase DNA binding protein 1-like gene (CHD1L), promoted cell migration, invasion and metastasis by activating Cdc42. Suppression of ARHGEF9 expression by RNAi abolished the *in vivo* invasiveness and metastasis of HCC cells, confirming the significance of GEF in regulating HCC cell aggressiveness (Chen et al., 2010).

### GTPases Activating Proteins(GAPs)

GAPs inactivate Rho by catalyzing the hydrolysis of GTP, thus the conversion of active GTP-bound Rho GTPase to the inactive GDP-bound state. The involvement of GAPs in HCC is best exemplified by deleted in liver cancer 1 (DLC-1). DLC-1 was first identified in primary HCC as a rat p122RhoGAP homolog. The gene is located on chromosome 8p21.3-22, a region that is frequently deleted in HCC (Yuan et al., 1998). Genomic deletion and epigenetic silencing of DLC-1 in HCC have been reported as frequent events (Ng et al., 2000; Wong et al., 2003). DLC-1 exerts its GAP activity on RhoA and to a lesser extent to Cdc42 (Healy et al., 2008; Wong et al., 2003). The inhibitory effects on HCC cell proliferation, motility and invasiveness of DLC-1 have been demonstrated in a number of studies using DLC-1 overexpressing approach (Kim et al., 2007; Wong et al., 2005; Zhou et al., 2004). The tumor suppressive role of DLC-1 was elegantly demonstrated by a knockdown approach using a "mosaic" mouse model. Knockdown of DLC-1 in p53-/- liver progenitors cells dramatically promoted tumor formation, whereas ectopic expression of DLC-1 in Ras expressing cells substantially reduced the growth of tumor(Xue et al., 2008b). Vast evidences have confirmed DLC-1 as a *bona fide*tumor suppressor in HCC, however the underlying mechanisms remain elusive by the time. Active research has been carried out to mechanistically address the tumor suppressive functions of DLC-1. In this perspective, several lines of evidences have shown that the tumor suppressive effect of DLC-1 was attributed to its RhoGAP activity. DLC-1 antagonizes RhoA and the downstream effectors in HCC, affecting the rearrangement of actin cytoskeleton and therefore the formations of stress fibers and focal adhesions (Kim et al., 2007; Wong et al., 2008; Xue et al., 2008b; Zhou et al., 2008). Localization of DLC-1 also determines its tumor suppressive functions (Figure 4). DLC-1 interacted with numerous tensin family members and localized to focal adhesions. Mutations of focal adhesion targeting residues S440 and Y442 of DLC-1 precluded the protein from localizing to focal adhesion and resulted in the loss of its tumor suppressive functions (Chan et al., 2009; Liao et al., 2007; Qian et al., 2007; Yam et al., 2006). Besides, DLC1 also utilizes 375-385 residues to interact with tensin2 phosphotyrosine binding (PTB) domain (Chan *et al.*, 2009). Interestingly, DLC1 has been reported to shuttle between cytoplasm and nucleus where it acts as an apoptosis inducer (Yuan *et al.*, 2007). Other than cellular localization, post-translational modification of DLC-1 is crucial to its functions as well. Ko *et al.* pinpointed a serine residue S567 of DLC-1 to be phosphorylated by Akt, most importantly, S567 phosphorylation is required for DLC-1 to function as a tumor suppressor in HCC (Ko et al., 2010). A homolog of DLC-1, DLC-2, was identified as a tumor suppressor gene. DLC-2 gene located on chromosome 13q12.3, a region that is frequently deleted in HCC as well. The expression pattern and functions of DLC-2 are similar to that of DLC-1. DLC-2 is underexpressed in HCC and possesses RhoGAP activity to RhoA and Cdc42, expression of DLC-2 was found to suppress HCC cell proliferation and motility (Ching et al., 2003; Leung et al., 2005).

## *Guanine Nucleotide Hydrolysis Dissociation Inhibitors(GDIs)*

Three GDIs have been identified, RhoGDIα, RhoGDIβ and RhoGDIγ, which are specifically expressed in different organs. GDIs modulate Rho GTPase signaling via three mechanisms. Firstly, GDIs hamper the dissociation of GDP from Rho GTPase, thus maintaining Rho inactive. Secondly, GDIs can inhibit both the intrinsic and GAP-catalyzed GTP hydrolysis of GTP-bound GTPase, thereby precluding the interaction of active Rho GTPase with the downstream effectors. Thirdly, GDIs regulate the shuttling of Rho GTPases between cytosol and membranes. By forming high-affinity complexes with GDIs, Rho GTPases remain as soluble cytosolic proteins and cannot interact with the membrane-associated GEFs (DerMardirossian and Bokoch, 2005). The role of GDIs in HCC remains largely unidentified. Expression profiling revealed a downregulation of RhoGDIβ in HBV and HCV positive HCC (Blanc et al., 2005; Li et al., 2005), an association with HCC tissues that harbor β-catenin activating mutations was observed (Boyault et al., 2007). Recent study has demonstrated the regulation of RhoGDI by miRNA. Ding *et al.* found that miR-151, a miRNA frequently amplified in HCC, targeted RhoGDIα directly and suppressed its expression, which consequently resulted in the activation of Rho GTPases and enhanced the *in vitro* and *in vivo* motility and invasiveness of HCC cells (Ding et al., 2010a).

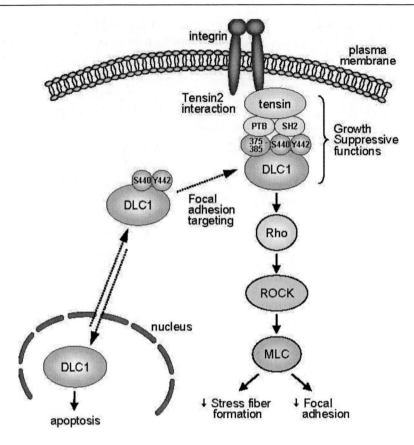

Figure 4. Subcellular localization of DLC1 determines its biological functions. Y442 and S440 residues are critical for the focal adhesion localization of DLC1. At the focal adhesions, DLC1 interacted with tensin2 through SH2 and PTB binding domains, utilizing different binding sites. A stretch of residues 375-385 interacts with PTB domain of tensin2 while Y442 and S440A residues bind SH2 domain of tensin2. The formation of this binding complex is important for DLC1 to exert growth suppressive function. DLC1 also shuttles between cytoplasm and nucleus continuously. DLC1 localized in nucleus was reported to induce apoptosis.

## Effectors of Rho GTPases

### *Rho-Kinase (ROCK)*

ROCK, ROCK1 and ROCK 2, is a family of protein serine/threonine kinases that are activated upon binding to Rho and function as a downstream effector (Leung et al., 1996). ROCK1 and ROCK2 are functionally redundant on actomyosin bundle assembly, ablation of either gene yielded similar effect on cell motility (Thumkeo et al., 2005). ROCK phosphorylates downstream target MLC (myosin light chain) and induces the actin-myosin-mediated contractile force, therefore making ROCK a key regulator on cell motility and adhesion (Riento and Ridley, 2003). The implication of the Rho/ROCK pathway in HCC has been demonstrated by various studies. In rat hepatoma cells MM1, activation of the Rho/ROCK pathway is essential for the motility and invasiveness, whereas perturbation of the Rho/ROCK pathway by ROCK inhibitor Y27632 substantially suppressed tumor invasion (Itoh et al., 1999). Treatment of ROCK inhibitor could also effectively prevent post-liver transplantation tumor recurrence in a rat hepatoma model (Ogawa et al., 2007). Expression of dominant negative ROCK1 in a highly metastatic HCC cell line Li7 could suppress the *in vitro* cell motility and *in vivo* metastatic ability significantly (Genda et al., 1999). Introduction of the Rho GAP protein DLC-1 also exerted a negative regulatory effect on the Rho/ROCK/MLC2 pathway (Wong et al., 2008). The role of ROCK2 in HCC has also been addressed. ROCK2 was found overexpressed in primary HCC and associated with tumor microsatellite formation. Functional studies further revealed the positive regulatory role of ROCK2 in HCC motility and invasiveness (Wong et al., 2009).

### P21-Activated Protein Kinase (PAK)

PAK is a family of protein serine/threonine kinases functioning as the downstream effectors of Rac and Cdc42. Three major isoforms of PAKs, namely PAK1, PAK2 and PAK3, have been implicated in cytoskeletal regulation, cell motility, cell cycle progression and growth signaling (Bokoch, 2003). Overexpression of PAK1 was reported in HCC and was associated with metastatic features (Chen et al., 2002; Ching et al., 2007). The positive regulation of PAK1 on HCC cell motility was demonstrated, furthermore, activation of c-Jun NH2-terminal kinase(JNK) and the subsequent phosphorylation of paxillin were observed in PAK1 induced HCC cell motility, suggesting the involvement of the Rac/PAK/JNK/paxillin pathway in HCC metastasis (Ching et al., 2007).

# Conclusion

Hepatocarcinogenesis is a complex process thatinvolves diverse molecular perturbations, which orchestrate to deregulate theprincipal signaling pathways in HCC. Accumulating evidences have highlighted the crucial involvement of the growth factors regulated pathways and Rho-ROCK signaling cascade in HCC. Besides, cross-talks among these pathways have further complicated their roles and integrated signal transduction in HCC. In this review, we particularly summarize the basic molecular studies and clinical association of the key players along these pathways in HCC. More intensive understanding of these pathways is awaited for the betterment of clinical treatment of HCC.

# Acknowledgments

Financial support: This work was supported by the Hong Kong Research Grants Council (HKU7798/07M, HKU7833/10M), The University of Hong Kong Seed Funding Programme for Basic Research and Outstanding Young Researcher Award (to J.W.P. Yam).

# References

Adams TE, McKern NM, Ward CW (2004). Signalling by the type 1 insulin-like growth factor receptor: interplay with the epidermal growth factor receptor. *Growth Factors* 22: 89-95.

Alexia C, Fallot G, Lasfer M, Schweizer-Groyer G, Groyer A (2004). An evaluation of the role of insulin-like growth factors (IGF) and of type-I IGF receptor signalling in hepatocarcinogenesis and in the resistance of hepatocarcinoma cells against drug-induced apoptosis. *Biochem Pharmacol* 68: 1003-15.

Baker M, Mackenzie IR, Pickering-Brown SM, Gass J, Rademakers R, Lindholm C *et al* (2006). Mutations in progranulin cause tau-negative frontotemporal dementia linked to chromosome 17. *Nature* 442: 916-9.

Berasain C, Garcia-Trevijano ER, Castillo J, Erroba E, Lee DC, Prieto J *et al* (2005). Amphiregulin: an early trigger of liver regeneration in mice. *Gastroenterology* 128: 424-32.

Birchmeier C, Birchmeier W, Gherardi E, Vande Woude GF (2003). Met, metastasis, motility and more. *Nat Rev Mol Cell Biol* 4: 915-25.

Blanc JF, Lalanne C, Plomion C, Schmitter JM, Bathany K, Gion JM *et al* (2005). Proteomic analysis of differentially expressed proteins in hepatocellular carcinoma developed in patients with chronic viral hepatitis C. *Proteomics* 5: 3778-89.

Boccaccio C, Ando M, Tamagnone L, Bardelli A, Michieli P, Battistini C *et al* (1998). Induction of epithelial tubules by growth factor HGF depends on the STAT pathway. *Nature* 391: 285-8.

Bokoch GM (2003). Biology of the p21-activated kinases. *Annu Rev Biochem* 72: 743-81.

Borlak J, Meier T, Halter R, Spanel R, Spanel-Borowski K (2005). Epidermal growth factor-induced hepatocellular carcinoma: gene expression profiles in precursor lesions, early stage and solitary tumours. *Oncogene* 24: 1809-19.

Bottaro DP, Rubin JS, Faletto DL, Chan AM, Kmiecik TE, Vande Woude GF *et al* (1991). Identification of the hepatocyte growth factor receptor as the c-met proto-oncogene product. *Science* 251: 802-4.

Boyault S, Rickman DS, de Reynies A, Balabaud C, Rebouissou S, Jeannot E *et al* (2007). Transcriptome classification of HCC is related to gene alterations and to new therapeutic targets. *Hepatology* 45: 42-52.

Cariani E, Lasserre C, Seurin D, Hamelin B, Kemeny F, Franco D *et al* (1988). Differential expression of insulin-like growth factor II mRNA in human primary liver cancers, benign liver tumors, and liver cirrhosis. *Cancer Res* 48: 6844-9.

Castillo J, Erroba E, Perugorria MJ, Santamaria M, Lee DC, Prieto J *et al* (2006). Amphiregulin contributes to the transformed phenotype of human hepatocellular carcinoma cells. *Cancer Res* 66: 6129-38.

Chan LK, Ko FC, Ng IO, Yam JW (2009). Deleted in liver cancer 1 (DLC1) utilizes a novel binding site for Tensin2 PTB domain interaction and is required for tumor-suppressive function. *PLoS One* 4: e5572.

Chang CS, Huang SM, Lin HH, Wu CC, Wang CJ (2007). Different expression of apoptotic proteins between HBV-infected and non-HBV-infected hepatocellular carcinoma. *Hepatogastroenterology* 54: 2061-8.

Chen L, Chan TH, Yuan YF, Hu L, Huang J, Ma S *et al* (2010). CHD1L promotes hepatocellular carcinoma progression and metastasis in mice and is associated with these processes in human patients. *J Clin Invest* 120: 1178-91.

Chen X, Cheung ST, So S, Fan ST, Barry C, Higgins J *et al* (2002). Gene expression patterns in human liver cancers. *Mol Biol Cell* 13: 1929-39.

Chen YW, Boyartchuk V, Lewis BC (2009). Differential roles of insulin-like growth factor receptor- and insulin receptor-mediated signaling in the phenotypes of hepatocellular carcinoma cells. *Neoplasia* 11: 835-45.

Cheung ST, Cheung PF, Cheng CK, Wong NC, Fan ST (In press). Granulin-epithelin precursor and ATP-dependent binding cassette (ABC)B5 regulate liver cancer cell chemoresistance. *Gastroenterology.*

Cheung ST, Wong SY, Lee YT, Fan ST (2006). GEP associates with wild-type p53 in hepatocellular carcinoma. *Oncol Rep* 15: 1507-11.

Cheung ST, Wong SY, Leung KL, Chen X, So S, Ng IO *et al* (2004). Granulin-epithelin precursor overexpression promotes growth and invasion of hepatocellular carcinoma. *Clin Cancer Res* 10: 7629-36.

Ching YP, Leong VY, Lee MF, Xu HT, Jin DY, Ng IO (2007). P21-activated protein kinase is overexpressed in hepatocellular carcinoma and enhances cancer metastasis involving c-Jun NH2-terminal kinase activation and paxillin phosphorylation. *Cancer Res* 67: 3601-8.

Ching YP, Wong CM, Chan SF, Leung TH, Ng DC, Jin DY *et al* (2003). Deleted in liver cancer (DLC) 2 encodes a RhoGAP protein with growth suppressor function and is underexpressed in hepatocellular carcinoma. *J Biol Chem* 278: 10824-30.

Chung YH, Kim JA, Song BC, Lee GC, Koh MS, Lee YS *et al* (2000). Expression of transforming growth factor-alpha mRNA in livers of patients with chronic viral hepatitis and hepatocellular carcinoma. *Cancer* 89: 977-82.

Connolly EC, Van Doorslaer K, Rogler LE, Rogler CE (2010). Overexpression of miR-21 promotes an in vitro metastatic phenotype by targeting the tumor suppressor RHOB. *Mol Cancer Res* 8: 691-700.

Cooper AB, Wu J, Lu D, Maluccio MA (2007). Is autotaxin (ENPP2) the link between hepatitis C and hepatocellular cancer? *J Gastrointest Surg* 11: 1628-34; discussion 1634-5.

Daveau M, Scotte M, Francois A, Coulouarn C, Ros G, Tallet Y *et al* (2003). Hepatocyte growth factor, transforming growth factor alpha, and their receptors as combined markers of prognosis in hepatocellular carcinoma. *Mol Carcinog* 36: 130-41.

Delpuech O, Trabut JB, Carnot F, Feuillard J, Brechot C, Kremsdorf D (2002). Identification, using cDNA macroarray analysis, of distinct gene expression profiles associated with pathological and virological features of hepatocellular carcinoma. *Oncogene* 21: 2926-37.

DerMardirossian C, Bokoch GM (2005). GDIs: central regulatory molecules in Rho GTPase activation. *Trends Cell Biol* 15: 356-63.

Desbois-Mouthon C, Baron A, Blivet-Van Eggelpoel MJ, Fartoux L, Venot C, Bladt F *et al* (2009). Insulin-like growth factor-1 receptor inhibition induces a resistance mechanism via the epidermal growth factor receptor/HER3/AKT signaling pathway: rational basis for cotargeting insulin-like growth factor-1 receptor and epidermal growth factor receptor in hepatocellular carcinoma. *Clin Cancer Res* 15: 5445-56.

Desbois-Mouthon C, Cacheux W, Blivet-Van Eggelpoel MJ, Barbu V, Fartoux L, Poupon R et al (2006). Impact of IGF-1R/EGFR cross-talks on hepatoma cell sensitivity to gefitinib. *Int J Cancer* 119: 2557-66.

Ding J, Huang S, Wu S, Zhao Y, Liang L, Yan M et al (2010a). Gain of miR-151 on chromosome 8q24.3 facilitates tumour cell migration and spreading through downregulating RhoGDIA. *Nat Cell Biol* 12: 390-9.

Ding W, You H, Dang H, Leblanc F, Galicia V, Lu SC et al (2010b). Epithelial-to-mesenchymal transition of murine liver tumor cells promotes invasion. *Hepatology*.

Ding X, Yang LY, Huang GW, Wang W, Lu WQ (2004). ADAM17 mRNA expression and pathological features of hepatocellular carcinoma. *World J Gastroenterol* 10: 2735-9.

Drucker C, Parzefall W, Teufelhofer O, Grusch M, Ellinger A, Schulte-Hermann R et al (2006). Non-parenchymal liver cells support the growth advantage in the first stages of hepatocarcinogenesis. *Carcinogenesis* 27: 152-61.

Eriksson T, Frisk T, Gray SG, von Schweinitz D, Pietsch T, Larsson C et al (2001). Methylation changes in the human IGF2 p3 promoter parallel IGF2 expression in the primary tumor, established cell line, and xenograft of a human hepatoblastoma. *Exp Cell Res* 270: 88-95.

Fabregat I, Roncero C, Fernandez M (2007). Survival and apoptosis: a dysregulated balance in liver cancer. *Liver Int* 27: 155-62.

Feng JQ, Guo FJ, Jiang BC, Zhang Y, Frenkel S, Wang DW et al (2010). Granulin epithelin precursor: a bone morphogenic protein 2-inducible growth factor that activates Erk1/2 signaling and JunB transcription factor in chondrogenesis. *FASEB J* 24: 1879-92.

Fournier TM, Kamikura D, Teng K, Park M (1996). Branching tubulogenesis but not scatter of madin-darby canine kidney cells requires a functional Grb2 binding site in the Met receptor tyrosine kinase. *J Biol Chem* 271: 22211-7.

Fukui K, Tamura S, Wada A, Kamada Y, Sawai Y, Imanaka K et al (2006). Expression and prognostic role of RhoA GTPases in hepatocellular carcinoma. *J Cancer Res Clin Oncol* 132: 627-33.

Genda T, Sakamoto M, Ichida T, Asakura H, Kojiro M, Narumiya S et al (1999). Cell motility mediated by rho and Rho-associated protein kinase plays a critical role in intrahepatic metastasis of human hepatocellular carcinoma. *Hepatology* 30: 1027-36.

Guirouilh J, Castroviejo M, Balabaud C, Desmouliere A, Rosenbaum J (2000). Hepato-carcinoma cells stimulate hepatocyte growth factor secretion in human liver myofibroblasts. *Int J Oncol* 17: 777-81.

Guirouilh J, Le Bail B, Boussarie L, Balabaud C, Bioulac-Sage P, Desmouliere A et al (2001). Expression of hepatocyte growth factor in human hepatocellular carcinoma. *J Hepatol* 34: 78-83.

Guo F, Lai Y, Tian Q, Lin EA, Kong L, Liu C (2010). Granulin-epithelin precursor binds directly to ADAMTS-7 and ADAMTS-12 and inhibits their degradation of cartilage oligomeric matrix protein. *Arthritis Rheum* 62: 2023-36.

Hakem A, Sanchez-Sweatman O, You-Ten A, Duncan G, Wakeham A, Khokha R et al (2005). RhoC is dispensable for embryogenesis and tumor initiation but essential for metastasis. *Genes Dev* 19: 1974-9.

He Z, Ong CH, Halper J, Bateman A (2003). Progranulin is a mediator of the wound response. *Nat Med* 9: 225-9.

Healy KD, Hodgson L, Kim TY, Shutes A, Maddileti S, Juliano RL *et al* (2008). DLC-1 suppresses non-small cell lung cancer growth and invasion by RhoGAP-dependent and independent mechanisms. *Mol Carcinog* 47: 326-37.

Heasman SJ, Ridley AJ (2008). Mammalian Rho GTPases: new insights into their functions from in vivo studies. *Nat Rev Mol Cell Biol* 9: 690-701.

Hisaka T, Yano H, Haramaki M, Utsunomiya I, Kojiro M (1999). Expressions of epidermal growth factor family and its receptor in hepatocellular carcinoma cell lines: relationship to cell proliferation. *Int J Oncol* 14: 453-60.

Ho JC, Ip YC, Cheung ST, Lee YT, Chan KF, Wong SY *et al* (2008). Granulin-epithelin precursor as a therapeutic target for hepatocellular carcinoma. *Hepatology* 47: 1524-32.

Hopfner M, Huether A, Sutter AP, Baradari V, Schuppan D, Scherubl H (2006). Blockade of IGF-1 receptor tyrosine kinase has antineoplastic effects in hepatocellular carcinoma cells. *Biochem Pharmacol* 71: 1435-48.

Hoque M, Mathews MB, Pe'ery T (2010). Progranulin (granulin/epithelin precursor) and its constituent granulin repeats repress transcription from cellular promoters. *J Cell Physiol* 223: 224-33.

Hoque M, Tian B, Mathews MB, Pe'ery T (2005). Granulin and granulin repeats interact with the Tat.P-TEFb complex and inhibit Tat transactivation. *J Biol Chem* 280: 13648-57.

Iizuka N, Tsunedomi R, Tamesa T, Okada T, Sakamoto K, Hamaguchi T *et al* (2006). Involvement of c-myc-regulated genes in hepatocellular carcinoma related to genotype-C hepatitis B virus. *J Cancer Res Clin Oncol* 132: 473-81.

Inui Y, Higashiyama S, Kawata S, Tamura S, Miyagawa J, Taniguchi N *et al* (1994). Expression of heparin-binding epidermal growth factor in human hepatocellular carcinoma. *Gastroenterology* 107: 1799-804.

Ito Y, Takeda T, Sakon M, Tsujimoto M, Higashiyama S, Noda K *et al* (2001). Expression and clinical significance of erb-B receptor family in hepatocellular carcinoma. *Br J Cancer* 84: 1377-83.

Itoh K, Yoshioka K, Akedo H, Uehata M, Ishizaki T, Narumiya S (1999). An essential part for Rho-associated kinase in the transcellular invasion of tumor cells. *Nat Med* 5: 221-5.

Jorissen RN, Walker F, Pouliot N, Garrett TP, Ward CW, Burgess AW (2003). Epidermal growth factor receptor: mechanisms of activation and signalling. *Exp Cell Res* 284: 31-53.

Kaposi-Novak P, Lee JS, Gomez-Quiroz L, Coulouarn C, Factor VM, Thorgeirsson SS (2006). Met-regulated expression signature defines a subset of human hepatocellular carcinomas with poor prognosis and aggressive phenotype. *J Clin Invest* 116: 1582-95.

Kim SO, Park JG, Lee YI (1996). Increased expression of the insulin-like growth factor I (IGF-I) receptor gene in hepatocellular carcinoma cell lines: implications of IGF-I receptor gene activation by hepatitis B virus X gene product. *Cancer Res* 56: 3831-6.

Kim TY, Lee JW, Kim HP, Jong HS, Jung M, Bang YJ (2007). DLC-1, a GTPase-activating protein for Rho, is associated with cell proliferation, morphology, and migration in human hepatocellular carcinoma. *Biochem Biophys Res Commun* 355: 72-7.

Kiso S, Kawata S, Tamura S, Higashiyama S, Ito N, Tsushima H *et al* (1995). Role of heparin-binding epidermal growth factor-like growth factor as a hepatotrophic factor in rat liver regeneration after partial hepatectomy. *Hepatology* 22: 1584-90.

Kiso S, Kawata S, Tamura S, Miyagawa J, Ito N, Tsushima H *et al* (1999). Expression of heparin-binding epidermal growth factor-like growth factor in the hepatocytes of fibrotic rat liver during hepatocarcinogenesis. *J Gastroenterol Hepatol* 14: 1203-9.

Kiss A, Wang NJ, Xie JP, Thorgeirsson SS (1997). Analysis of transforming growth factor (TGF)-alpha/epidermal growth factor receptor, hepatocyte growth Factor/c-met,TGF-beta receptor type II, and p53 expression in human hepatocellular carcinomas. *Clin Cancer Res* 3: 1059-66.

Ko FC, Chan LK, Tung EK, Lowe SW, Ng IO, Yam JW (2010). Akt Phosphorylation of Deleted in Liver Cancer 1 Abrogates Its Suppression of Liver Cancer Tumorigenesis and Metastasis. *Gastroenterology*.

Lai AZ, Abella JV, Park M (2009). Crosstalk in Met receptor oncogenesis. *Trends Cell Biol* 19: 542-51.

Lee HS, Huang AM, Huang GT, Yang PM, Chen PJ, Sheu JC *et al* (1998). Hepatocyte growth factor stimulates the growth and activates mitogen-activated protein kinase in human hepatoma cells. *J Biomed Sci* 5: 180-4.

Lee KH, Kim JR (2009). Hepatocyte growth factor induced up-regulations of VEGF through Egr-1 in hepatocellular carcinoma cells. *Clin Exp Metastasis* 26: 685-92.

Lee TK, Man K, Ho JW, Wang XH, Poon RT, Sun CK *et al* (2005). Significance of the Rac signaling pathway in HCC cell motility: implications for a new therapeutic target. *Carcinogenesis* 26: 681-7.

Lee TK, Poon RT, Yuen AP, Man K, Yang ZF, Guan XY *et al* (2006). Rac activation is associated with hepatocellular carcinoma metastasis by up-regulation of vascular endothelial growth factor expression. *Clin Cancer Res* 12: 5082-9.

Lee YI, Han YJ, Lee SY, Park SK, Park YJ, Moon HB *et al* (2003). Activation of insulin-like growth factor II signaling by mutant type p53: physiological implications for potentiation of IGF-II signaling by p53 mutant 249. *Mol Cell Endocrinol* 203: 51-63.

Lesko E, Majka M (2008). The biological role of HGF-MET axis in tumor growth and development of metastasis. *Front Biosci* 13: 1271-80.

Leung T, Chen XQ, Manser E, Lim L (1996). The p160 RhoA-binding kinase ROK alpha is a member of a kinase family and is involved in the reorganization of the cytoskeleton. *Mol Cell Biol* 16: 5313-27.

Leung TH, Ching YP, Yam JW, Wong CM, Yau TO, Jin DY *et al* (2005). Deleted in liver cancer 2 (DLC2) suppresses cell transformation by means of inhibition of RhoA activity. *Proc Natl Acad Sci U S A* 102: 15207-12.

Li C, Tan YX, Zhou H, Ding SJ, Li SJ, Ma DJ *et al* (2005). Proteomic analysis of hepatitis B virus-associated hepatocellular carcinoma: Identification of potential tumor markers. *Proteomics* 5: 1125-39.

Li XR, Ji F, Ouyang J, Wu W, Qian LY, Yang KY (2006). Overexpression of RhoA is associated with poor prognosis in hepatocellular carcinoma. *Eur J Surg Oncol* 32: 1130-4.

Liao YC, Si L, deVere White RW, Lo SH (2007). The phosphotyrosine-independent interaction of DLC-1 and the SH2 domain of cten regulates focal adhesion localization and growth suppression activity of DLC-1. *J Cell Biol* 176: 43-9.

Lin SB, Hsieh SH, Hsu HL, Lai MY, Kan LS, Au LC (1997). Antisense oligodeoxy-nucleotides of IGF-II selectively inhibit growth of human hepatoma cells overproducing IGF-II. *J Biochem* 122: 717-22.

Liu AX, Rane N, Liu JP, Prendergast GC (2001). RhoB is dispensable for mouse development, but it modifies susceptibility to tumor formation as well as cell adhesion and growth factor signaling in transformed cells. *Mol Cell Biol* 21: 6906-12.

Liu S, Yu M, He Y, Xiao L, Wang F, Song C *et al* (2008). Melittin prevents liver cancer cell metastasis through inhibition of the Rac1-dependent pathway. *Hepatology* 47: 1964-73.

Liu Y, Xi L, Liao G, Wang W, Tian X, Wang B *et al* (2007). Inhibition of PC cell-derived growth factor (PCDGF)/granulin-epithelin precursor (GEP) decreased cell proliferation and invasion through downregulation of cyclin D and CDK4 and inactivation of MMP-2. *BMC Cancer* 7: 22.

Lund P, Schubert D, Niketeghad F, Schirmacher P (2004). Autocrine inhibition of chemotherapy response in human liver tumor cells by insulin-like growth factor-II. *Cancer Lett* 206: 85-96.

Ma PC, Maulik G, Christensen J, Salgia R (2003). c-Met: structure, functions and potential for therapeutic inhibition. *Cancer Metastasis Rev* 22: 309-25.

Ma S, Lee TK, Zheng BJ, Chan KW, Guan XY (2008). CD133+ HCC cancer stem cells confer chemoresistance by preferential expression of the Akt/PKB survival pathway. *Oncogene* 27: 1749-58.

Matsumoto K, Nakamura T (1992). Hepatocyte growth factor: molecular structure, roles in liver regeneration, and other biological functions. *Crit Rev Oncog* 3: 27-54.

Michalopoulos GK, DeFrances MC (1997). Liver regeneration. *Science* 276: 60-6.

Moon WS, Park HS, Yu KH, Park MY, Kim KR, Jang KY *et al* (2006). Expression of betacellulin and epidermal growth factor receptor in hepatocellular carcinoma: implications for angiogenesis. *Hum Pathol* 37: 1324-32.

Nakamura T, Nawa K, Ichihara A (1984). Partial purification and characterization of hepatocyte growth factor from serum of hepatectomized rats. *Biochem Biophys Res Commun* 122: 1450-9.

Neaud V, Faouzi S, Guirouilh J, Le Bail B, Balabaud C, Bioulac-Sage P *et al* (1997). Human hepatic myofibroblasts increase invasiveness of hepatocellular carcinoma cells: evidence for a role of hepatocyte growth factor. *Hepatology* 26: 1458-66.

Ng IO, Liang ZD, Cao L, Lee TK (2000). DLC-1 is deleted in primary hepatocellular carcinoma and exerts inhibitory effects on the proliferation of hepatoma cell lines with deleted DLC-1. *Cancer Res* 60: 6581-4.

Nussbaum T, Samarin J, Ehemann V, Bissinger M, Ryschich E, Khamidjanov A *et al* (2008). Autocrine insulin-like growth factor-II stimulation of tumor cell migration is a progression step in human hepatocarcinogenesis. *Hepatology* 48: 146-56.

Ogawa T, Tashiro H, Miyata Y, Ushitora Y, Fudaba Y, Kobayashi T *et al* (2007). Rho-associated kinase inhibitor reduces tumor recurrence after liver transplantation in a rat hepatoma model. *Am J Transplant* 7: 347-55.

Ohtsu H, Dempsey PJ, Eguchi S (2006). ADAMs as mediators of EGF receptor transactivation by G protein-coupled receptors. *Am J Physiol Cell Physiol* 291: C1-10.

Ong CH, Bateman A (2003). Progranulin (granulin-epithelin precursor, PC-cell derived growth factor, acrogranin) in proliferation and tumorigenesis. *Histol Histopathol* 18: 1275-88.

Ortiz C, Caja L, Sancho P, Bertran E, Fabregat I (2008). Inhibition of the EGF receptor blocks autocrine growth and increases the cytotoxic effects of doxorubicin in rat hepatoma cells: role of reactive oxygen species production and glutathione depletion. *Biochem Pharmacol* 75: 1935-45.

Osada S, Kanematsu M, Imai H, Goshima S (2008). Clinical significance of serum HGF and c-Met expression in tumor tissue for evaluation of properties and treatment of hepatocellular carcinoma. *Hepatogastroenterology* 55: 544-9.

Ou C, Wu FX, Luo Y, Cao J, Zhao YN, Yuan WP *et al* (2005). [Expression and significance of epidermal growth factor receptor variant type III in hepatocellular carcinoma]. *Ai Zheng* 24: 166-9.

Pan FY, Zhang SZ, Xu N, Meng FL, Zhang HX, Xue B *et al* (2010). beta-catenin signaling involves HGF-enhanced HepG2 scattering through activating MMP-7 transcription. *Histochem Cell Biol*.

Park BC, Huh MH, Seo JH (1995). Differential expression of transforming growth factor alpha and insulin-like growth factor II in chronic active hepatitis B, cirrhosis and hepatocellular carcinoma. *J Hepatol* 22: 286-94.

Park WS, Dong SM, Kim SY, Na EY, Shin MS, Pi JH *et al* (1999). Somatic mutations in the kinase domain of the Met/hepatocyte growth factor receptor gene in childhood hepatocellular carcinomas. *Cancer Res* 59: 307-10.

Pizarro GO, Zhou XC, Koch A, Gharib M, Raval S, Bible K *et al* (2007). Prosurvival function of the granulin-epithelin precursor is important in tumor progression and chemoresponse. *Int J Cancer* 120: 2339-43.

Pollak MN, Schernhammer ES, Hankinson SE (2004). Insulin-like growth factors and neoplasia. *Nat Rev Cancer* 4: 505-18.

Qian X, Li G, Asmussen HK, Asnaghi L, Vass WC, Braverman R *et al* (2007). Oncogenic inhibition by a deleted in liver cancer gene requires cooperation between tensin binding and Rho-specific GTPase-activating protein activities. *Proc Natl Acad Sci U S A* 104: 9012-7.

Qin J, Diaz-Cueto L, Schwarze JE, Takahashi Y, Imai M, Isuzugawa K *et al* (2005). Effects of progranulin on blastocyst hatching and subsequent adhesion and outgrowth in the mouse. *Biol Reprod* 73: 434-42.

Riento K, Ridley AJ (2003). Rocks: multifunctional kinases in cell behaviour. *Nat Rev Mol Cell Biol* 4: 446-56.

Royal I, Park M (1995). Hepatocyte growth factor-induced scatter of Madin-Darby canine kidney cells requires phosphatidylinositol 3-kinase. *J Biol Chem* 270: 27780-7.

Scharf JG, Schmidt-Sandte W, Pahernik SA, Ramadori G, Braulke T, Hartmann H (1998). Characterization of the insulin-like growth factor axis in a human hepatoma cell line (PLC). *Carcinogenesis* 19: 2121-8.

Scheving LA, Stevenson MC, Taylormoore JM, Traxler P, Russell WE (2002). Integral role of the EGF receptor in HGF-mediated hepatocyte proliferation. *Biochem Biophys Res Commun* 290: 197-203.

Schirmacher P, Held WA, Yang D, Chisari FV, Rustum Y, Rogler CE (1992). Reactivation of insulin-like growth factor II during hepatocarcinogenesis in transgenic mice suggests a role in malignant growth. *Cancer Res* 52: 2549-56.

Sedlaczek N, Hasilik A, Neuhaus P, Schuppan D, Herbst H (2003). Focal overexpression of insulin-like growth factor 2 by hepatocytes and cholangiocytes in viral liver cirrhosis. *Br J Cancer* 88: 733-9.

Serrero G, Ioffe OB (2003). Expression of PC-cell-derived growth factor in benign and malignant human breast epithelium. *Hum Pathol* 34: 1148-54.

Sohda T, Yun K, Iwata K, Soejima H, Okumura M (1996). Increased expression of insulin-like growth factor 2 in hepatocellular carcinoma is primarily regulated at the transcriptional level. *Lab Invest* 75: 307-11.

Stefano JT, Correa-Giannella ML, Ribeiro CM, Alves VA, Massarollo PC, Machado MC *et al* (2006). Increased hepatic expression of insulin-like growth factor-I receptor in chronic hepatitis C. *World J Gastroenterol* 12: 3821-8.

Su Q, Liu YF, Zhang JF, Zhang SX, Li DF, Yang JJ (1994). Expression of insulin-like growth factor II in hepatitis B, cirrhosis and hepatocellular carcinoma: its relationship with hepatitis B virus antigen expression. *Hepatology* 20: 788-99.

Suzuki K, Hayashi N, Yamada Y, Yoshihara H, Miyamoto Y, Ito Y *et al* (1994). Expression of the c-met protooncogene in human hepatocellular carcinoma. *Hepatology* 20: 1231-6.

Tan TL, Fang N, Neo TL, Singh P, Zhang J, Zhou R *et al* (2008). Rac1 GTPase is activated by hepatitis B virus replication--involvement of HBX. *Biochim Biophys Acta* 1783: 360-74.

Tang DJ, Dong SS, Ma NF, Xie D, Chen L, Fu L *et al* (2010). Overexpression of eukaryotic initiation factor 5A2 enhances cell motility and promotes tumor metastasis in hepatocellular carcinoma. *Hepatology* 51: 1255-63.

Thumkeo D, Shimizu Y, Sakamoto S, Yamada S, Narumiya S (2005). ROCK-I and ROCK-II cooperatively regulate closure of eyelid and ventral body wall in mouse embryo. *Genes Cells* 10: 825-34.

Toyoda H, Komurasaki T, Uchida D, Takayama Y, Isobe T, Okuyama T *et al* (1995). Epiregulin. A novel epidermal growth factor with mitogenic activity for rat primary hepatocytes. *J Biol Chem* 270: 7495-500.

Ueki T, Fujimoto J, Suzuki T, Yamamoto H, Okamoto E (1997). Expression of hepatocyte growth factor and its receptor, the c-met proto-oncogene, in hepatocellular carcinoma. *Hepatology* 25: 619-23.

van Hengel J, D'Hooge P, Hooghe B, Wu X, Libbrecht L, De Vos R *et al* (2008). Continuous cell injury promotes hepatic tumorigenesis in cdc42-deficient mouse liver. *Gastroenterology* 134: 781-92.

Vejchapipat P, Tangkijvanich P, Theamboonlers A, Chongsrisawat V, Chittmittrapap S, Poovorawan Y (2004). Association between serum hepatocyte growth factor and survival in untreated hepatocellular carcinoma. *J Gastroenterol* 39: 1182-8.

Wang D, Dou K, Xiang H, Song Z, Zhao Q, Chen Y *et al* (2007). Involvement of RhoA in progression of human hepatocellular carcinoma. *J Gastroenterol Hepatol* 22: 1916-20.

Wang H, Jiang H, Zhou M, Xu Z, Liu S, Shi B *et al* (2009). Epidermal growth factor receptor vIII enhances tumorigenicity and resistance to 5-fluorouracil in human hepatocellular carcinoma. *Cancer Lett* 279: 30-8.

Wang R, Ferrell LD, Faouzi S, Maher JJ, Bishop JM (2001). Activation of the Met receptor by cell attachment induces and sustains hepatocellular carcinomas in transgenic mice. *J Cell Biol* 153: 1023-34.

Wang W, Yang LY, Huang GW, Lu WQ, Yang ZL, Yang JQ *et al* (2004). Genomic analysis reveals RhoC as a potential marker in hepatocellular carcinoma with poor prognosis. *Br J Cancer* 90: 2349-55.

Wang X, DeFrances MC, Dai Y, Pediaditakis P, Johnson C, Bell A *et al* (2002). A mechanism of cell survival: sequestration of Fas by the HGF receptor Met. *Mol Cell* 9: 411-21.

Webber EM, FitzGerald MJ, Brown PI, Bartlett MH, Fausto N (1993). Transforming growth factor-alpha expression during liver regeneration after partial hepatectomy and toxic injury, and potential interactions between transforming growth factor-alpha and hepatocyte growth factor. *Hepatology* 18: 1422-31.

Webber EM, Wu JC, Wang L, Merlino G, Fausto N (1994). Overexpression of transforming growth factor-alpha causes liver enlargement and increased hepatocyte proliferation in transgenic mice. *Am J Pathol* 145: 398-408.

Werner H, Roberts CT, Jr. (2003). The IGFI receptor gene: a molecular target for disrupted transcription factors. *Genes Chromosomes Cancer* 36: 113-20.

Wheeler AP, Ridley AJ (2004). Why three Rho proteins? RhoA, RhoB, RhoC, and cell motility. *Exp Cell Res* 301: 43-9.

Wong CC, Wong CM, Ko FC, Chan LK, Ching YP, Yam JW *et al* (2008). Deleted in liver cancer 1 (DLC1) negatively regulates Rho/ROCK/MLC pathway in hepatocellular carcinoma. *PLoS One* 3: e2779.

Wong CC, Wong CM, Tung EK, Man K, Ng IO (2009). Rho-kinase 2 is frequently overexpressed in hepatocellular carcinoma and involved in tumor invasion. *Hepatology* 49: 1583-94.

Wong CM, Lee JM, Ching YP, Jin DY, Ng IO (2003). Genetic and epigenetic alterations of DLC-1 gene in hepatocellular carcinoma. *Cancer Res* 63: 7646-51.

Wong CM, Yam JW, Ching YP, Yau TO, Leung TH, Jin DY *et al* (2005). Rho GTPase-activating protein deleted in liver cancer suppresses cell proliferation and invasion in hepatocellular carcinoma. *Cancer Res* 65: 8861-8.

Wu F, Yang LY, Li YF, Ou DP, Chen DP, Fan C (2009). Novel role for epidermal growth factor-like domain 7 in metastasis of human hepatocellular carcinoma. *Hepatology* 50: 1839-50.

Xue F, Takahara T, Yata Y, Xia Q, Nonome K, Shinno E *et al* (2008a). Blockade of Rho/Rho-associated coiled coil-forming kinase signaling can prevent progression of hepatocellular carcinoma in matrix metalloproteinase-dependent manner. *Hepatol Res* 38: 810-817.

Xue W, Krasnitz A, Lucito R, Sordella R, Vanaelst L, Cordon-Cardo C *et al* (2008b). DLC1 is a chromosome 8p tumor suppressor whose loss promotes hepatocellular carcinoma. *Genes Dev* 22: 1439-44.

Yam JW, Ko FC, Chan CY, Jin DY, Ng IO (2006). Interaction of deleted in liver cancer 1 with tensin2 in caveolae and implications in tumor suppression. *Cancer Res* 66: 8367-72.

Yamagamim H, Moriyama M, Matsumura H, Aoki H, Shimizu T, Saito T *et al* (2002). Serum concentrations of human hepatocyte growth factor is a useful indicator for predicting the occurrence of hepatocellular carcinomas in C-viral chronic liver diseases. *Cancer* 95: 824-34.

Yang W, Lv S, Liu X, Liu H, Hu F (2010). Up-regulation of Tiam1 and Rac1 Correlates with Poor Prognosis in Hepatocellular Carcinoma. *Jpn J Clin Oncol*.

Yoshioka K, Nakamori S, Itoh K (1999). Overexpression of small GTP-binding protein RhoA promotes invasion of tumor cells. *Cancer Res* 59: 2004-10.

Yuan BZ, Jefferson AM, Millecchia L, Popescu NC, Reynolds SH (2007). Morphological changes and nuclear translocation of DLC1 tumor suppressor protein precede apoptosis in human non-small cell lung carcinoma cells. *Exp Cell Res* 313: 3868-80.

Yuan BZ, Miller MJ, Keck CL, Zimonjic DB, Thorgeirsson SS, Popescu NC (1998). Cloning, characterization, and chromosomal localization of a gene frequently deleted in human liver cancer (DLC-1) homologous to rat RhoGAP. *Cancer Res* 58: 2196-9.

Zhang YC, Wang XP, Zhang LY, Song AL, Kou ZM, Li XS (2006). Effect of blocking IGF-I receptor on growth of human hepatocellular carcinoma cells. *World J Gastroenterol* 12: 3977-82.

Zhou X, Thorgeirsson SS, Popescu NC (2004). Restoration of DLC-1 gene expression induces apoptosis and inhibits both cell growth and tumorigenicity in human hepatocellular carcinoma cells. *Oncogene* 23: 1308-13.

Zhou X, Zimonjic DB, Park SW, Yang XY, Durkin ME, Popescu NC (2008). DLC1 suppresses distant dissemination of human hepatocellular carcinoma cells in nude mice through reduction of RhoA GTPase activity, actin cytoskeletal disruption and down-regulation of genes involved in metastasis. *Int J Oncol* 32: 1285-91.

In: Liver Cancer: Causes, Diagnosis and Treatment
Editor: Benjamin J. Valverde

ISBN: 978-1-61209-115-0
© 2011 Nova Science Publishers, Inc.

*Chapter V*

# Health-related Quality of Life in Patients with Liver Cancer

### *Sheng-Yu Fan*
Department of Psychology, University of Sheffield, UK

## Abstract

Liver cancer is one of most common cancers in the world and is associated with considerable impact on not only physical but also psychosocial functioning. Health-related quality of life (HRQOL) is increasingly seen to be an important endpoint in health care. The aims of this chapter are to consider issues in the definition and measurement of HRQOL, as applied specifically to patients with liver cancer. HRQOL in patients with liver cancer can be considered both from a generic viewpoint in comparison with the general population, and in terms of disease-specific issues. In this regard, pain, fatigue, nausea, jaundice, weight loss, and body image need to be considered. Current research suggests that patients with liver cancer have substantially compromised HRQOL compared with the healthy population, both in physical and psychological dimensions. Suggestions are made for improving assessment of HRQOL in this population, and the timing and evaluation of programs to improve HRQOL over the course of treatment.

## Introduction

Liver cancer is the sixth most common cancer worldwide in terms of numbers of cases (626,000 or 5.7% of new cancer cases), and the third most common cause of death from cancer (598,000) due to the poor prognosis [1]. The largest concentrations of patients occur in Asia and sub-Saharan Africa [2-3]. There are risks of long-term developmental progression from hepatitis, cirrhosis to liver caner. There are various treatments including surgery, local ablative therapy, hepatic artery transcatheter treatment, and systemic treatment [4-5]. The five-year survival rate in patients who can receive surgery is 60-70%, and the prognosis for those who receive non-surgical treatment is relatively lower [6-7]. As survival rates improve, health-related quality of life (HRQOL) has become of increasing importance for patients with liver cancer.

# Health-related Quality of Life

It is important to consider not only the survival of cancer patients but also their well-being [8]. Liver cancer causes not only uncomfortable symptoms but also has implications for patients' psychosocial functioning. Quality of life has been used interchangeably with a number of different terms, such as health status, well-being, life satisfaction, and happiness [9]. HRQOL is a specific term which combines the concepts of health and quality of life.

Health has been defined not only as the absence of disease or infirmity but also a state of complete physical, mental and social well-being [10]. HRQOL is a reflection of the way that individuals perceive and react to their health status and nonmedical aspects of their lives, which include (i) health-related factors, such as physical, functional, emotional, and mental well-being; (ii) non-health-related elements, such as job, family, friends, and other life circumstances [11].

There are several characteristics of HRQOL. First, it broadens our understanding beyond the focus on disease or symptoms to include function and ability to take part in everyday work and social life [12]. It also encompasses feelings of mental and physical well-being, physical fitness, adjustment and efficiency of mind and body [13]. Second, HRQOL is a multi-dimensional concept, including an individual's physical health, psychological state, level of independence, social relationships, and their relationships to salient features of their environment [14]. Third, it is a dynamic concept representing individual responses to the physical, mental, and social effects of illness which influence the extent to which personal satisfaction with life circumstances can be achieved [15]. In short, HRQOL is an integrative index that encompasses consequences for the daily lives of individuals, including health perceptions, functional status, symptoms, and individuals' preferences and values [16].

HRQOL covers all aspects of health and performance status, and consequently it is more informative than medical indices such as survival rate, modality rate, or functional index [17]. HRQOL measures can be an important endpoint in health care and clinical trials, for example evaluating the effects of interventions [18] and making decisions about optimal treatments [19]. HRQOL includes both subjective and objective components, where objective functioning is important in defining an individual's degree of health or ability, and individual's subjective perceptions translate the objective functioning into the HRQOL experienced [20].

The assessment of HRQOL can be made using *generic* or *disease-specific* measures. Generic instruments include heath profiles and utility measures, which contain the dimensions of physical, emotional, social functioning, as well as global perceptions of health and well-being [21]. The advantage of generic measures are that they allow comparison with a healthy population, in order to understand the overall impact of disease. A disease specific measure focuses on the special area of primary interest, where the instrument may be specific to the disease (e.g. cancer or heart disease), to a population of patients (e.g. children or elderly), to a certain function (e.g. sleeping or eating), or to a problem (e.g. pain) [22]. It can detect the detailed changes or impairments caused by the specific disease.

# Measurements of Health-related Quality of Life in Patients with Liver Cancer

There are widely used international generic HRQOL measures that have been used to assessed the HRQOL in patients with liver cancer [23], including the Short-Form 36 (SF-36) [24-25], World Health Organization Quality of Life assessment (WHOQOL) [26], the Functional Assessment of Cancer Therapy-Generic (FACT-G) [27], European Organization for Research and Treatment for Cancer Quality of Life Questionnaire Core-30 (EORTC-QLQ-C30) [28].

For disease-specific measures, the FACT group developed the Functional Assessment of Cancer Therapy- Hepatobiliary (FACT-Hep) for patients with hepatobiliary cancer, such as metastatic colorectal cancer, hepatocellular carcinoma (HCC), pancreatic cancer, and cancers of the gallbladder and bile duct [29]; whereas the EORTC group developed the European Organization for Research and Treatment of Cancer (EORTC) QLQ-HCC18 for patients with HCC [30]. In addition, the FACT Hepatobiliary Symptom Index (FHSI) is a simplified index which was extracted from FACT-Hep for clinical screening [31]. The disease specific items of three measurements are presented in Table 1.

It is recommended that generic measures need supplementation with disease-specific measures to address positive and negative clinically important changes [22]. A standard measurement instrument with well-established psychometric characteristics and disease specificity is necessary to assess HRQOL in patients with liver cancer. The generic measure includes physical, psychological, and social components of life. Meanwhile, a cancer-specific instrument is necessary to combine a core questionnaire for use in a particular cancer with a module questionnaire which assesses specific issues in cancer patient subgroups [32]. The EORTC QLQ-HCC18 and the FACT-Hep have to accompany the EORTC QLQ-30, FACT-G respectively to measure HRQOL in patients with liver cancer. According to the liver cancer specific questionnaires, the disease-specific concerns include pain, fatigue, nausea, jaundice, weight loss, and body image.

# HRQOL in Patients with Liver Cancer: A Systematic Review

For the purposes of this article, we updated our recent systematic review that combined liver cancer and HRQOL relevant keywords, to understand the HRQOL in patients with liver cancer [23]. Literature searches form February 2009 till July 2010 revealed one additional study that met the inclusion criteria [33]. The aims were broadly similar to the original review: to determine the differences in HRQOL between patients with liver cancer and a healthy population, the effects of treatment on HRQOL, the relationships between physical variables and HRQOL, the relationships between psychological variables and HRQOL, in addition we extend the aims to include studies that addressed the effects of psychological interventions.

**Table 1. Liver cancer specific measures of HRQOL and symptoms assessed**

| Tool | EORTC QLQ-HCC18 (number of items: 18) | FACT-Hep (number of items: 18) | FHSI (number of items: 8) |
|---|---|---|---|
| Item | Shoulder pain | Back pain | Pain |
| | Abdomen pain | Discomfort or pain in stomach | Discomfort or pain in stomach |
| | Worry weight too light | Losing weight | |
| | Feel full just beginning eating | Digest food well | Pain in back |
| | Fever | Diarrhea | Losing weight |
| | Worry eyes and skin becoming yellow | Fever | Fatigue |
| | | Fatigue | Lack of energy |
| | Thirsty | Bothered by jaundice or yellow skin | Jaundice or yellow color to skin |
| | Abdominal swelling | | |
| | Worry figure of abdomen | Dry Mouth | Nausea |
| | Vitality is not like anticipate | Swelling or cramps in my stomach | |
| | Difficulty finishing things | Unhappy about change in appearance | |
| | Feel itch | | |
| | Trouble tasting | Able to do my usual activities | |
| | Feel cold | Itching | |
| | Lost the muscle in arms or legs | Change in food tastes | |
| | Worry nutrition | Chills | |
| | Need to sleep in daytime | Control of bowels | |
| | Influences on sexual life | Bothered by constipation | |
| | | Good appetite | |

**Table 2. The original and pooled mean (SD) of FACT-G subscale**

| | n | PWB | EWB | FWB | SFWB | Overall |
|---|---|---|---|---|---|---|
| Pooled | 978 | 21.73 (5.94) | 16.13 (4.73) | 16.92 (6.23) | 19.61 (5.16) | 74.02 (14.90) |
| Norm[a] (GP) | 1075 | 22.70 (5.40) | 19.90 (4.80) | 18.50 (6.80) | 19.10 (6.80) | 80.10 (18.10) |
| Norm[a] (cancer) | 2236 | 21.30 (6.00) | 18.70 (4.50) | 18.90 (6.80) | 22.10 (5.30) | 80.90 (17.00) |

PWB: Physical well-being; EWB: Emotional well-being; FWB: Functional well-being; SFWB: Social/family well-being; Overall: HRQOL (PWB+EWB+FWB+SFWB); GP: General population. a: data from Brucker, Yost, Cashy, Webster, & Cella, 2005 (43).

## The Difference in HRQOL between Patients with Liver Cancer and Healthy Population

We found the FACT-G was the most widely used instrument to measure HRQOL in patients with liver cancer [23]. We therefore pooled together the results of 11 studies which used FACT-G [29, 33-42], and compared the results with the norms for healthy populations and patients with other cancers [43]. Patients with HCC had worse physical well-being (t=-

3.86, p<.001), emotional well-being (t=-17.91, p<.001), functional well-being (t=-5.49, p<.001), and overall HRQOL (t=-8.29, p<.001) than norms for the general population. In addition, patients with HCC had worse emotional well-being (t=-14.38, p<.001), functional well-being (t=-8.06, p<.001), social/family well-being (t=-12.48, p<.001), and overall HRQOL (t=-11.44, p<.001) than patients with other cancers (see Table 2).

## The Effects of Treatment on HRQOL

Following hepatic resection, HRQOL declined during 2-10 weeks after the liver operation, but increased to preoperative level at 3-4 months, and was higher than the preoperative level at 9 months [36, 44]. Significant improvement was found in physical well-being [36]. Following transcatheter arterial embolization (TAE) or transcatheter arterial chemoembolization (TACE) treatment, HRQOL in patients who received TAE or TACE was lower at 3 months than pre-treatment [39, 41], and was higher at 6 months than at 3 months, but did not return to baseline [39]. Patients treated with 90-Yttrium microspheres had better HRQOL than patients who received Cisplatin through hepatic arterial infusion [37]. In addition, patients treated with radiofrequency ablation (RFA) or TACE-RFA had better HRQOL than those treated with only TACE [42].

## The Relationships between Physical Variables and HRQOL

There were significant positive correlations between liver function and HRQOL. Patients with better Child-Pugh classification [35, 38, 42], higher albumin [45-46], lower serum bilirubin [45], and lower serum cholinesterase [47] had better HRQOL. Severe symptoms were negatively associated with patients' HRQOL [33], including pain [35, 41, 44, 46, 48], sleep disorder [49], fatigue [41, 46], nausea [46], and sexual problem [50]. In addition, patients with worse performance status [46], advanced stage [51] or tumour recurrence [42, 44, 47] had worse HRQOL.

## The Relationships between Psychological Variables and HRQOL

HRQOL was negatively correlated with depression [33, 46, 48], uncertainty [35], and chance health locus of control [52]; and was positively correlated with satisfaction with medical services [53]. Patients who reported uncertainty about disease, treatment, and the future, and felt controlled by chance had worse HRQOL.

## The Effects of Psychological Interventions

Three studies used randomized control trial designs to investigate the effects of psychological interventions on HRQOL, including education, cognitive behavioural therapy, emotional support, and relaxation [54-56]. In all cases, the results revealed the positive benefits for patients with liver cancer.

As shown in previous studies [23, 57-58], our work supports findings that patients with liver cancer have worse HRQOL in terms of physical condition, emotional status, and functional ability. They have worse HRQOL than patients with chronic liver disease, especially in physical aspects. Physical well-being may be impaired due to severe symptoms or treatment side effects, especially pain, loss of appetite, difficulties digesting, and fatigue. In addition, liver cancer also causes great impact on patients' psychological well-being.

Liver operation, hepatic artery transcatheter treatment, and radiation therapy can improve patients' HRQOL. However, the recovery rate varies depending on patients' physical condition and treatment. Various factors may influence the change pattern. The recovery rate of patients treated by resection is better than those treated by TAE/TACE. The HRQOL in patients treated by resection improves over that before treatment, but the HRQOL in patients treated with TAE/TACE does not return back to the baseline level. A potential explanation is that patients who receive resection are at an earlier stage and have better liver function. Liver function is another significant factor associated with HRQOL.

Meanwhile, increasing severity of liver disease based on the Child-Pugh classification is strongly correlated with decreased physical component of HRQOL [59]. Patients with less severe symptoms have better HRQOL. The large-size tumour may compress the adjacent stomach, the gross ascite may cause a feeling of abdominal swelling, hepatic dysfunction may reduce appetite, and the multiple symptoms may lead to poor tolerance to intervention [60].

Liver cancer has a great impact on physical health and psychological well-being, even the stigma of death, and patients' normal life trajectory is challenged. Psychosocial variables also play an important role in determining HRQOL. HRQOL is negatively correlated with depression, uncertainty, chance health locus of control; and positively correlated with satisfaction with medical services. In addition, psychosocial interventions may reduce negative feelings and enhance HRQOL. However, these studies incorporated multiple components of interventions and the sample sizes were small, it is necessary to focus on the specific intervention and extend sample size.

# Future Studies and Application

In clinical practice, routine screening of HRQOL could enhance the quality of care, by allowing detection of how the disease and treatment affect HRQOL and the effects of interventions. Future work is needed to facilitate understanding of the determinants of physical and psychosocial factors on HRQOL in patients with liver cancer. First HRQOL can be a good indicator of the effects of treatment, and it is important to investigate any changes in HRQOL after a specific treatment. Second is the influence of physical variables on HRQOL. Patients with different stages, liver functions, and symptoms may have various levels of HRQOL. Studies can focus on whether patients with different liver functions but under the same treatment may have different HRQOL, as well as the predictors of HRQOL when patients received a specific treatment. The evaluation of treatment effects on patients' HRQOL need to include controls to account for disease stages, liver function, and recurrence. Third is the effect of psychological variables on HRQOL and the interaction between physical variables and psychological variables. Physical variables alone can not explain the change of HRQOL, but psychological variables also play important roles in formulating patients' HRQOL. Therefore, future studies must focus on the interaction between physical and psychological variables, as well as whether psychological interventions can improve HRQOL in patients with liver cancer and the effective components of interventions.

# Conclusion

In summary, the assessment of HRQOL in patients with liver cancer must include generic and disease-specific measures. The generic measure includes physical, psychological, and social dimensions; and the disease-specific items include pain, fatigue, nausea, jaundice, weight loss, and body image. Liver cancer has a negative impact on patients' HRQOL, mainly on physical, emotional, and functional well-being. Medical variables, such as disease stage, treatment, liver function, and symptoms play an important role in determining HRQOL. Psychological variables, such as depression, uncertainty, and locus of control also are related to HRQOL and may influence patients' interpretation of HRQOL. Because of relatively high incidence of HCC, and improving survival rates, more attention is needed to evaluate the HRQOL of these patients. Future studies would benefit from a theoretical framework to understand the effects of physical and psychological factors and the impact on HRQOL.

# References

[1]     Parkin, D.M., Bray, F., Ferlay, J., Pisani, P. *Global cancer statistics*, 2002. CA Cancer J Clin 2005;55:74-108.

[2]     El-Serag, H.B. Hepatocellular carcinoma: an epidemiologic view. *J Clin Gastroenterol* 2002;35(5 Suppl 2):S72-78.

[3]     McGlynn, K.A., Tsao, L., Hsing, A.W., Devesa, S.S., Fraumeni, J.F.J. International trends and patterns of primary liver cancer. *Int J Cancer* 2001; 94:290-296.

[4]     Bruix, J., Sherman, M. Management of hepatocellular carcinoma. *Hepatology* 2005; 42:1208-36.

[5]     Lau, WY. Primary liver tumors. *Semin Surg Oncol* 2000;19:135-144.

[6]     Cance, W.G., Stewart ,A.K., Menck, H.R. The National Cancer Data Base Report on treatment patterns for hepatocellular carcinomas: improved survival of surgically resected patients, 1985-1996. *Cancer* 2000; 88:912-920.

[7]     Llovet, J.M. Updated treatment approach to hepatocellular carcinoma. *J Gastroenterol* 2005; 40:225-235.

[8]     de Haes, J.C., van Knippenberg, F.C. The quality of life of cancer patients: a review of the literature. *Soc Sci Med* 1985; 20:809-817.

[9]     Bergner, M. Quality of life, health status, and clinical research. *Med Care* 1989;27(3 Suppl):S148-156.

[10]   WHO. Preamble to the Constitution of the World Health Organization as adopted by the International Health Conference 1948; New York.

[11] Gill, T.M., Feinstein, A.R. A critical appraisal of the quality of quality-of-life measurements. *JAMA* 1994;272:619-626.

[12] Seedhouse, D. *Health: the foundations of achievement.* Chichester: John Wiley; 1986.

[13] Bowling, A. Health-related quality of life: conceptual meaning, use and measurement. In: Bowling A, editor. *Measuring disease: a review of disease-specific quality of life measurement scale.* 2 ed. Buckingham: Open university press; 2001. p. 1-22.

[14] Sajid, M.S., Tonsi, A., Baig, M.K. Health-related quality of life measurement. *Int J Health Care Qual Assur* 2008;.21:365-373.

[15] Holmes, S, Dickerson, J. The quality of life: design and evaluation of a self-assessment instrument for use with cancer patients. *Int J Nurs Stud* 1987;.24:15-24.

[16] Clancy, C.M., Eisenberg, J.M. Outcomes research: measuring the end results of health care. *Science* 1998;.282:245-246.

[17] Bonnetain, F., Paoletti, X., Collette, S., Doffoel, M., Bouche, O., Raoul, J.L., Rougier, P., Masskouri, F., Barbare, J.C., Bedenne, L. Quality of life as a prognostic factor of overall survival in patients with advanced hepatocellular carcinoma: Results from two French clinical trials. *Qual Life Res* 2008;17:831-843.

[18] Osoba, D. What has been learned from measuring health-related quality of life in clinical oncology. *Eur J Cancer* 1999;35:1565-1570.

[19] Kiebert, G.M., Curran, D., Aaronson, N.K. Quality of life as an endpoint in EORTC clinical trials. *Stat Med* 1998;17:561-569.

[20] Testa, M.A., Simonson, D.C. Assesment of quality-of-life outcomes. *N Engl J Med* 1996;334:835-840.

[21] Anderson, R.T., Aaronson, N.K., Wilkin, D. Critical review of the international assessments of health-related quality of life. *Qual Life Res* 1993;2:369-395.

[22] Guyatt, G.H., Feeny, D.H., Patrick, D.L. Measuring health-related quality of life. *Ann Intern Med* 1993; 118:622-629.

[23] Fan, S.Y., Eiser, C., Ho, M.C. Health-related quality of life in patients with hepatocellular carcinoma: a systematic review. *Clin Gastroenterol Hepatol* 2010; 8:559-564.

[24] McHorney, C.A., Ware, J.E., Jr., Raczek, A.E. The MOS 36-Item Short-Form Health Survey (SF-36): II. Psychometric and clinical tests of validity in measuring physical and mental health constructs. *Med Care* 1993; 31:247-263.

[25] Ware J.E., Jr., Sherbourne, C.D. The MOS 36-item short-form health survey (SF-36). I. Conceptual framework and item selection. *Med Care* 1992; 30:473-483.

[26] WHO group. The World Health Organization Quality of Life Assessment (WHOQOL): development and general psychometric properties. *Soc Sci Med* 1998;46:1569-1585.

[27] Cella, D.F., Tulsky, D.S., Gray, G., Sarafian, B., Linn, E., Bonomi, A., Silberman, M., Yellen, S.B., Winicour, P., Brannon, J., Eckberg, K., Purl, S., Blendowsk,i C., Goodman, M., Barnicle, M., Stewart, I., McHale, M., Bonomi, P., Kaplan, E., Taylor, S., Thomas, C., Harris, J. The Functional Assessment of Cancer Therapy scale: development and validation of the general measure. *J Clin Oncol* 1993;11:570-579.

[28] Aaronson, N.K., Ahmedzai, S., Bergman, B., Bullinger, M., Cull, A., Duez, N.J., Filiberti, A., Flechtner, H., Fleishman, S.B., de Haes, J.C., Kaasa, S., Klee, M., Osoba, D., Razavi D., Rofe P.B., Schraub S., Sneeuw K., Sullivan M., Takeda, F. The European Organization for Research and Treatment of Cancer QLQ-C30: a quality-of-

life instrument for use in international clinical trials in oncology. *J Natl Cancer Inst* 1993;85:365-376.

[29] Heffernan N, Cella D, Webster K, Odom L, Martone M, Passik S, Bookbinder M, Fong Y, Jarnagin W, Blumgart L. Measuring health-related quality of life in patients with hepatobiliary cancers: the Functional Assessment of Cancer Therapy-Hepatobiliary questionnaire. *J Clin Oncol* 2002;20: 2229-2239.

[30] Blazeby JM, Currie E, Zee BC, Chie WC, Poon RT, Garden OJ. Development of a questionnaire module to supplement the EORTC QLQ-C30 to assess quality of life in patients with hepatocellular carcinoma, the EORTC QLQ-HCC18.. *Eur J Cancer* 2004; 40:2439-2444.

[31] Yount S, Cella D, Webster K, Heffernan N, Chang CH, Odom L, van Gool R. Assessment of patient-reported clinical outcome in pancreatic and other hepatobiliary cancer: the FACT Hepatobiliary Symptom Index. *J Pain Symptom Manage* 2002;24:32-44.

[32] Pallis AG, Mouzas IA. Instruments for quality of life assessment in patients with gastrointestinal cancer. *Anticancer Res* 2004;24:2117-2121.

[33] Ryu E, Kim K, Cho MS, Kwon IG, Kim HS, Fu MR. Symptom clusters and quality of life in Korean patients with hepatocellular carcinoma. *Cancer Nurs* 2010;33:3-10.

[34] Fielding R, Wong WS. Quality of life as a predictor of cancer survival among Chinese liver and lung cancer patients. *Eur J Cancer* 2007;43:1723-1730.

[35] Lai H, Lin S, Yeh S. Exploring uncertainty, quality of life and related factors in patients with liver cancer. *Chinese Journal of Nursing* 2007;54:41-52.

[36] Poon RT, Fan ST, Yu WC, Lam BK, Chan FY, Wong J. A prospective longitudinal study of quality of life after resection of hepatocellular carcinoma. *Arch Surg* 2001;136:693-699.

[37] Steel JL, Baum A, Carr B. Quality of life in patients diagnosed with primary hepatocellular carcinoma: hepatic arterial infusion of Cisplatin versus 90-Yttrium microspheres. *Psychooncology* 2004;13:73-79.

[38] Steel JL, Chopra K, Olek MC, Carr BI. Health-related quality of life: Hepatocellular carcinoma, chronic liver disease, and the general population. *Qual Life Res* 2007;16:203-215.

[39] Steel JL, Eton DT, Cella D, Olek MC, Carr BI. Clinically meaningful changes in health-related quality of life in patients diagnosed with hepatobiliary carcinoma. *Ann Oncol* 2006;17:304-312.

[40] Steel JL, Geller DA, Carr BI. Proxy rating of health related quality of life in patients with hepatocellular carcinoma. *Qual Life Res* 2005;14:1025-1033.

[41] Sun V, Ferrell B, Juarez G, Wagman LD, Yen Y, Chung V. Symptom concerns and quality of life in hepatobiliary cancers. *Oncol Nurs Forum* 2008;35:E45-52.

[42] Wang YB, Chen MH, Yan K, Yang W, Dai Y, Yin SS. Quality of life after radiofrequency ablation combined with transcatheter arterial chemoembolization for hepatocellular carcinoma: Comparison with transcatheter arterial chemoembolization alone. *Qual Life Res* 2007;16:389-397.

[43] Brucker PS, Yost K, Cashy J, Webster K, Cella D. General population and cancer patient norms for the Functional Assessment of Cancer Therapy-General (FACT-G). *Eval Health Prof* 2005;28:192-211.

[44] Chen L, Liu Y, Li GG, Tao SF, Xu Y, Tian H. Quality of life in patients with liver cancer after operation: a 2-year follow-up study. *Hepatobiliary Pancreat Dis Int* 2004;3:530-533.

[45] Kondo Y, Yoshida H, Tateishi R, Shiina S, Mine N, Yamashiki N, Sato S, Kato N, Kanai F, Yanase M, Yoshida H, Akamatsu M, Teratani T, Kawabe T, Omata M. Health-related quality of life of chronic liver disease patients with and without hepatocellular carcinoma. *J Gastroenterol Hepatol* 2007;22:197-203.

[46] Shun SC, Chiou JF, Lai YH, Yu PJ, Wei LL, Tsai JT. Changes in quality of life and its related factors in liver cancer patients receiving stereotactic radiation therapy. *Support Care Cancer* 2008;16:1059-1065.

[47] Ueno S, Tanabe G, Nuruki K, Yoshidome S, Kubo F, Kihara K, Aoki D, Aikou T. Quality of life after hepatectomy in patients with hepatocellular carcinoma: implication of change in hepatic protein synthesis. *Hepatogastroenterology* 2002;49:492-496.

[48] Wong WS, Fielding R. Eating ability predicts subsequent quality of life in Chinese patients with breast, liver, lung, or nasopharyngeal carcinoma: A longitudinal analysis. *Acta Oncol* 2008;47:71-80.

[49] Bianchi G, Loguercio C, Sgarbi D, Abbiati R, Brunetti N, De Simone T, Zoli M, Marchesini G. Reduced quality of life of patients with hepatocellular carcinoma. *Dig Liver Dis* 2003;35:46-54.

[50] Steel JL, Hess SA, Tunke L, Chopra K, Carr BI. Sexual functioning in patients with hepatocellular carcinoma. *Cancer* 2005;104:2234-2243.

[51] Zhao JB, Li YH, Chen Y, Zeng QL, He XF, Wei ZH, Luo P, Shan H, Zhou G, Li X. Evaluation of quality of life before and after interventional therapy in patients with primary hepatocellular carcinoma. *Chinese Journal of Radiology* 2002;36:873-876.

[52] Tsai L, Chien N, Chan C, Lin C, Lan S. Factors associated with quality of life among patients with liver cancer in a teaching hospital. *Tzu Chi Nursing Journal* 2007;6:80-91.

[53] Wong WS, Fielding R. The association between patient satisfaction and quality of life in Chinese lung and liver cancer patients. *Med care* 2008;46:293-302.

[54] Guo YM. Effects of emotional intervention and Chinese medicated diet in improving the quality of life in patients with liver cancer after chemotherapy. *Chinese Journal of Clinical Rehabilitation* 2005;9:30-31.

[55] Lin ML, Tsang YM, Hwang SL. Efficacy of a stress management program for patients with hepatocellular carcinoma receiving transcatheter arterial embolization. *J Formos Med Assoc* 1998;2:113-117.

[56] Steel JL, Nadeau K, Olek M, Carr BI. Preliminary results of an individually tailored psychosocial intervention for patients with advanced hepatobiliary carcinoma. *J Psychosoc Oncol* 2007;25:19-42.

[57] Gutteling JJ, de Man RA, Busschbach JJ, Darlington AS. Overview of research on health-related quality of life in patients with chronic liver disease. *Neth J Med* 2007;65:227-234.

[58] Martin LM, Sheridan MJ, Younossi ZM. The impact of liver disease on health-related quality of life: a review of the literature. *Curr Gastroenterol Rep* 2002;4:79-83.

[59] Arguedas MR, DeLawrence TG, McGuire BM. Influence of hepatic encephalopathy on health-related quality of life in patients with cirrhosis. *Dig Dis Sci* 2003;48:1622-1626.

[60] Yeo W, Mo FK, Koh J, Chan AT, Leung T, Hui P, Chan L, Tang A, Lee JJ, Mok TSK, Lai PBS, Johnson PJ, Zee B. Quality of life is predictive of survival in patients with unresectable hepatocellular carcinoma. *Ann Oncol* 2006;17:1083-1089.

In: Liver Cancer: Causes, Diagnosis and Treatment
Editor: Benjamin J. Valverde

ISBN 978-1-61209-115-0
© 2011 Nova Science Publishers, Inc.

*Chapter VI*

# Diagnosing Liver Cancer; A Multi-modal Approach

*Marco L.H. Gruwel*[1,2,*], *Eilean McKenzie-Matwiy*[1] *and Erika Lattová*[3,4]

[1]NRC-CNRC, Institute for Biodiagnostics, 435 Ellice Avenue, Winnipeg, MB, R3B 1Y6 Canada.
[2]Department of Medical Microbiology, University of Manitoba, Winnipeg, MB, R3E 0W3 Canada.
[3]Department of Chemistry, University of Manitoba, Winnipeg, MB, R3T 2N2 Canada.
[4]The Institute of Chemistry, Centre for Glycomics, Slovak Academy of Sciences, 842 38 Bratislava, Slovakia

## Abstract

Liver cancer is the $3^{rd.}$ leading cause of death world wide for which the WHO estimates at least 550,000 fatalities per year. In many cases chronic Hepatitis B infection results in the development of hepatocellular carcinoma. As Hepatitis B infection is endemic in China and other parts of Asia, a large part of the world population has the potential to develop liver cancer. The high morbidity rate of liver cancer is related to the late diagnosis when treatment is no longer effective. Diagnosis is usually performed using standard imaging modalities including ultrasonography (US), magnetic resonance imaging (MRI), computed tomography (CT) and positron emission tomography (PET), used for the detection of focal liver lesions. Diagnosis by imaging is usually limited by the skill of the operator (US), the detection limit of the lesion size (MRI, CT) or the cost factor (PET). People at risk, those chronically infected

---

*E-mail address: marco.gruwel@nrc-cnrc.gc.ca

with Hepatitis B (and C), are often screened for liver cancer using the serum $\alpha$-1 fetoprotein level as a liver cancer biomarker. Unfortunately, the current diagnostic use of the alpha-fetoprotein serum level is limited due to numerous complications. Liver cancer patients, or patients at risk, will thus benefit from a better, accurate diagnosis which allows for effective, timely treatment and provides a higher survival rate. Mass spectrometry (MS) has the potential to become a major clinical test for liver cancer biomarkers providing a rapid, accurate and the most sensitive screening procedure. When increases in biomarkers occur, MR imaging and spectroscopy can be used to screen the liver of patients for lesions to localize the tumor and initiate treatment planning. Post-translational modifications in proteins have been shown to associate with cancer diseases and MS analysis of human and animal sera revealed alterations in N-glycans between healthy individuals and those with hepatocellular carcinoma. MALDI-MS, in combination with MS/MS, helped to identify N-glycan structures in a woodchuck model of hepatocellular carcinoma of which some showed elevated levels in animals with liver cancer. $^{31}$P MR spectroscopy showed elevated levels of phosphomonoesters, particularly phosphocholine, in selectively imaged voxels within the tumor.

**Keywords:** hepatocellular carcinoma, glycosylation, magnetic resonance imaging, magnetic resonance spectroscopy, mass spectrometry.

# 1. Introduction

Hepatocellular carcinoma (HCC), or primary liver cancer, is liver cancer that originates within the liver and does not form from other metastasized forms of cancer. HCC is an aggressive tumor with a poor long-term prognosis, making it one of the leading causes of cancer-related deaths worldwide. Most cases of HCC are secondary to hepatitis B (HBV) or C (HCV) viral infection. Risk factors such as alcohol, Aflotoxin B1, hemochromatosis and liver cirrhosis are also known to induce HCC. Individuals chronically infected with hepatitis B are 100 times more likely to develop progressive liver diseases such as cirrhosis and HCC than uninfected people, with men more likely to develop HCC than women [1–4]. HCC is now the fourth most common cancer worldwide, causing an estimated 600,000 by 2008 (WHO, 2008), most of which were in developing countries [4]. Transmission of the hepatitis B virus occurs from exposure to contaminated blood and body fluids, including reusing tattoo and piercing needles, sharing syringes, razors, or toothbrushes, via contaminated blood transfusions, or through *in utero* transmission to the developing fetus by an infected mother. Rates of HCC due to chronic hepatitis B infection have been declining with the introduction of vaccines and with screening of donated blood and blood products [2,5].

Initial symptoms of HCC in people are variable for numerous reasons. In many areas of the world in which the HCC incident rate is high due to chronic infection with HBV or HCV, there is a confounding limited access to general health care. In these areas screening examinations for patients with HCC is generally not available. As a result, diagnosis often occurs at an advanced stage of HCC development for which treatment often is very difficult. On the other hand, in areas where people do have access to health care, HCC usually develops more slowly which could complicate early diagnosis. To date, diagnosis of HCC is not possible using a single, routine blood test, however, diagnosis is usually performed using blood tests, imaging modalities or a combination of these two, and in some cases by biopsy. A number of serum biomarkers have been proposed of which $\alpha$-1 fetoprotein (AFP) is the most commonly used serum test [6,7]. After discovery by Abelev *et al.* [8] in the early sixties, a quantitative serum assay was introduced in 1971 [9]. Although used as a marker for HCC, AFP is known not to be elevated in all patients with HCC while patients with cirrhosis or hepatic inflamation often show elevated levels of AFP [6]. Recently, Lok *et al.* showed that neither des-$\gamma$-carboxy prothrombin (DCP) nor AFP could be used as an optimal biomarker for HCC [10].

HCC is often diagnosed using a blood test in combination with an imaging modality. Imaging studies can provide information of tumor size, the number of tumors and tumor perfusion. The role of the different imaging modalities (CT, MRI, US and PET) has been discussed by Oliva *et al.* [11]. Patients with chronic liver disease (HBV, HCV) at risk for developing HCC usually undergo periodic screening with US while a typical metastases examination involves contrast-enhanced CT or MRI for patients with fatty liver, or unable to handle contrast *i.v.*. Although US presents a fast, cost-effective way to screen the liver, it does have sub-optimal sensitivity and specificity, especially in case complicated by cirrhosis [12]. Vascular anatomy is usually studied in a separate examination using MR or CT angiography. A combined PET-CT study allows for the anatomical detection of "hotspots", however, PET exams are associated with higher costs and limited availability [13]. PET is less accurate than contrast-enhanced MRI [11], however, dual-isotope ($^{18}$F-FDG, $^{11}$C-Acetate) PET studies increased the overall HCC sensitivity [14].

Biopsy is rarely required for diagnosis, especially for patients with risk factors (chronic HBV or HCV infection and cirrhosis) and carries the risk of potential seeding of tumor in the needle tract.

## 2. Current Clinical Diagnostic Criteria

The American Association for the Study of Liver Diseases (AASLD; *http://www.aasld.org*) recommends that the diagnosis of HCC can be made through combination of radiology, biopsy and AFP serology [15]. The sensitivity of MRI to detect HCC is 81%, compared to CT's 68% [16]. Intravenous contrast agents like gadolinium can be used to increase the sensitivity. If a patient has lesions greater than 2cm in diameter that show arterial phase enhancement, venous phase wash-out during contrast enhanced MRI or computed tomography, and elevated AFP ($>200$ng$\cdot$mL$^{-1}$), the positive predictive value of HCC increases to 95% [15]. Lesions smaller than 2cm are more difficult to diagnose as they may not have the typical wash-out characteristics of the larger HCCs, they may not cause an elevation in AFP, and biopsy results may not be conclusive due to the small sample-size of the biopsy relative to the size of the whole organ [15]. Patients with suspected tumors smaller than 2cm that lack the typical contrast enhancement patterns of HCC are recommended to undergo screening with ultrasound, CT or MRI regularly to ensure that the suspected lesion is not changing size [15]. US guided biopsy of a suspected lesion smaller than 2cm may help improve the diagnosis of HCC, however, small and early HCC may lack histological features that differentiate HCC from other lesions such as dysplastic nodules [15]. Combining imaging features already known to be specific to HCC, with the biochemical information specific to the growth of the tumor would improve diagnosis of HCC.

The diagnosis of HCC does not accurately predict the stage of the disease or the clinical outcome. Different methods of staging the disease have been developed (Okuda, Child-Pugh, MELD, BCLC [17]) but they are more accurate in determining patients with end stage HCC and poor prognosis [15]. Patients with 1 isolated HCC or up to 3 tumors smaller than 3cm each, typically respond well to treatment (resection, transplant, or ablation) and have a 5-year survival rate between 50-75% [15]. Having more than 3 tumors, but without metastasis to other organs, has a 3-year life expectancy of 50% [15]. Patients with metastasizing HCC have a 1-year life expectancy of 50% [15].

Biopsies may cause patient discomfort with the possibility of bleeding, and may not sample from the lesion of interest because of difficulty in obtaining accurate images to use as a guide for the biopsy [15]. There is some concern that the biopsy may cause seeding or spreading cancerous tissue to new areas of the liver during the biopsy procedure [15]. Biopsies only sample 1/50,000 of the liver's total volume, which can not accurately represent the entire liver [18]. Multi-voxel $^{31}$P-Magnetic Resonance Spectroscopy (MRS) like 2D-CSI [19] can sample larger areas non-invasively with less risk to the patient [18]. Changes to the liver phosphorus spectrum are being correlated to liver disorders including HCC, steatosis, cirrhosis, hemachromatosis, regeneration after hepatectomy, transplant rejection and response to chemotherapy [20–25].

Results from human studies of HCC depend on whether the patients have other liver disorders including cirrhosis (either alcoholic or viral in origin), fatty livers, chronic infection with other viruses, and inherited liver disorders. Data analysis is further complicated if the HCC is a primary malignancy or secondary due to metastasis from another tumor elsewhere in the body [26].

## 3.  Improving HCC Diagnosis

A major bottleneck in the diagnosis of HCC is its late detection, using AFP as a cancer marker, for a large portion of the world's population. Most often at this stage, HCC is well developed and treatment is very limited. In order to provide an effective treatment for HCC, early diagnosis is thus a must. Therefore the imaging modalities used for HCC detection should provide images with a higher spatial resolution in order to provide early detection. In addition, highly sensitive and simple techniques based on the detection of specific HCC biomarkers should be developed. Such an approach requires a two-pronged, multi-modal process, one involving the biochemical detection of biomarkers and another involving the spatial localization of HCC development. Recent developments in this research area make use of the Woodchuck as the preferred animal model for the study of HCC [19, 27, 28]. Sofar this work has culminated in the the development and application of new techniques in MS [27, 28] and MR spectroscopic imaging [19], using an increase in some oligosaccharide structures in serum and phosphatidylcholine (PC) in the liver, respectively, as potential biomarkers for early cancer detection. In the next subsection an introduction to the Woodchuck model for HCC is given, followed by subsections on improvements in HCC detection using a multi-modal approach.

## 3.1. Animal Model for HCC

With the discovery that a significant number of captive woodchucks at the Penrose Research Centre in Philadelphia, PA developed HCC due to woodchuck hepatitis virus (WHV) infection [29, 30], the woodchuck has become the preferred animal model of HCC since 1979. WHV is a previously unknown DNA virus with significant homology to HBV [31, 32]. In addition to immunological studies for both acute and chronic infection by Hepadnavirus, woodchucks have been used for imaging studies using ultrasound [33, 34], PET [35], MRI and MR spectroscopy (MRS) [19, 36–39].

Neonatal woodchucks inoculated three days after birth with $5 \cdot 10^6$ $WID_{50}$ of WHV7P1, a lab-adapted WHV strain, have been used to create a predictable model of infection [40]. The outcome of an infection, whether the woodchuck will develop chronic or acute infection, can be accurately predicted based on serum analysis at week 14 [40, 41]. At week 14, the incubation phase of the infection, WHV DNA in woodchucks resolving the infection has begun to decline while it is still increasing in chronic infected woodchucks. This increase in viral load is due to chronic infected woodchucks having a defective Th1, or cytotoxic T cell-mediated immune response to the virus [41]. From 14 weeks onward, woodchucks which resolved their WHV infection have undetectable serum concentrations of WHV surface antigen and liver enzymes similar to uninfected woodchucks of the same age [40, 41] and developed anti-WHV-core antibodies and by week 14, have begun to develop anti-WHV-surface antibodies which protects from future infections [41]. Histological examination of tissue obtained from chronic infected woodchucks indicates bile duct proliferation, regions of necrosis and degenerating hepatocytes, and lower levels of inflammation [40]. Human tissue would be scored as having moderate hepatitis if it were examined at this point in the infection [40]. At fifteen months post-infection, chronic infected woodchucks have significant concentrations of WHV DNA and WHV surface antigen in the blood and liver tissue and continue to have mild and persistent inflammation in the liver, detectable by slight elevations in ALT and sorbitol dehydrogenase [42]. The infection will persist until the eventual death of the woodchuck at approximately 2.5-3 years post-infection due to irreversible liver damage and HCC.

Woodchucks that are chronically infected with WHV have nearly a 100% chance of developing HCC within 29-56 months post-infection [30]. Infected woodchucks that have an acute infection and develop both protective neutralizing antibodies and specific T lymphocytes have an 80% survival rate greater than 60 months [30]. A chronic infection is due primarily to a deficient Th1 response to the virus [42]. An appropriate immune response should have created multi-specific Th1 cytotoxic T-lymphocytes towards many different viral antigens, especially against WHV-core, as well as stimulated a Th2 immune response that would have created neutralizing antibodies.

HCC development in humans is a multi-step process requiring many years of persistent infection. The severity of the disease and the development of HCC also depends on the strain of HBV that an individual is infected with [43]. Rates of HCC are higher in countries where HBV is endemic and the number of individuals with chronic hepatitis is significantly higher [2, 4, 44]. The relative risk of developing HCC with chronic infection is 100 times greater than without infection [1, 45, 46].

Unlike human HCC, woodchuck HCC is not metastatic and not associated with cirrhosis

[31,47]. In humans, HCC develops more in males than in females, whereas in woodchucks, there is no sex preference [3, 4, 32]. The tumours that develop in woodchucks are well differentiated from surrounding liver parenchyma by fibrotic connective tissue [31,32,46]. The tumours can range in size from 1-10 cm and begin to develop from foci of a few altered hepatocytes after the first year of active hepatitis [29, 31, 32]. Within the tumour are regions of necrosis, low levels of WHV protein expression, inflammation, and bile duct proliferation [31,32,46].

The mechanism of carcinogenesis is unknown as WHV does not contain any known oncogenes. It is speculated that carcinogenesis may result from integration of a viral genomic section that upregulates the expression of the hepatocyte's regulatory genes [47–49]. The severity of liver disease due to chronic infection is also determined by the extent of inflammation due to host response to the disease. A more aggressive immune response to the virus correlates to greater liver damage and increases the potential for tumourgenesis.

## 3.2.  MR Spectroscopic Imaging of the Liver

In comparison to US and CT, MRI has proven to be more reliable when focal liver lesions have to be detected and characterized [50]. This greater potential is based on a superior amount of diagnostic information available, using $T_1$ and $T_2$-weighted MR-sequences including the possibility of multiple acquisitions after injection of contrast media. Presently, conclusive HCC detection by means of MR or CT is restricted to a $2 \times 2 \times 2 cm^3$ detection-size limit due to restricted vascular pattern recognition [15]. Smaller lesions are very difficult to biopsy as needle placement will be problematic. In addition the difference between dysplasia and well differentiated HCC becomes more difficult to judge with decreasing size. As the success rate of HCC treatment increases significantly with its early detection, a need for higher spatial resolution is warranted. Multi-voxel [31]P-Magnetic Resonance Spectroscopy (MRS) [19] can be performed with a comparable or better resolution of $1.5 \times 2 \times 1.5 cm^3$. [31]P MRS provides a direct, non-invasive, metabolic finger print of a selected area within the liver [24, 26, 51], and could be used for this purpose. [31]P MRS has been used studying diffuse and chronic liver disease [25,26,52], viral hepatitis [18,53] and liver metabolism in patients with a distant malignant tumour [54, 55]. Most of these experiments were performed on relative large sections of the liver, strictly for the study of overall liver metabolism. However, altered [31]P metabolism can also be used as an additional diagnostic tool for the detection of HCC.

Woodchucks infected with WHV were used to study the development of HCC using both MRI and [31]P MRS (2D-CSI) [19]. MR observations were correlated to serum analysis of aspartate aminotransferase (AST), γ-glutamate transferase (GGT), conjugated bilirubin, total protein, and globulin. Although GGT and AST levels do not correlate to the extent of tumor growth, these can be used as a serum marker for the degree of liver injury due to the tumor [48,56]. All infected woodchucks developed HCC within $986 \pm 26$ days post-infection. Uninfected woodchucks survived for 1100 or more days without HCC development [32, 46]. Unlike human hepatitis, WHV is rarely cirrhotic [32]; consequently, the differences in the [31]P-MR spectra were not due to fibrosis.

All MRS experiments were performed in a 7-T horizontal-bore magnet (Magnex, UK) equipped with an Avance DRX Bruker console. The animal was positioned in the center of

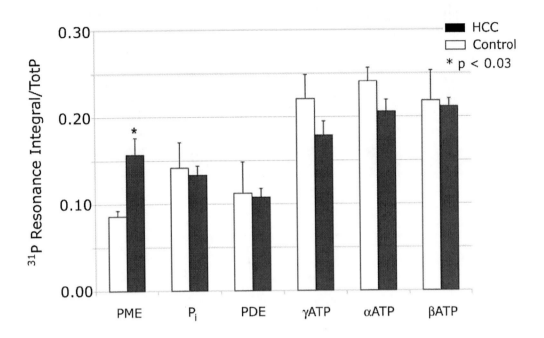

Figure 1. Comparing control and HCC $^{31}$P levels. PME is significantly elevated in the chronically infected woodchucks with HCC (n=11) than in the uninfected woodchucks (n=6) with normal livers. Other phosphorus containing molecules detected by $^{31}$P-MRS were not significantly different between HCC and control livers. All calculations reported as mean ± standard error.

a doubly tunable quadrature volume coil tuned to 300 and 121.5 MHz for proton imaging and phosphorus spectroscopy, respectively [57]. Using a $^1$H scout image, the position of a 20-mm axial slab for $^{31}$P 2D-CSI was determined which incorporated the largest portion of liver tissue without artifacts from the diaphragm and stomach. The $^{31}$P-MR spectra were acquired using a field of view (FOV) of $24 \times 24$ cm$^2$, a sweep width of 7 kHz, a data matrix of 1024 spectroscopic points, a TR of 1000 ms, and 16 averages.

Resonances from phosphomonoesters (PME) (7.1 ppm), P$_i$ (4.7 ppm), phosphodiesters(PDE) (2.5 ppm), and three resonances of $\alpha$(-7.5 ppm), $\beta$(-16.0 ppm), and $\gamma$-NTP (-2.1 ppm) were detected in spectra from control woodchucks and those with advanced HCC. Ratios of phosphorus-containing metabolites to the total phosphorus signal (TotP) were calculated for each woodchuck in two consecutive monthly imaging sessions prior to euthanasia. The $^{31}$P MR spectra of chronically infected woodchucks with advanced HCC had a statistically significant increase in $\frac{PME}{TotP}$ compared to controls (Figure 1). Woodchucks with HCC had an average $\frac{PME}{TotP}$ of $0.157 \pm 0.01$ while control woodchucks had a $\frac{PME}{TotP}$ of $0.086 \pm 0.003$ (p<0.03). Other phosphorus containing molecules were not significantly different between control and animals with HCC.

The observed PME signal contains contributions from adenosine monophosphate, phos-

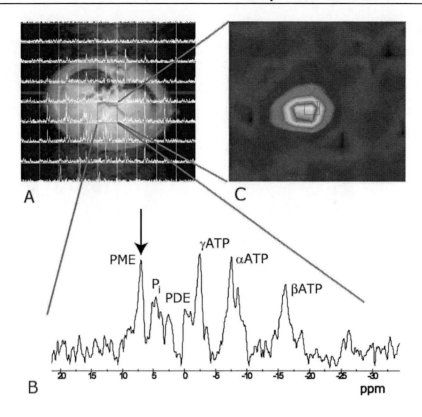

Figure 2. A) 2D-CSI data set with each $^{31}$P-MRS spectrum overlayed on the axial scout image. A voxel of interest is highlighted by the red square and the corresponding $^{31}$P MR spectrum shown in B). The voxel dimensions are $1.5 \times 1.5$ cm$^2$ in plane, using a 2.0 cm thick slab. The arrow indicates the spectral region (frequency) selected for display in the metabolite map for the whole FOV shown in C). C) Metabolite map showing the relative amounts of PME over the entire 2D-CSI data using a false colour map.

phocholine (PC) and phosphoethanolamine (PE), the precursors to phosphatidylcholine and phosphatidylethanolamine used in the cell membranes [26,53]. Glycerophosphocholine and glycerophosphoethanolamine, along with adenosine diphosphate, contribute to the PDE signal [53]. The increase in the $\frac{PME}{TotP}$ in the livers of infected animal is similar to previously reported studies using $^{31}$P-MRS to compare the $^{31}$P spectrum of HCC in humans [58,59]. An increase in $\frac{PME}{TotP}$ is an indication of cellular proliferation and cell membrane synthesis. The advantage to phosphorus spectroscopy is that it can simultaneously provide information about cellular growth and degradation, as well as tissue energetics. A characteristic feature of many solid tumours is the significant increase in PME resonances, found between 7.2-8.0 ppm in the $^{31}$P spectrum [19,22,26]. The PME peak is composed of signals from PC and PE that represent increased cell membrane synthesis, typical of the unregulated cellular proliferation found in cancer and liver regeneration [22,59]. The resonances associated with the PDE peak, found between 3.0-3.5 ppm, result from the membrane degradation

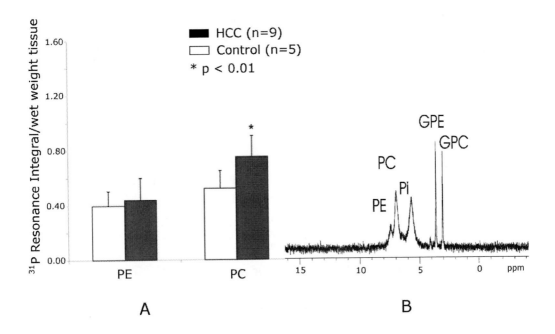

Figure 3. A) Significant elevations in PC but not PE were detected by $^{31}$P high resolution NMR of woodchuck liver samples with known HCC development compared to cancer-free control animals. All results are reported as the mean of the integrals from the three samples ± standard deviation per gram of tissue (wet weight). Results were considered significant using a 2-tailed Student's t-test (p<0.05) with a Levene's test for variance (Statistica©6.1, StatSoft Inc.) B) Typical $^{31}$P NMR spectrum of a woodchuck with HCC.

products GPC and GPE. The three resonances at -1.5 ppm, -6.5 ppm and -16 ppm represent the three phosphate groups of nucleotide triphosphate ($\gamma$, $\alpha$, and $\beta$ respectively). The individual contributions from each nucleotide triphosphate can not be separated by phosphorus spectroscopy; therefore the NTP resonance represents the sum of all contributions from these molecules. A reduction in PDE and an increase in $\frac{P_i}{\beta-NTP}$ have been linked to necrosis [26, 60]. Livers of infected woodchucks showed similar ratios of $\frac{PDE}{TotP}$ and $\frac{P_i}{TotP}$ to the control animals (Figure 1), which would infer that the tumour develops as a result of cellular proliferation without necrosis.

To confirm that increases in PME resonance detected *in vivo* are due to tumour growth, and not due to compensating regeneration, PCA extraction performed on carefully selected frozen liver tissue samples excised at necropsy from the woodchucks that underwent 2D-CSI. Samples of HCC were taken from the largest tumour of the chronically infected woodchucks (n=9) while samples of uninfected woodchucks were taken from the largest lobe of the liver (n=5). The extracted samples were analyzed *ex vivo* using high resolution $^{31}$P-NMR. *In vivo*, the PME resonance appears as a broad single peak at 6.9-7.2 ppm but is actually composed of resonances from PC and PE, which can be differentiated using high resolution $^{31}$P-NMR spectroscopy. The same technique can be used to resolve the PDE resonance, a broad peak located at 3.0 ppm, into its composing resonances of glycerophosphocholine (GPC) and glycerophosphoethanolamine (GPE). $^{31}$P-NMR analysis was performed on an 8.4T Bruker Avance spectrometer using a one-pulse sequence with inverse gated decoupling at 145.865 MHz, a sweep width of 11574.07 Hz, a number of scans of 1024, a repetition time of 5 s with a total acquisition time of 75 minutes using a 5 mm multinuclear probehead. An external reference of phenylphosphate (PPA) (8.8mM) in $D_2O$ within a sealed glass capillary tube was used as an external reference for the peak assignment. Peaks were assigned as follwos; PPA 18.5 ppm, PE 7.2 ppm, PC 6.8 ppm, $P_i$ 5.8 ppm, GPE 4.0 ppm, GPC 3.4 ppm, $\alpha$-NTP -7.3 ppm [51]. Results are shown in Figure 3. Samples obtained from HCC had significantly elevated PC ($0.753\pm0.151$ $vs.$ $0.521\pm0.129$, p<0.01) control samples, but not PE (p=0.63). There was no significant difference in GPE and GPC levels between HCC and control livers ($0.313\pm0.239$ $vs.$ $0.212\pm0.08$, p=0.39 and $0.128\pm0.065$ $vs.$ $0.101\pm0.04$, p=0.42, respectively), indicating that there is no significant amount of necrosis within the HCC of the woodchucks studied [22].

## 3.3. Glycomics as a Potential Tool for the Development of HCC Biomarkers

Over the last years, major advances in sensitive high throughout technologies have been made in the field of proteomics and offer much promise in the search for molecular markers of early stage cancers [61]. Literature reports that many biomolecular changes occur during the outbreak of disease and most of them are associated with the post-translational modification (PTM) of proteins. Glycosylation is one mode of PTMs and its importance is reflected by a large number of glycosylated proteins employed in a myriad of biological processes [62–65].

The two most abundant types of oligosaccharides of cell surfaces and secreted glycoproteins are classified by the nature of their linkage to the protein: the N-glycans with N-acetylglucosamine linked at asparagine in the consensus sequence Asn-X-Ser/Thr and O-glycans with N-acetylgalactosamine linked at serine or threonine residues [66]. The structural variability of glycans is dictated by a panel of highly specific glycosyltransferases and glycosidases present in the endoplasmic reticulum and Golgi apparatus of the cell [67]. Alterations in the expression of these enzymes result in changes of the glycomic profile found on its glycoprotein. The associations between oligosaccharide structures and various biological functions, including cell adhesion and cancer metastasis is well known [68]. Numerous glycoproteins were found to be potentially important as biomarkers in various diseases.

Since serum contains a large group of glycoproteins synthesized by organs in the body, including the liver and plasma cells, extensive research has been performed on specific glycoprotein isolated from serum. AFP is one of most common diagnostic markers monitoring HCC. This glycoprotein consists of 591 amino acids with a single carbohydrate chain linked at asparagine-233 [69]. Although the exact biological function of AFP is still unclear, it is suggested to function as a transport molecule for several different ligands such as bilirubin, fatty acids, flavonoids, phytoestrogens, retinoids, including drugs and other compounds [70, 71]. AFP was separated into several glycoforms based on a different affinity towards lectins by means of lectin-electrophoretic techniques [72, 73]. Concanavalin A affinity electrophoresis of serum AFP results in one band or a multiple of bands used as a diagnostic marker for HCC [74]. According to their banding capacity three types of glycoforms were identified and one of them with an additional fucose residue attached at the 6-position of N-acetylglucosamine of the reducing terminus. The latter being suspected to be produced by cancer cells [75, 76]. Although the AFP serum level is used as a tumor marker for HCC, there is a very high number of cases with false results, leading to the search for alternative biomarkers of HCC.

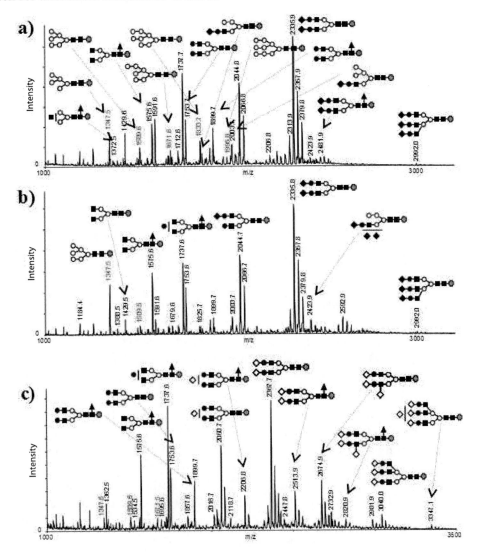

Figure 4. Representative MALDI-mass spectra of glycan fractions obtained after solid phase extraction on STRATA-XC cartridges followed by derivatization with phenylhydrazine, from the serum of: a) a woodchuck with HCC (GGT = 83 IU/L ; b) a control woodchuck (GGT = 7 IU/L); and c) a healthy mouse used as control sample to verify the absence of sialylated biantennary fucosylated glycans in woodchuck sera not caused by an approach used for the analysis of glycans. N-glycans corresponding to high-mannose structures are red coloured. Symbols: ▲ Fucose; ● Galactose; ○ Manose; ■ N-acetylglucosamine; ♦ N-acetylneuraminic acid; ◊ N-glycolylneuraminic acid.

GP73 is a 73 kDa human glycoprotein with unknown functions, localized in the Golgi apparatus [77]. Earlier results indicated that this protein can be upregulated in response to infection by viruses such as HBV and HCV. Increased expression of GP73 in hepatocytes appeared to be a general feature of advanced liver disease with supposed regulation via distinct pathways that involve hepatotropic viruses or cytokines [78]. Further research of GP73 isolated from animal sera of woodchucks chronically infected with WHV confirmed the specific association of this glycoprotein with the development of HCC [27]. The 2DE electrophoretic profile of animal serum depleted of Ig molecules showed several proteins to be hyperfucosylated (e.g. $\alpha$-acid glycoprotein, AFP, $\alpha$-1-antitrypsin, $\alpha$-1-antichymotrypsin). Among them, GP73 has become the centre of interest. Using a mass spectrometric approach (MS/MS), it was demonstrated that GP73 is N-glycosylated on at least two out of the potential three sites. Most of the glycans are bi-antennary with a core fucose, with a smaller fraction of tri- and tetra-antennary structures also occurring [79].

In an effort to get a better understanding of the fucosylation levels of a liver-specific protein in the bile and serum, the oligosaccharide structures of $\alpha$-1-antitrypsin (AAT), $\alpha$-1-acid-glycoprotein (AGP) and Haptoglobin (Hp) were analyzed using a combination of high performance liquid chromatography (HPLC) and MALDI-TOF MS analyses [80]. The results demonstrated that fucosylation is a possible signal for the secretion of glycoproteins into bile ducts in the liver and a disruption in this system might involve an increase of fucosylated AFP in the serum of patients with HCC.

The results discussed above have initiated the development of novel fucosylated biomarkers for the early detection of HCC based on a combination of AFP with GP73, fucosylated kininogen and $\alpha$-1-antitrypsin [81]. The analysis of serum from 113 patients with cirrhosis and 164 serum samples from patients with cirrhosis and HCC showed greater performance and less false positive results than the currently used AFP marker.

The liver-specific glycoprotein hemopexin produced mainly by the hepatocyte and present in serum in a concentration sufficient for purification $(0.4\text{-}1.5\text{g}\cdot\text{L}^{-1})$ was recently shown to be an ideal candidate to represent the liver-specific glycoproteome and a possible marker for liver-specific changes [82, 83]. Hemopexin carries five N-linked oligosaccharides on its N-terminus and is a type II acute phase protein [84]. This glycoprotein isolated from sera of 49 healthy volunteers was compared versus samples from 81 patients divided into the categories of fibrosis, cirrhosis and HCC with cirrhosis. It was observed that the number of branching $\alpha$-1,3-fucosylated multi-antennary glycans on hemopexin were increased in the HCC group compared with the cirrhosis without HCC, whereas non-modified biantennary glycans decreased progressively across groups from fibrosis to the cirrhosis and HCC groups [83].

In an effort to develop a simpler noninvasive method for the discovery of new diagnostic cancer biomarkers, attempts based on a direct release of N-linked oligosaccharides from a serum sample have been made. In 2004, Callewart *et al.* demonstrated the importance of the total serum N-glycome profile using a slab gel-based DNA sequencer in monitoring the progression of chronic liver disease [85]. This method was optimized by the labeling of N-glycans with 8-aminopyrene-1,3,6- trisulfonic acid (APTS) followed by analysis on the capillary electrophoresis-based DNA sequencer [86]. Prior to derivatization with APTS, glycans were desialylated to simplify the final N-glycan profile. This so called *GlycoFibreTest* is based on the ratio between bisecting N-acetylglucosamine modified agalacto glycans and tri-antennary glycans. Using a sensitive matrix-assisted laser desorption ionization (MALDI) mass spectrometric method, 26 oligosaccharide structures were analyzed from serum samples of healthy donors and patients suffering from cirrhosis or chronic hepatitis C [87]. The increase of the number of glycans with a bisecting N-acetylglucosamine residue and core fucosylation in sera of patients with cirrhosis was a good indicator for pursuing this approach. Our analysis of N-glycans enzymatically released from total serum samples of woodchucks, using a highly sensitive MALDI technique showed a total of forty structures in the sera of woodchucks with HCC and in healthy controls [28]. However, to our surprise, we mainly observed an increase in the level of oligomannose structures in total serum samples of woodchucks with GGT values of 50-98 IU (Figure 4). High-mannose glycans have been described on the β-chain of the C4 protein secreted by human hepatoma-derived cells [88] and the serum level of this protein varied in patients with autoimmune diseases [89]. While the increase of fucosylated biantennary glycans was observed in woodchucks with GGT levels higher than 100 IU [27], the high-mannose structures showed to be elevated even in sera samples with GGT levels below 100 IU, and thus providing to be a better candidate for early HCC detection [28].

Although all published results devoted to glycan changes in association with HCC, including others not discussed here, are still not of limited values, they underscore the significance of serum as a noninvasive prognostic biomarker. The availability of already published data will likely result in more challenging research in the field of HCC biomarkers.

# 4. Perspectives

In this work we have focused on the use of different diagnostic and analytical technologies for the early detection of HCC. The previous paragraphs have shown that the woodchuck animal model for HCC can be a tremendous help in the development of new HCC biomarkers. Early detection of HCC is not only dependent on the development of new technologies but rather the optimal integration and use of these technologies into a patient-friendly multi-modal diagnostic test. The role of any multi-modal imaging technology ideally should provide the exact localization, extent, and metabolic activity of the target disease,

Research based on MS analysis of serum samples, studied at the level of glycomics, offers information to better understand the molecular pathogenesis of disease. Detailed studies of glycosylation provide a promising key in the search for an appropriate biomarker to facilitate early detection of the disease. However, especially for the liver, biomarkers for disease can be detected in serum but these markers do not provide any information on the spatial location within the organ. For the latter detection, 3D imaging modalities such as MR are required. In a previous paragraph we have shown the use of spectroscopic imaging using 2D-CSI (Figure 2) to provide a means of early HCC detection based on an increase in PMEs in the spectrum, as a form of molecular imaging. The combination of Mass Spec and MRI could possibly develop into a patient-friendly multi-modal diagnostic test for HCC.

The development of multi-modal technologies based on PET, MRI, and optical imaging is the single biggest focus in many imaging and cancer centres worldwide. Recently PET and MRI have been combined to provide a way to trace metabolites, using PET, on an

## References

[1] Beasley RP, Hwang LY, Lin CC, Chien CS. Hepatocellular carcinoma and hepatitis B virus. A prospective study of 22 707 men in Taiwan. *Lancet.* 1981;2(8256):1129–1133.

[2] Chang MH, Chen CJ, Lai MS, Hsu HM, Wu TC, Kong MS, et al. Universal hepatitis B vaccination in Taiwan and the incidence of hepatocellular carcinoma in children. Taiwan Childhood Hepatoma Study Group. *N Engl J Med.* 1997;336(26):1855–1859.

[3] El-Serag HB, Mason AC. Rising incidence of hepatocellular carcinoma in the United States. *N Engl J Med.* 1999;340(10):745–750.

[4] Pisani P, Parkin DM, Bray F, Ferlay J. Estimates of the worldwide mortality from 25 cancers in 1990. *Int J Cancer.* 1999;83(1):18–29.

[5] Alter H. Discovery of non-A, non-B hepatitis and identification of its etiology. *Am J Med.* 1999;107(6B):16S–20S.

[6] Gomaa AI, Khan SA, Leen ELS, Waked I, Taylor-Robinson SD. Diagnosis of hepatocellular carcinoma. *World J Gastroenterol.* 2009;15(11):1301–1314.

[7] Sakamoto M. Early HCC: diagnosis and molecular markers. *J Gastroenterol.* 2009;44 Suppl 19:108–111.

[8] Abelev GI, Perova SD, Khramkova NI, Postnikova ZA, Irlin IS. Production of embryonal alpha-globulin by transplantable mouse hepatomas. *Transplantation.* 1963;1:174–180.

[9] Ruoslahti E, Seppälä M, Pihko H, Vuopio P. Studies of carcino-fetal proteins. II. Biochemical comparison of -fetoprotein from human fetuses and patients with hepatocellular cancer. *Int J Cancer.* 1971;8(2):283–288.

[10] Lok AS, Sterling RK, Everhart JE, Wright EC, Hoefs JC, Bisceglie AMD, et al. Des-gamma-carboxy prothrombin and alpha-fetoprotein as biomarkers for the early detection of hepatocellular carcinoma. *Gastroenterology.* 2010;138(2):493–502.

[11] Oliva MR, Saini S. Liver cancer imaging: role of CT, MRI, US and PET. *Cancer Imaging.* 2004;4 Spec No A:S42–S46.

[12] Vogl TJ, Eichler K, Zangos S, Mack M, Hammerstingl R. [Hepatocellular carcinoma: Role of imaging diagnostics in detection, intervention and follow-up]. *Rofo.* 2002;174(11):1358–1368.

[13] Kinkel K, Lu Y, Both M, Warren RS, Thoeni RF. Detection of hepatic metastases from cancers of the gastrointestinal tract by using noninvasive imaging methods (US, CT, MR imaging, PET): a meta-analysis. *Radiology*. 2002;224(3):748–756.

[14] Park JW, Kim JH, Kim SK, Kang KW, Park KW, Choi JI, et al. A prospective evaluation of 18F-FDG and 11C-acetate PET/CT for detection of primary and metastatic hepatocellular carcinoma. *J Nucl Med*. 2008;49(12):1912–1921.

[15] Bruix J, Sherman M, Practice Guidelines Committee AAftSoLD. Management of hepatocellular carcinoma. *Hepatology*. 2005;42(5):1208–1236.

[16] Willatt JM, Hussain HK, Adusumilli S, Marrero JA. MR Imaging of hepatocellular carcinoma in the cirrhotic liver: challenges and controversies. *Radiology*. 2008;247(2):311–330.

[17] Shouval D. HCC: what's the score. *Gut*. 2002;50(6):749–750.

[18] Lim AKP, Patel N, Hamilton G, Mylvahan K, Kuo YT, Goldin RD, et al. 31P MR spectroscopy in assessment of response to antiviral therapy for hepatitis C virus-related liver disease. *AJR Am J Roentgenol*. 2007;189(4):819–823.

[19] McKenzie EJ, Jackson M, Sun J, Volotovskyy V, Gruwel MLH. Monitoring the development of hepatocellular carcinoma in woodchucks using 31P-MRS. *MAGMA*. 2005;18(4):201–205.

[20] Bell JD, Bhakoo KK. Metabolic changes underlying 31P MR spectral alterations in human hepatic tumours. *NMR Biomed*. 1998;11(7):354–359.

[21] Cox IJ, Sharif A, Cobbold JFL, Thomas HC, Taylor-Robinson SD. Current and future applications of in vitro magnetic resonance spectroscopy in hepatobiliary disease. *World J Gastroenterol*. 2006;12(30):4773–4783.

[22] Khan SA, Cox IJ, Hamilton G, Thomas HC, Taylor-Robinson SD. In vivo and in vitro nuclear magnetic resonance spectroscopy as a tool for investigating hepatobiliary disease: a review of H and P MRS applications. *Liver Int*. 2005;25(2):273–281.

[23] Meyerhoff DJ, Karczmar GS, Valone F, Venook A, Matson GB, Weiner MW. Hepatic cancers and their response to chemoembolization therapy. Quantitative image-guided 31P magnetic resonance spectroscopy. *Invest Radiol*. 1992;27(6):456–464.

[24] Solga SF, Horska A, Clark JM, Diehl AM. Hepatic 31P magnetic resonance spectroscopy: a hepatologist's user guide. *Liver Int*. 2005;25(3):490–500.

[25] Taylor-Robinson SD, Sargentoni J, Bell JD, Saeed N, Changani KK, Davidson BR, et al. In vivo and in vitro hepatic 31P magnetic resonance spectroscopy and electron microscopy of the cirrhotic liver. *Liver*. 1997;17(4):198–209.

[26] Cox IJ, Menon DK, Sargentoni J, Bryant DJ, Collins AG, Coutts GA, et al. Phosphorus-31 magnetic resonance spectroscopy of the human liver using chemical shift imaging techniques. *J Hepatol*. 1992;14(2-3):265–275.

[27] Block TM, Comunale MA, Lowman M, Steel LF, Romano PR, Fimmel C, et al. Use of targeted glycoproteomics to identify serum glycoproteins that correlate with liver cancer in woodchucks and humans. *Proc Natl Acad Sci U S A*. 2005;102(3):779–784.

[28] Lattová E, McKenzie EJ, Gruwel MLH, Spicer V, Goldman R, Perreault H. Mass spectrometric study of N-glycans from serum of woodchucks with liver cancer. *Rapid Commun Mass Spectrom*. 2009;23(18):2983–2995.

[29] Bellezza CA, Concannon PW, Hornbuckle WE, Roth L, Tennant B. Laboratory Animal Medicine. 2nd ed. Fox JG, Anderson LC, Loew FM, Quimby FW, editors. Academic Press; 2002.

[30] Tennant BC. *Handbook of animal models of infection: Experimental models in antimicrobial chemotherapy.* Zak O, Sande MA, editors. Academic Press, London UK; 1999.

[31] Buendia MA. *Viruses And Cancer: Fifty-First Symposium For The Society For General Microbiology,* Held At The University Of Cambridge, March 1. Minson A NJ, M M, editors. Cambridge University Press; 1994.

[32] Michalak TI. The Woodchuck Animal Model of Hepatitis B. *Viral Hepatitis Reviews*. 1998;4(3):139–165.

[33] Lisi D, Kondili LA, Ramieri MT, Giuseppetti R, Bruni R, Rocca CD, et al. Ultrasonography in the study of hepatocellular carcinoma in woodchucks chronically infected with WHV. *Lab Anim*. 2003;37(3):233–240.

[34] Nada T, Moriyasu F, Kono Y, Suginoshita Y, Matsumura T, Kobayashi K, et al. Sonographic detection of tumor blood flow using a new contrast agent in woodchuck hepatomas. *J Ultrasound Med*. 1997;16(7):485–491.

[35] Salem N, MacLennan GT, Kuang Y, Anderson PW, Schomisch SJ, Tochkov IA, et al. Quantitative evaluation of 2-deoxy-2[F-18]fluoro-D-glucose-positron emission tomography imaging on the woodchuck model of hepatocellular carcinoma with histological correlation. *Mol Imaging Biol*. 2007;9(3):135–143.

[36] McKenzie EJ, Jackson M, Turner A, Gregorash L, Harapiak L. Chronic care and monitoring of woodchucks (Marmota monax) during repeated magnetic resonance imaging of the liver. *J Am Assoc Lab Anim Sci*. 2006 Mar;45(2):26–30.

[37] Ohtomo SJSY K, Itai Y. [Iron oxide-enhanced MR imaging of hepatocellular carcinoma of woodchuck]. *Nippon Igaku Hoshasen Gakkai Zasshi*. 1991;51(5):433–435.

[38] Pützer BM, Stiewe T, Rödicker F, Schildgen O, Rühm S, Dirsch O, et al. Large nontransplanted hepatocellular carcinoma in woodchucks: treatment with adenovirus-mediated delivery of interleukin 12/B7.1 genes. *J Natl Cancer Inst*. 2001;93(6):472–479.

[39] Tennant BC, Toshkov IA, Peek SF, Jacob JR, Menne S, Hornbuckle WE, et al. Hepatocellular carcinoma in the woodchuck model of hepatitis B virus infection. *Gastroenterology.* 2004;127(5 Suppl 1):S283–S293.

[40] Cote PJ, Toshkov I, Bellezza C, Ascenzi M, Roneker C, Graham LA, et al. Temporal pathogenesis of experimental neonatal woodchuck hepatitis virus infection: increased initial viral load and decreased severity of acute hepatitis during the development of chronic viral infection. *Hepatology.* 2000;32(4 Pt 1):807–817.

[41] Wang Y, Menne S, Baldwin BH, Tennant BC, Gerin JL, Cote PJ. Kinetics of viremia and acute liver injury in relation to outcome of neonatal woodchuck hepatitis virus infection. *J Med Virol.* 2004;72(3):406–415.

[42] Wang Y, Menne S, Jacob JR, Tennant BC, Gerin JL, Cote PJ. Role of type 1 versus type 2 immune responses in liver during the onset of chronic woodchuck hepatitis virus infection. *Hepatology.* 2003;37(4):771–780.

[43] Liu CJ, Kao JH, Chen DS. Therapeutic implications of hepatitis B virus genotypes. *Liver Int.* 2005;25(6):1097–1107.

[44] Ni YH, Chang MH, Huang LM, Chen HL, Hsu HY, Chiu TY, et al. Hepatitis B virus infection in children and adolescents in a hyperendemic area: 15 years after mass hepatitis B vaccination. *Ann Intern Med.* 2001;135(9):796–800.

[45] Hann HWL, Lee J, Bussard A, Liu C, Jin YR, Guha K, et al. Preneoplastic markers of hepatitis B virus-associated hepatocellular carcinoma. *Cancer Res.* 2004;64(20):7329–7335.

[46] Tennant BC. Animal models of hepadnavirus-associated hepatocellular carcinoma. *Clin Liver Dis.* 2001;5(1):43–68.

[47] Bruni R, Conti I, Villano U, Giuseppetti R, Palmieri G, Rapicetta M. Lack of WHV integration nearby N-myc2 and in the downstream b3n and win loci in a considerable fraction of liver tumors with activated N-myc2 from naturally infected wild woodchucks. *Virology.* 2006;345(1):258–269.

[48] Jacob JR, Sterczer A, Toshkov IA, Yeager AE, Korba BE, Cote PJ, et al. Integration of woodchuck hepatitis and N-myc rearrangement determine size and histologic grade of hepatic tumors. *Hepatology.* 2004;39(4):1008–1016.

[49] Radaeva S, Li Y, Hacker HJ, Burger V, Kopp-Schneider A, Bannasch P. Hepadnaviral hepatocarcinogenesis: in situ visualization of viral antigens, cytoplasmic compartmentation, enzymic patterns, and cellular proliferation in preneoplastic hepatocellular lineages in woodchucks. *J Hepatol.* 2000;33(4):580–600.

[50] Ward J, Robinson PJ, Guthrie JA, Downing S, Wilson D, Lodge JPA, et al. Liver metastases in candidates for hepatic resection: comparison of helical CT and gadolinium- and SPIO-enhanced MR imaging. *Radiology.* 2005;237(1):170–180.

[51] Bell JD, Cox IJ, Sargentoni J, Peden CJ, Menon DK, Foster CS, et al. A 31P and 1H-NMR investigation in vitro of normal and abnormal human liver. *Biochim Biophys Acta.* 1993;1225(1):71–77.

[52] Dezortova M, Taimr P, Skoch A, Spicak J, Hajek M. Etiology and functional status of liver cirrhosis by 31P MR spectroscopy. *World J Gastroenterol.* 2005;11(44):6926–6931.

[53] Lim AKP, Patel N, Hamilton G, Hajnal JV, Goldin RD, Taylor-Robinson SD. The relationship of in vivo 31P MR spectroscopy to histology in chronic hepatitis C. *Hepatology.* 2003;37(4):788–794.

[54] Dagnelie PC, Sijens PE, Kraus DJ, Planting AS, van Dijk P. Abnormal liver metabolism in cancer patients detected by (31)P MR spectroscopy. *NMR Biomed.* 1999;12(8):535–544.

[55] Leij-Halfwerk S, van den Berg JW, Sijens PE, Wilson JH, Oudkerk M, Dagnelie PC. Altered hepatic gluconeogenesis during L-alanine infusion in weight-losing lung cancer patients as observed by phosphorus magnetic resonance spectroscopy and turnover measurements. *Cancer Res.* 2000;60(3):618–623.

[56] Hornbuckle WE, Graham ES, Roth L, Baldwin BH, Wickenden C, Tennant BC. Laboratory assessment of hepatic injury in the woodchuck (Marmota monax). *Lab Anim Sci.* 1985;35(4):376–381.

[57] Tomanek B, Volotovskyy V, Gruwel MLH, McKenzie E, King SB. Double-frequency birdcage volume coil for 4.7T and 7T. *Concepts in Magnetic Resonance Part B, Magnetic Resonance Engineering.* 2005;26(1):16–22.

[58] Glazer GM, Smith SR, Chenevert TL, Martin PA, Stevens AN, Edwards RH. Image localized 31P magnetic resonance spectroscopy of the human liver. *NMR Biomed.* 1989;1(4):184–189.

[59] Taylor-Robinson SD, Sargentoni J, Bell JD, Thomas EL, Marcus CD, Changani KK, et al. In vivo and in vitro hepatic phosphorus-31 magnetic resonance spectroscopy and electron microscopy in chronic ductopenic rejection of human liver allografts. *Gut.* 1998;42(5):735–743.

[60] Corbin IR, Ryner LN, Singh H, Minuk GY. Quantitative hepatic phosphorus-31 magnetic resonance spectroscopy in compensated and decompensated cirrhosis. *Am J Physiol Gastrointest Liver Physiol.* 2004;287(2):G379–G384.

[61] Krueger KE, Srivastava S. Posttranslational protein modifications: current implications for cancer detection, prevention, and therapeutics. *Mol Cell Proteomics.* 2006;5(10):1799–1810.

[62] Crocker PR, Feizi T. Carbohydrate recognition systems: functional triads in cell-cell interactions. *Curr Opin Struct Biol.* 1996;6(5):679–691.

[63] Varki A, Cummings R, Esko J, Freeze H, Hart G, Marth J, editors. *Essentials of Glycobiology.* Cold Spring Harbor Laboratory Press; 1999.

[64] Yarema KJ, Bertozzi CR. Characterizing glycosylation pathways. *Genome Biol.* 2001;2(5):REVIEWS0004.

[65] Bertozzi CR, Kiessling LL. Chemical glycobiology. *Science.* 2001;291(5512):2357–2364.

[66] Schachter H. Biosynthetic controls that determine the branching and microheterogeneity of protein-bound oligosaccharides. *Biochem Cell Biol.* 1986;64(3):163–181.

[67] Rademacher TW, Parekh RB, Dwek RA. Glycobiology. *Annu Rev Biochem.* 1988;57:785–838.

[68] Zhao Y, Sato Y, Isaji T, Fukuda T, Matsumoto A, Miyoshi E, et al. Branched N-glycans regulate the biological functions of integrins and cadherins. *FEBS J.* 2008;275(9):1939–1948.

[69] Yoshima H, Mizuochi T, Ishii M, Kobata A. Structure of the asparagine-linked sugar chains of alpha-fetoprotein purified from human ascites fluid. *Cancer Res.* 1980;40(11):4276–4281.

[70] Deutsch HF. Chemistry and biology of alpha-fetoprotein. *Adv Cancer Res.* 1991;56:253–312.

[71] Mizejewski GJ. Alpha-fetoprotein structure and function: relevance to isoforms, epitopes, and conformational variants. *Exp Biol Med (Maywood).* 2001;226(5):377–408.

[72] Alpert E, Drysdale JW, Isselbacher KJ, Schur PH. Human -fetoprotein. Isolation, characterization, and demonstration of microheterogeneity. *J Biol Chem.* 1972;247(12):3792–3798.

[73] Kerckaert JP, Bayard B, Biserte G. Microheterogeneity of rat, mouse and human alpha1-fetoprotein as revealed by polyacrylamide gel electrophoresis and by crossed immuno-affino-electrophoresis with different lectins. *Biochim Biophys Acta.* 1979;576(1):99–108.

[74] Saitoh S, Ikeda K, Koida I, Suzuki Y, Kobayashi M, Tsubota A, et al. Diagnosis of hepatocellular carcinoma by concanavalin A affinity electrophoresis of serum alpha-fetoprotein. *Cancer.* 1995;76(7):1139–1144.

[75] Aoyagi Y, Isemura M, Suzuki Y, Sekine C, Soga K, Ozaki T, et al. Fucosylated alpha-fetoprotein as marker of early hepatocellular carcinoma. *Lancet.* 1985;2(8468):1353–1354.

[76] Aoyagi Y, Isemura M, Suzuki Y, Sekine C, Soga K, Ozaki T, et al. Change in fucosylation of alpha-fetoprotein on malignant transformation of liver cells. *Lancet.* 1986;1(8474):210.

[77] Kladney RD, Bulla GA, Guo L, Mason AL, Tollefson AE, Simon DJ, et al. GP73, a novel Golgi-localized protein upregulated by viral infection. *Gene.* 2000;249(1-2):53–65.

[78] Kladney RD, Cui X, Bulla GA, Brunt EM, Fimmel CJ. Expression of GP73, a resident Golgi membrane protein, in viral and nonviral liver disease. *Hepatology.* 2002;35(6):1431–1440.

[79] Norton PA, Comunale MA, Krakover J, Rodemich L, Pirog N, D'Amelio A, et al. N-linked glycosylation of the liver cancer biomarker GP73. *J Cell Biochem.* 2008;104(1):136–149.

[80] Nakagawa T, Uozumi N, Nakano M, Mizuno-Horikawa Y, Okuyama N, Taguchi T, et al. Fucosylation of N-glycans regulates the secretion of hepatic glycoproteins into bile ducts. *J Biol Chem.* 2006;281(40):29797–29806.

[81] Wang M, Long RE, Comunale MA, Junaidi O, Marrero J, Bisceglie AMD, et al. Novel fucosylated biomarkers for the early detection of hepatocellular carcinoma. *Cancer Epidemiol Biomarkers Prev.* 2009;18(6):1914–1921.

[82] Comunale MA, Wang M, Hafner J, Krakover J, Rodemich L, Kopenhaver B, et al. Identification and development of fucosylated glycoproteins as biomarkers of primary hepatocellular carcinoma. *J Proteome Res.* 2009;8(2):595–602.

[83] Debruyne EN, Vanderschaeghe D, Vlierberghe HV, Vanhecke A, Callewaert N, Delanghe JR. Diagnostic value of the hemopexin N-glycan profile in hepatocellular carcinoma patients. *Clin Chem.* 2010;56(5):823–831.

[84] Takahashi N, Takahashi Y, Putnam FW. Complete amino acid sequence of human hemopexin, the heme-binding protein of serum. *Proc Natl Acad Sci U S A.* 1985;82(1):73–77.

[85] Callewaert N, Vlierberghe HV, Hecke AV, Laroy W, Delanghe J, Contreras R. Non-invasive diagnosis of liver cirrhosis using DNA sequencer-based total serum protein glycomics. *Nat Med.* 2004;10(4):429–434.

[86] Vanderschaeghe D, Laroy W, Sablon E, Halfon P, Hecke AV, Delanghe J, et al. GlycoFibroTest is a highly performant liver fibrosis biomarker derived from DNA sequencer-based serum protein glycomics. *Mol Cell Proteomics.* 2009;8(5):986–994.

[87] Morelle W, Flahaut C, Michalski JC, Louvet A, Mathurin P, Klein A. Mass spectrometric approach for screening modifications of total serum N-glycome in human diseases: application to cirrhosis. *Glycobiology.* 2006;16(4):281–293.

[88] Chan AC, Atkinson JP. Oligosaccharide structure of human C4. *J Immunol.* 1985;134(3):1790–1798.

[89] Wu YL, Higgins GC, Rennebohm RM, Chung EK, Yang Y, Zhou B, et al. Three distinct profiles of serum complement C4 proteins in pediatric systemic lupus erythematosus (SLE) patients: tight associations of complement C4 and C3 protein levels in SLE but not in healthy subjects. *Adv Exp Med Biol.* 2006;586:227–247.

[90] Hofmann M, Pichler B, Schölkopf B, Beyer T. Towards quantitative PET/MRI: a review of MR-based attenuation correction techniques. *Eur J Nucl Med Mol Imaging*. 2009;36 Suppl 1:S93–104.

In: Liver Cancer: Causes, Diagnosis and Treatment
Editor: Benjamin J. Valverde

ISBN: 978-1-61209-115-0
©2011 Nova Science Publishers, Inc.

*Chapter VII*

# Cost Effectiveness Analysis
# of Liver Transplantation

## *Haruhisa Fukuda[1] and Hirohisa Imai[2]*
[1]Institute for Health Economics and Policy, Japan
[2] National Institute of Public Health, Department of Epidemiology,
Wako, Japan

For patients with end-stage liver disease (ESLD), liver transplantation is an established therapy. The efficacy of deceased donor liver transplantation (DDLT) has been verified in various studies, and the procedure is a socially acceptable medical technique. On the other hand, one current challenge is the increase in the number of DDLT cases, causing longer waiting periods for available organs, a situation that has been recognized as a social issue. Living donor liver transplantation (LDLT) is performed as an alternative.

However, liver transplantation is a costly medical procedure. Thus, it is difficult to determine whether a novel technique should be covered by health insurance solely from the perspective of its effectiveness, given the intense pressure to reduce medical costs. Health economics assessment (HEA) takes into account both economics and effectiveness. Therefore, such assessment should be carried out and the results should be presented and understood by the public before a new technique is accepted.

This chapter summarizes past findings regarding cost, effectiveness, and cost-effectiveness, and offers points to consider when conducting an adequate HEA. After reading this chapter, readers will be able to perform cost-effectiveness analyses adequately not only for liver transplantation but also for other health technologies.

This chapter consists of the following 7 sections. Section 1 shows trends in the number of liver transplantation cases and current survival data. Costs associated with liver transplantation are discussed in Section 2. We conduct a systematic review and present the cost estimates of liver transplantation. Additionally, we examine the quality of cost studies and discuss the costing and reporting methods that enable the readers to make appropriate decisions. Furthermore, from the viewpoint of international comparisons, we compare a breakdown of the costs of liver transplantation. With regard to effectiveness, we provide an introduction to the methods used to assess utility. We also list past publications that have estimated utility scores. Section 4 provides a systematic review of the cost-effectiveness of liver transplantation and examines whether liver transplantation is cost-effective. Section 5 examines cost-utility analyses for LDLT conducted in Japan. There are very few reports of such studies. In Section 6, we discuss practical aspects of undertaking cost-effectiveness analyses: which cost items should be included in a cost analysis and how cost-effectiveness should be judged are the major issues addressed in this section. We also examine ethical issues in resource allocation that a cost-effectiveness analysis alone is unable to deal with. Finally, in Section 7, we conclude the chapter with some further recommendations on how to conduct cost-effectiveness analyses.

# 1. Current Status of Liver Transplantation

## 1.1. Number of Liver Transplantations Cases

The first human liver transplantation was performed at the University of Colorado by Starzl in 1963. The number of liver transplantation cases increased from the 1980s to the 1990s, and over 5000 patients per year received liver transplants after 2001. Liver transplantation has been widely performed in advanced countries, with the cumulative number of cases totaling approximately 103,000 in the US as of August 23, 2010 [1] and approximately 88,000 in the EU as of June 2009 [2]. Liver transplantation has been accepted as an established therapy for ESLD patients. By the end of 2008, there were approximately 5,300 cases of liver transplantation reported in Japan.

However, there are significant differences in the number ratio of LDLT cases to DDLT cases in Western countries versus that in Japan. DDLT is the major liver transplantation performed in the US and Europe. For a period of time however, the US has steered toward an increase in the number of LDLT cases. The lack of deceased donors owing to an increase in the number of DDLT cases is expected to be solved with the use of living donors. The proportion of LDLT cases was 10.1% (524 cases) of all liver transplantation cases (5195) (Table 1) in 2001. However, once a dead case is reported, the number of LDLT cases has decreased rapidly to ensure donor safety. As a result, LDLT accounted for fewer than 4% of all cases in 2009 [1]. Also in Europe, deceased donors are commonly used in liver transplantation and the proportion of LDLT cases was only 3.9% [2]. In contrast, 400-500 liver transplantations per year are performed in Japan, and most of them are LDLT [3]. This represents a large difference between Western countries and Japan.

**Table 1. Trends of number of liver transplantation cases**

| | | Total | 2010 | 2009 | 2008 | 2007 | 2006 | 2005 | 2004 | 2003 | 2002 | 2001 | 2000 |
|---|---|---|---|---|---|---|---|---|---|---|---|---|---|
| USA | Total | 103,427 | 2,634 | 6,320 | 6,319 | 6,494 | 6,651 | 6,444 | 6,171 | 5,673 | 5,332 | 5,196 | 5,000 |
| | CDLT | 99,301 | 2,510 | 6,101 | 6,070 | 6,228 | 6,363 | 6,121 | 5,848 | 5,351 | 4,969 | 4,672 | 4,595 |
| | CDLT, % | 96.0% | 95.3% | 96.5% | 96.1% | 95.9% | 95.7% | 95.0% | 94.8% | 94.3% | 93.2% | 89.9% | 91.9% |
| Europe | Total | 87,964 | - | 4,646 | 5,638 | 5,490 | 5,481 | 5,422 | 5,096 | 5,142 | 4,948 | 4,821 | 4,587 |
| Japan | Total | 5,250 | - | - | 477 | 443 | 510 | 566 | 554 | 442 | 441 | 423 | 333 |
| | CDLT | 61 | - | - | 13 | 10 | 5 | 4 | 3 | 2 | 7 | 6 | 6 |
| | CDLT, % | 1.2% | - | - | 2.7% | 2.3% | 1.0% | 0.7% | 0.5% | 0.5% | 1.6% | 1.4% | 1.8% |

## 1.2. Survival Rates in Liver Transplantation

Table 2 shows survival rates by country. The US and countries in the Europe have similar survival rates for patients who have undergone DDLT. The 1- and 5-year survival rates are 87.3% and 73.4% in the US, [1], and 83% and 71% in the Europe, respectively [2]. On the other hand, the 1-year and 5-year survival rates of LDLT are 83.2% and 76.8% in Japan [3]. They are 91.7% and 77.7% in the US respectively [1], which is not significantly different from those in Japan.

**Table 2. Survival rates in liver transplantation**

| Country | DD or LD | n | Survival rates | | | |
|---|---|---|---|---|---|---|
| | | | 1 year | 3 year | 5 year | 10 year |
| US [1] | DD | 10,533 | 87.3 | — | 73.4 | 58.7 |
| | LD | 592 | 91.7 | — | 77.7 | 70.7 |
| Europe [2] | Total | 63,221 | 83 | — | 71 | 61 |
| Japan [3] | DD | 61 | 77.0 | 75.3 | 72.1 | 68.3 |
| | LD | 5,189 | 83.2 | 79.1 | 76.8 | 72.8 |

DD: deceased donor liver transplantation.
LD: living donor liver transplantation.

# 2. Cost of Liver Transplantation

## 2.1. Systematic Review of Liver Transplantation Costs

Liver transplantation is an established treatment for patients with ESLD. However, liver transplantation involves high medical costs because of multiple diagnostic procedures, a surgery lasting many hours, a long hospital stay with intensive care, and long-term immunosuppressive therapy. Under the current cost-containment policy, it is imperative for both insurers and policy makers to determine how much a liver transplantation costs. Thus, in this section, we aim to conduct a systematic review of published studies in which the costs of liver transplantation that have been estimated.

Using the MEDLINE database, we conducted a literature search up to June 30, 2010. For search keywords we used "Liver Transplantation" [MESH] AND "Costs and Cost Analysis" [MESH], and as a result, we retrieved 310 papers. We identify papers that potentially provide therapeutic cost estimations of liver transplantation through titles and abstracts, and examined the entire texts of the papers. Furthermore, we analyzed the references cited in the studies obtained in the MEDLINE search. When screening was reasonably complete, we selected 38 papers that actually provided cost estimates of liver transplantation for the use in our review [4–41].

Table 3 provides an overview of 89 studies conducted between 1990 and 2009 that assessed the costs of liver transplantation. All reported costs were converted to US dollars for the year 2009. Because of differences in purchasing power parity (PPP) and the year of study between the articles, we adjusted the cost estimates using the PPP for gross domestic product

(GDP) between the US and other countries, and the consumer price index (CPI) for the US. PPP for GDP is reported by OECD and CPI was provided by the US Bureau of Labor Statistics (http://www.bls.gov/cpi/). A major finding from the included studies was the large variation in cost estimates because of the variety of cost scope used in the studies, which prevented meaningful comparison between them. Thus, readers seeking estimates of liver transplantation costs must pay close attention when interpreting such estimates. Although some studies included costs from pretransplantation to post-transplantation, the majority estimated and reported costs only for the liver transplantation operation itself. However, even focusing solely on the liver transplantation itself, to increase comparability between the publications, the reported costs per case ranged from US$59,396 to US$312,665.

## Table 3. Costs of liver transplantation

| First author | Country | Study duration | n | Cost estimates (US$, 2009) | | | |
|---|---|---|---|---|---|---|---|
| | | | | Pre | Operataion | Post | Total |
| Buchanan [4] | USA | 2002.3-2007.8 | 990 | 135,155 | 312,665 | 79,257 | 552,204 |
| Markley [5] | USA | 2004.1-2006.2 | 166 | excl. | 117,254 | excl. | 117,254 |
| Passarani [6] | Italy | 2001.6-2003.11 | 12 | 239,124[a] | | excl. | 239,124 |
| Englesbe [7] | USA | 2002.7-2005.6 | 240 | excl. | 214,032 | excl. | 214,032 |
| Ishida [8] | Japan | 1999.1-2001.12 | 11 | 8,962 | 190,532[b] | | 199,494 |
| Kogure [9] | Japan | 2001.9-2005.1 | 17 | excl. | 107,544[b] | | 107,544 |
| Washburn [10] | USA | 2002.2-2004.5 | 222 | excl. | 85,542[b] | | 85,542 |
| Kraus [11] | Germany | 2003.6-2003.9 | 38 | excl. | 62,234 | excl. | 62,234 |
| Oostenbrink [12] | Netherlands | 1995.1-2001.8 | 179 | 189,144[c] | | | 189,144 |
| Reed [13] | USA | Unknown | 888 | excl. | 198,420 | excl. | 198,420 |
| Brand [14] | USA | 1996.11-1997.12 | 26 | 90,142 | 207,326[b] | | 297,467 |
| Cole [15] | USA | 1997.1-2002.1 | 47 | excl. | 127,906 | 196,667 | 324,572 |
| Filipponi [16] | Italy | 1997.1-2000.12 | 252 | excl. | 119,288[b] | | 119,288 |
| Longworth [17] | UK | 1995.12-1996.12 | 208 | 128,236[c] | | | 128,236 |
| Trotter [18] | USA | 1997.8-2000.6 | 67 | 9,831 | 127,210 | 43,112 | 180,153 |
| Azoulay [19] | France | 1986.9-1999.9 | 139 | excl. | 116,627[b] | | 116,627 |
| Sagmeister [20] | Switzerland | 1995.1-2000.10 | 51 | excl. | 81,477 | 12,350 | 93,827 |
| Taylor [21] | Canada | 1991.1-1992.12 | 119 | 676 | 67,861 | 6,046 | 110,307 |
| Skeike [22] | Norway | 1998.1-1998.7 | 8 | excl. | 77,783 | excl. | 77,783 |
| Best [23] | USA | 1993.1-1999.12 | 1621 | 13,071 | 179,425 | 51,204 | 243,699 |
| Bucuvalas [24] | USA | 1994.3-1999.4 | 83 | excl. | 194,684[b] | | 194,684 |
| Nair [25] | USA | 1994.1-1996.12 | 121 | excl. | 151,168 | excl. | 151,168 |
| Schnitzler [26] | USA | 1990.4-1994.6 | 683 | excl. | 269,768 | excl. | 269,768 |
| van Agthoven [27] | Netherlands | 1993.1-1997.11 | 100 | 32,828 | 122,727[b] | | 155,554 |
| Freeman [28] | USA | Unknown | 37 | excl. | 82,378[b] | | 82,378 |
| Gilbert [29] | USA | 1991.1-1996.12 | 144 | 43,467 | 209,673[b] | | 253,139 |
| Rufat [30] | France | 1994.1-1995.12 | 71 | 13,448 | 79,431[b] | | 92,879 |
| Showstack [31] | USA | 1991.1-1994.7 | 711 | excl. | 286,379 | excl. | 286,379 |
| Brown [32] | USA | 1992.6-1993.6 | 111 | excl. | 299,501 | excl. | 299,501 |
| Geevarghese [33] | USA | 1991.2-1996.3 | 100 | excl. | 153,633 | excl. | 153,633 |
| Russo [34] | USA | 1991.9-1996.12 | 130 | excl. | 148,230 | excl. | 148,230 |
| Schulak [35] | USA | 1984.7-1996.6 | 935 | excl. | 123,923 | excl. | 123,923 |
| Brown [36] | USA | 1992.7-1993.6 | 111 | excl. | 299,501 | excl. | 299,501 |
| Smith [37] | USA | 1990.1-1992.12 | 91 | excl. | 309,530[b] | | 309,530 |
| Pageaux [38] | France | 1989.3-1991.12 | 39 | excl. | 120,084[b] | | 120,084 |
| Evans [39] | USA | 1988.1-1988.12 | unknown | excl. | 216,460 | excl. | 216,460 |
| Burroughs [40] | UK | 1988.10-1989.10 | 23 | excl. | 59,396 | 5,281 | 64,677 |
| Bonsel [41] | Netherlands | 1979.3-1987.9 | 76 | 39,781 | 137,002 | 88,027 | 264,810 |

excl.: excluded.

[a]: Total costs of pretransplantation and operation.

[b]: Total costs of operation and posttransplantation.

[c]: Total costs of pretransplantation, operation and posttransplantation.

## 2.2. International Comparison of Cost Estimates

The US carried out the majority of studies on liver transplantation cost analysis, accounting for 57.9% (22 of 38 papers). Studies were also conducted in the Netherlands (3) France (3), the UK (2), Italy (2), Japan (2), Germany (1), Norway (1), Switzerland (1), and Canada (1). An analysis of the number of papers published by continent showed 25 in North America, 13 in Europe, and 2 in Asia (both in Japan).

A comparison of the reported cost estimates (2009 US$) showed that the cost of liver transplantation in the US was higher than that in other countries. (Figure 1). As for the costs of pretransplantation, there seems to be no significant difference in median cost between the US and Europe (US: US$43,467 versus Europe: US$32,828). However, the cost studies conducted in the US showed large variations in cost estimates (min: US$43,467 versus max: US$135,155). Although liver transplantation itself performed in the US would cost in an estimated ranged from US$117,254 to US$312,665, the costs of liver transplantation reported from Europe ranged from US$59,396 to US$137,002.

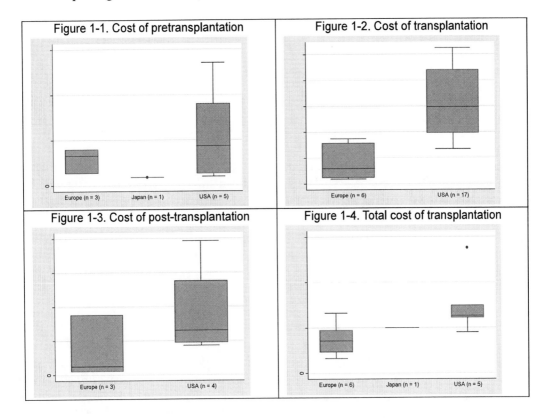

Figure 1. International comparison of liver transplantation costs.

The median cost estimate from the US is about 2.5 times that from Europe (US: US$198,420 versus Europe: US$79,630). Regarding post-transplantation costs, there is also a large difference between the US and European values, namely US$65,231 (median) and US$12,350 (median), respectively. When the total costs of liver transplantation, including pretransplantation, transplantation itself, and post-transplantation, were compared, the highest cost estimates are from the US, followed by Japan and Europe. For Japan, however, there is only one reported study in which cost estimates for LDLT were investigated.

We examined whether the breakdown of costs for liver transplantation differed between the US and Europe. Table 4 shows the results by publication and area. Of the 38 publications that estimated costs of liver transplantation, we identified seven studies that included professional fees in the cost estimates and reported the breakdown of those costs; there were five studies from Europe and two from the US. Although the study conducted by Gilvert *et al.* [29] did not report professional fees in their cost estimates, they may have been included in other cost components.

**Table 4. Comparison of breakdown of costs of liver transplantation: Europe vs. US**

| Region | Europe | | | | | USA | |
|---|---|---|---|---|---|---|---|
| First author | Oostenbrink [12] | van Aghoven [27] | Burroughs [40] | Filipponi [16] | Rufat [30] | Gilbert [29] | Evans [39] |
| Country | Netherlands | Netherlands | UK | Italy | France | USA | USA |
| Professional fees | 13.6% | 38.8% | 32.5% | 18.9% | 29.4% | — | 16.7% |
| Hospitalization | 36.5% | 16.8% | — | 18.7% | 18.9% | 34.9% | 9.4% |
| Transplantation | 7.6% | 6.6% | 6.0% | 1.3% | 2.9% | 14.8% | 20.3% |
| Medication | 8.8% | 10.9% | 8.5% | 15.1% | 16.5% | 5.9% | 6.5% |
| Diagnostic | 20.4% | 2.6% | 37.0% | 27.9% | 16.6% | 18.4% | 29.2% |
| Blood | — | 2.9% | 3.5% | — | 9.1% | 26.0% | 3.9% |
| Others | 13.1% | 21.4% | 12.5% | 18.1% | 6.6% | 0.0% | 14.0% |

7 studies that included professional fees in the costs estimates and reported the breakdown of costs.

There was a large difference in the proportion of total cost due to the liver transplantation itself between the US and Europe. The costs of transplantation accounted, on average, for less than 10% of the total cost in Europe but for 15-20% in the US. In terms of medications, although some studies from Europe reported that the costs of medications accounted for more than 10% of the total, studies from the US reported proportions of only 5-6%. Regarding diagnostics, however, the proportions ranged from 20% to 30% in studies from both Europe and the US.

## 2.3. Reasons Why the Cost Estimate Varies

As shown in Table 3 and Figure 1, cost estimate highly varied among publications, even within the same country. Why was there such a high variability in cost estimate among publications? The following factors account for such large differences in the cost of treatment and operations for the same disease within the same country among studies [42-44]:

[1] Severity of the disease
[2] Including scope and expense of items included in cost estimation
[3] Individual medical treatment per unit
[4] Cost estimation methodology

The above-mentioned factors greatly diminish the possibility of establishing any form of generalizability. Thus, reported cost estimates should not be directly applied to another researcher's findings, but instead as Cronbach advised, these estimates should be treated as "working assumptions" and applied indirectly [45]. That is, the working assumptions used in cost estimation should be considered in the context of where and how the estimates were intended to be used. In particular, regarding cost data, researchers should report the factors mentioned above.

## 2.4. Evaluation of the Quality of Cost Studies

Researchers must increase the transferability of their cost estimates for readers to be able to meaningfully extrapolate these estimates to studies in their own institutions or countries. Although past studies showed detailed information on disease severity, insufficient attention has been paid to the following three perspectives:

[1] Reporting the scope of costing explicitly
[2] Reporting unit costs explicitly
[3] Reporting costing methods explicitly

Table 5 shows the evaluation criteria for the transferability of cost studies

### Table 5. Evaluation criteria for transferability of cost studies

| Axis | Criteria |
|---|---|
| [1] Reporting the scope of costing explicitly | (A) All components of costs were described and data on costs in each component were reported |
| | (B) All components of costs were described but data on costs in each component were not reported |
| | (C) Only scope of costing was described but components of costs were not described |
| [2] Reporting unit costs explicitly | Unit costs were reported |
| | Unit costs were not reported |
| [3] Reporting costing methods explicitly | Microcosting |
| | Costs extracted from the hospital accounting system |
| | Costs calculated using cost-to-charge ratio |
| | Medicare Fee |
| | Charge |

As the first perspective, we assess whether estimates have clarified the scopes of costing, and we have established a hierarchy of three levels of transparency as follows:

A. All components of costs were described and data on costs in each component were reported.
B. All components of costs were described, but data on costs in each component were not reported.
C. Only the scope of costing was described, and components of costs were not described.

Cost studies that provide a clear description of the scope of costing and data on costs in each component (Level A) are the most valuable. Such studies enable readers to determine whether the estimates include cost items without exaggeration or omission (internal validity). Furthermore, because there is detailed information regarding costs in each component, the reader can comparatively evaluate the cost component in his or her own institution versus the institution where the original evaluation was conducted. It is thus possible to adjust for intrinsic differences and to allow the reader to apply these to his or her own institution (external validity). Cost studies that report all components of costs alone (Level B) enable readers to assess the internal validity of the cost estimates. However, readers would be unable to determine the potential applicability to their own settings. Cost studies that provide limited descriptions of the scope of costing (Level C) have little value, because readers would be unable to determine either internal or external validity.

As variations in unit costs are affected by country or hospital, it is desirable that cost estimates provide data on unit costs (as the second axis) explicitly. Because providing exact data on unit costs for all items used would be unnecessarily expensive, a cost study should provide unit costs for high-cost items. For readers, such data on unit costs contribute to being able to assess extrapolation of a cost study.

To report costing methods (the third axis) has two meanings. First, readers should be able to understand the viewpoint of the analysis reported. This is essential, because an item may be a cost from one viewpoint, but not from another. Second, readers should be able to understand the types of costs included in the analysis. Resource uses and their costs can be divided into resource use directly attributable to the patient, such as professional fees for intervention and medications, and resource use indirectly attributable to the patient, such as overhead costs. According to such information on costing methods, readers will be able to determine which cost components the cost study included and the degree of accuracy of the cost estimates.

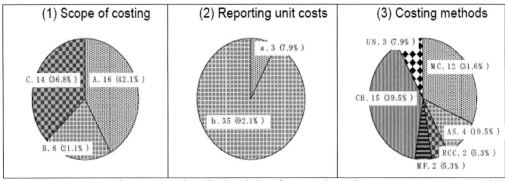

(1) A: All components of costs were described and data for costs in each component were reported, B: All components of costs were described but data for costs in each component were not reported, C: Only scope of costing was described but components of costs were not described.
(2) a: Unit costs were reported, b: Unit costs were not reported.
(3) MC: Microcosting, AS: Costs extracted from the hospital accounting system, RCC: Costs calculated using cost-to-charge ratio, MF: Medicare Fee, CH: Charge, UN: Unknown.

Figure 2. Results of cost study transferability.

Methods for estimating costs can be broadly categorized into five types: charges, costs calculated using the cost-to-charge ratio (RCC), Medicare fees, costs extracted from a hospital accounting system, and microcosting. Because the costing method used in a cost study likely depends on the study aim, there is no one answer as to which costing method is best for estimating costs. Moreover, some charges are determined politically and therefore have high usability only for other researchers in the same country subject to the same insurance/reimbursement payment systems. The ability to extrapolate such information to different countries is greatly reduced. Furthermore, because cost estimates using RCC include the influence of charge data, it is not desirable to extrapolate such information to different countries.

Results of the evaluation of transferability of cost studies are shown in Figure 2. The transferability of the scope of costing was graded from Levels A to C. There were 16 (42.1%) studies graded Level A, eight (21.1%) studies graded Level B, and 14 (36.8%) studies graded Level C. There were only three (7.9%) studies that showed unit cost data.

Regarding costing methods, in 15 (40%) studies, cost estimates were calculated using charges. This was followed by 12 (31.6%) publications with cost estimates calculated using microcosting methods, four (10.5%) publications using hospital accounting systems, two (5.3%) studies that used RCC, and two (5.3%) studies using Medicare fee information. There were also three (7.9%) studies with an unknown method of costing. When there is no information regarding costing methods in a cost study, readers are unable to determine the study viewpoint or costing scope, and thus the study loses its value.

# 3. Effectiveness of Liver Transplantation

Although several indicators can be used to assess the effectiveness of liver transplantation for ESLD, one of the most important indicators is survival rate. Given advances in medical technology, 1-year survival rates for liver transplantation now exceed 80% in developed countries and exceed 70% at 5 years. Now, improvement in health-related quality of life is an essential component to assess.

## 3.1. Methods to Assess Utility of Liver Transplantation

Methods to assess health-related quality of life can be categorized into two types: "health status assessment," which assesses the state of health and its influence on function and disability, and "utility assessment," which evaluates the value or desirability of a particular health state. In this section, we focus only on utility assessment. The most simple and straightforward instrument is the visual analog scale (VAS) method. Although VAS is strictly a rating rather than a utility measure, it is often used in utility assessment. A method fully consistent with expected utility theory is that of the standard gamble (SG). However, the SG approach involves respondents' understanding of the concept of probabilities, which is difficult for some people. Instead, the time trade-off approach was developed to avoid the concept of probabilities. These evaluation methods, however, are relatively time-consuming for assessments and involve cognitive effort by respondents. To minimize these problems, indirect measurement methods have been developed. Three instruments in common use today are the EuroQol (EQ-5D), Short Form Six Dimensions (SF-6D) and Health Utilities Index

(HUI). For each instrument, patients are asked to complete a simple questionnaire that defines their generic state of health, and the appropriate utility is determined from a scoring algorithm. In many studies, the utility scores of patients who underwent liver transplantation since the late 1990s have been examined and assessed using the following instruments: VAS [46,50], TTO [46], SG [46,50], SG-transformed VAS [51], EQ-5D [47-50,52,53], HUI [50], and SF-6D [47].

## 3.2. Utility in Liver Transplantation Patients

Researchers have assessed utility in patients who underwent liver transplantations, both pre- and post-transplantation (Table 6). For example, Sherman *et al.* evaluated utility in patients waiting for liver transplants [46]. They interviewed 10 patients and assessed utility scores using VAS, TTO, and SG instruments. The mean ± SE VAS score was 0.62 ± 0.06. In contrast, the mean ± SE TTO and SG scores were 0.81 ± 0.10 and 0.72 ± 0.10, respectively. These results showed that VAS yielded the lowest score, SG the middle score, and TTO the highest score. Three reported studies have shown the estimated utility scores using the EQ-5D instrument; the scores ranged from 0.462 to 0.53 [47-49]. Regarding the SF-6D instrument, in one reported study, the score was 0.606, which was higher than that using EQ-5D [47].

**Table 6. Utility scores for liver transplantation**

| First author | n | VAS | TTO | SG | SG-transformed VAS | HUI | EQ5D | SF6D |
|---|---|---|---|---|---|---|---|---|
| *Pre-liver transplantation* | | | | | | | | |
| Sherman[a] [46] | 10 | 0.62 | 0.81 | 0.72 | — | — | — | — |
| Longworth [47] | 183 | — | — | — | — | — | 0.517 | 0.606 |
| Ratcliffe [48] | 164 | — | — | — | — | — | 0.53 | — |
| Ratcliffe [49] | 279 | — | — | — | — | — | 0.462 | — |
| *Post-liver transplantation* | | | | | | | | |
| Chong[a] [50] | 30 | 0.65 | — | 0.73 | — | 0.7 | 0.69 | — |
| Siebert[a] [51] | 8 | — | — | — | 0.86 | — | — | — |
| Longworth [47] | 183 | — | — | — | — | — | 0.608 | 0.615 |
| Ratcliffe[b] [48] | 164 | — | — | — | — | — | 0.62 | — |
| Ratcliffe[b] [49] | 279 | — | — | — | — | — | 0.636 | — |
| Bryan [52] | 121 | — | — | — | — | — | 0.75 | — |
| Lewis[c] [53] | 12 | — | — | — | — | — | 0.74 | — |

a. Patients with hepatitis C only.
b. 3 months post-liver transplantation.
c. median.

In seven reported studies, post-transplantation was assessed utility scores. The most common method used was EQ-5D. Although the instrument and patient population varied, reported scores ranged from 0.6 to 0.7 [47-53]. Changes in utility scores of patients pre- and post-transplantation were reported in two studies [47,48]. In the study by Longworth and Bryan [47], the utility score determined by EQ-5D improved significantly from 0.517 to 0.608 ($p < 0.05$), whereas the mean SF-6D score at 12 months post-transplantation was not significantly different from the pretransplant score (0.606 vs. 0.615). In the study by Ratcliffe *et al.* [48], the EQ-5D scores at pre- and post-transplantation showed a statistically significant improvement from 0.53 to 0.62 ($p = 0.003$).

# 4. Cost Effectiveness of Liver Transplantation

In Sections 2 and 3, we provided an overview of studies examining cost and effectiveness, respectively. Although liver transplantation is a high-cost intervention benefiting relatively few people, currently, post-liver transplantation survival rates are high and patient utility significantly improves from pre- to post-transplantation. Next, in Section 4, we examine by cost-effectiveness analysis (CEA) whether liver transplantation is worth implementing.

Although liver transplantation is an expensive medical technique, it contributes to the prolongation of life and improvement of utility in patients with ESLD. However, not enough medical resources are available, and the balance between effectiveness and economics should be evaluated to be able to propose a method of resource allocation. Therefore, CEA and cost-utility analysis (CUA) are effective approaches. In Section 4, we analyze whether liver transplantation is a technique that provides a high cost-effectiveness.

The four HEA studies published from 1990 to 2002 were reviewed by Ishida and Imai *et al.*[54]. The studies include those conducted in the US [55], Netherlands [56], Switzerland [20], and Japan [57]. Life-year extension as an outcome index was used in three CEA studies and quality-adjusted life year (QALY) was used in one CUA study. Additionally, of these 4 studies, HEA was performed for DDLT in three studies and for LDLT in two studies.

In this section, we will first summarize the results of the incremental cost effectiveness ratio (ICER) and incremental cost utility ratio (ICUR) of liver transplantation by adding the recent papers to the review reported by Ishida and Imai *et al.*[54]. After that, we will determine whether liver transplantation is appropriate considering its cost. Additionally, to evaluate the HEA results on liver transplantation in each country, we will make an international comparison.

## 4.1. Systematic Review of Cost-Effectiveness Analyses of Liver Transplantation

Ishida and Imai *et al.* [54] reviewed papers published up to July 2003, and we updated their information by conducting a literature search for publications between August 2003 and June 30, 2010. Using the MEDLINE database, we searched for the keywords "Liver Transplantation" [MESH] AND "Costs and Cost Analysis" [MESH].

As a result, 39 papers were retrieved. We extracted papers that seemed likely to provide HEA studies of liver transplantation through titles and abstracts, and examined the entire texts of the selected papers. Owing to a close examination of the papers, four papers [20, 55-57] were identified in the publications up to June 30, 2010 in addition to the four papers [8,17,58,59] included in the review by Ishida and Imai *et al.*[54], making a total of eight HEA studies.

Detailed information on the HEA studies on liver transplantation included in our review are shown in Table 7. Of these studies, four were CEA studies using life-year extension as an outcome index, and the remaining four were CUA studies using QALY as an outcome index.

**Table 7. Results of cost-effectiveness analysis for liver transplantation patients**

| First author | Year Country | Number of transplantations | Time | DD or LD | Incremental Cost-Effectiveness Ratio (US$, 2009) | Cost-Effectiveness |
|---|---|---|---|---|---|---|
| Northup [58] | 2009 USA | 1635 | 00-09 | DD and DD + LD | [DD] 42,903 / QALY [DD + LD] 127,348 / QALY | Superior in cost-effectiveness to DD. |
| Ishida [8] | 2006 Japan | 11 | 99-01 | LD | [3 months follow-up] 721,643 / QALY [24 months follow-up] 112,300 / QALY | Superior in cost-effectiveness |
| Ouwens [59] | 2003 Netherlands | 81 | 78-87 | DD | 39,757 / LYG | Not mentioned |
| Longworth [17] | 2003 UK | 208 | 95-96 | DD | [PBC] 56,660 / QALY [PSC] 42,090 / QALY [ALC] 95,410 / QALY | Cost-effectiveness for PBC and PSC. Not superior for ALD. |
| Sagmeister [20] | 2002 Switzerland | 51 | 95-00 | DD and DD + LD | [DD] 15,442 / QALY [DD+LD] 16,184 / QALY | Superior in cost-effectiveness |
| Hisashige [57] | 1997 Japan | 180 | 90s | LD | [6 years follow-up] 130,659 / LYG [Follow-up to 80 years] ¥16,352 / LYG | Superior in cost-effectiveness |
| Bonsel [56] | 1990 Netherlands | 76 | 78-87 | DD | [1 LYG] 252,764 / LYG [5 LYG] 89,323 / LYG | Superior in cost-effectiveness |
| Kankaanpaa [55] | 1990 USA | 32 | 81-86 | DD | [Death within 1 year] 520,683 / LYG [Death after 1 year] 109,617 / LYG | Caution |

DD: deceased donor liver transplantation.
LD: living donor liver transplantation.
LYG: life-year gained.
QALY: quality-adjusted life year.
PBC: primary biliary cirrhosis, PSC: primary sclerosing cholangitis, ALD: alcoholic liver disease.

Northup *et al.* performed a CEA of DDLT and LDLT using a multistage Markov decision analysis with a 10-year time horizon [58]. All direct and indirect outpatient and inpatient costs, including those in the pretransplantation, perioperative, and post-transplantation time periods, were estimated using microcosting algorithms. The utility to the recipient at post-transplantation was derived from past studies. Mean costs per patient who underwent DDLT were estimated at US$180,804 and US$248,225 for a patient who was listed for DDLT with an LDLT available. The DDLT-only strategy cost an average of US$35,976/QALY. The incremental cost-effectiveness ratio of moving from the DDLT-only strategy to LDLT was approximately US$248,225. Given that an ICER of less than US$50,000 (US$59,627, after adjusting for inflation to 2009 US$)/QALY was accepted as cost-effective, then DDLT is a cost-effective treatment.

Ouens *et al.* conducted a CEA of 81 liver transplantation cases in the Netherlands from 1978 to 1987 [59]. The median follow-up after transplantation was approximately 1 year. Although estimates of treatment costs were based on data from the literature, costs included direct medical costs from pretransplantation to the follow-up period after transplantation. In the first 3 years of follow-up, direct medical costs per patient totaled US$145,726. They calculated QALYs using EQ-5D questionnaires. The costs per QALY gained for liver transplantation was US$39,757. Because the authors sought to compare cost-effectiveness between lung, heart, and liver transplantations, the study did not compare the cost-effectiveness of liver transplantation with a cost-effectiveness threshold.

Longworth *et al.* performed a CEA for patients with primary biliary cirrhosis (PBC), primary sclerosing cholangitis (PSC), and alcoholic liver disease (ALD), who were on a waiting list for liver transplantation over 27 months in England and Wales [17]. Costs were estimated over the 27 months from the time of listing using a microcosting approach. Total costs per transplantation ranged from US$103,637 to US$130,322. QALY was assessed using the EQ-5D classification system, administered by a postal questionnaire to participants. The mean costs per QALY gained were US$56,660, US$42,090, and US$94,410 for PBC, PSC, and ALD patients, respectively. Considering that the National Health Service (NHS) has decided that it can afford to pay a maximum of approximately £30,000 (US$59,193, after adjusting for inflation to 2009 US$) for an additional QALY, the authors proposed that liver transplantation was a cost-effectiveness treatment for patients with PBC and PSC, but not for ALD patients.

Sagmeister *et al.* [20] conducted a CEA using the Markov model. They compared the effectiveness, lifetime costs, and cost-effectiveness of DDLT with those of combined DDLT and LDLT for ESLD patients. For patients with DDLT, cost estimates included costs of transplantation, annual costs of decompensated cirrhosis, costs in the first year after transplantation, and costs for the following years after transplantation. For patients with LDLT, cost estimates included costs of transplantation, costs of lobectomy (for the donor), costs for donor evaluation, annual costs of decompensated cirrhosis, costs in the first year after transplantation, and costs for the following years after transplantation. However, the report provided insufficient information regarding costing methods. The cost of DDLT was estimated to be US$81,477. They derived the utility of health states in the model by a time trade-off technique and calculated QALYs. Marginal cost for one additional QALY gained per patient with ESLD treated by DDLT amounted to US$15,442 and that treated by combined DDLT and LDLT amounted to US$16,184. Given that the most frequently used threshold for cost-effectiveness in the US is US$50,000/QALY, both DDLT and combined DDLT and LDLT were cost-effective based on this criterion.

Hisashige *et al.* conducted a CEA of LDLT in 180 patients (mostly 1-2-year-old pediatric patients) with biliary atresia [57]. They evaluated direct medical costs and assessed life years gained as the outcome. While cost per life year gained by liver transplantation was estimated at US$130,659/LYG with a 6-year follow-up, it was US$16,352/LYG with follow-up to 80 years. Compared with the thresholds of cost-effectiveness established by Laupacis *et al.*[60] (See Section 6-2), LDLT was determined to be a cost-effective intervention. Indeed, they concluded that the longer the recipient survived, the more cost-effective it became.

In a study of 76 liver transplantation cases, Bonsel *et al.* analyzed the cost-effectiveness of liver transplantation during the 1978-1987 period [56]. Cost data were abstracted from the hospital administrative system and calculated costs per patient at various treatment stages, such as screening, waiting time, from the operation to 3 months, 4-12 months after the transplantation, and each post-transplantation year (from the $2^{nd}$ to the $5^{th}$ year). Life years gained was assessed as the effectiveness criterion. The total costs per transplantation, including 5 years of follow-up, amounted to US$475,112. Combining cost data and effectiveness data resulted in an ICER from US$252,764/LYG (1-year follow-up) to

US$89,323/LYG (5-year follow-up). With the 5-year follow-up results, they concluded that the cost-effectiveness of liver transplantation was acceptable.

Kankaanpaa conducted a CEA examining 32 liver transplant patients from 1981 to 1986 [55]. The cost figures included direct costs (charges for hospital facilities, pretransplantation work-up, and professional fees) and indirect costs (traveling costs, lodging costs, and rehabilitation costs). Direct costs were calculated using charges, and the professional charges included those for the transplantation itself, anesthesia, pretransplant hospitalization and work-up, and post-transplantation follow-up visits. The effectiveness data were obtained using life years gained. The cost study showed the average total cost of the first year to be US$562,635. Whereas the cost per life-year saved in seven patients who died within 1 year was calculated to be US$520,683/LYG, the cost per life-year saved in 25 patients who survived more than 1 year was calculated to be US$109,617/LYG. Kankaanpaa did not make a conclusion about the cost-effectiveness of liver transplantation in the paper.

The cost-utility analysis of LDLT conducted by Ishida *et al.* [8] is shown in Section 5.

## 4.2. International Comparison of Cost-Effectiveness Analyses

The following counties conducted HEA studies of liver transplantation: US (2) [55, 58], Europe (4) [17, 20, 56, 59], and Japan (2) [8, 57]. HEA studies were actively conducted in Europe, whereas more than half of the cost analysis studies on liver transplantation were carried out in the US.

In the US, Kankaanpaa [55] and Northup *et al.* [58] carried out cost-effectiveness analyses. Kankaanpaa calculated the costs per actuarial life-year saved as US$520,683/LYG and US$109,617/LYG for patients surviving < 1 year and surviving > 1 year, respectively. Although Kankaanpaa avoided a conclusion as to whether liver transplantation was cost-effective, such treatment resulting in more than 1-year survival seems to be cost-effective, as determined on the basis of thresholds frequently used in the US (however, the use of life-years gained rather than QALY makes this determination difficult). Moreover, Northup *et al.* concluded that DDLT is a cost-effective treatment with an ICER of less than US$50,000 per QALY. However, LDLT in combination with DDLT proved to be modestly more effective, but much more expensive, than the DDLT-only strategy per QALY saved.

Of the studies conducted in Europe, most have concluded that DDLT is a cost-effective technique. However, for patients with ADL, liver transplantation was considered not to be a cost-effective treatment. In contrast, the two reported cost-effectiveness studies conducted in Japan both focused on LDLT. Both studies [8,57] determined that LDLT is a cost-effective treatment. Consequently, liver transplantation is recognized as a therapeutic procedure that provides excellent cost-effectiveness regardless of country.

# 5. Cost Utility Analysis of LDLT in Japan

## 5.1. Background

Liver transplantation is the only treatment available for patients with ESLD. LDLT is becoming increasingly common in the face of shortages of deceased donors and concomitant rapid increases in the waiting time for DDLT. However, LDLT has not yet become fully accepted, as issues including donor safety [61-63], medical ethics [64-67], and economics remain somewhat controversial.

Survival rates for LDLT have improved for patients with ESLD [1,3] because of refinements in organ preservation, surgical technique and immunosuppressive therapies. Conversely, little has been done to clarify its cost-effectiveness. The lack of economic assessment of medical costs for LDLT may obstruct its social acceptance due to criticisms of high medical expenses under the current conditions of tight medical financing, and may thus hinder the utilization of precious medical resources. A published economic study of LDLT has shown costs below the suggested upper limit of cost-effectiveness (less than US$50,000) [20], but this study shows limitations regarding the use of hypothetical estimates of medical cost and health-related quality of life (HRQOL).

In Section 5, we examine the cost-utility of LDLT using trial-based cost estimates and utility scores, rather than model-based estimates, for patients with ESLD.

## 5.2. Methods

The study of Ishida *et al.* [8] comprises of both cost and utility analyses, based on the data from patients with ESLD treated at the Hokkaido University Hospital in Sapporo, Japan. The potential subjects in this study were patients aged 18 to 60 years old who fulfilled LDLT criteria (physical and mental examinations, written informed consent both patients and their families, etc.) and treated in the First Department of Surgery at the hospital between January 1999 and December 2001. All the participants in this study received written information about the goals and research methods of the study and they provided their written consent. The Ethics Committee of the School of Medicine, Hokkaido University, approved the study protocol.

Information regarding medical costs was derived from 11 participants. In cost-utility analysis, medical costs generally differ from medical charges [68]. Because no cost-charge ratio has been reported in Japan or in the hospital, medical charges were substituted for medical costs. These charges were based on the national fee schedule for each participant and the duration of estimation for medical costs was from the first day of preoperative evaluation for LDLT to 24 months post-LDLT. The schedule contained the data under 2 headings: hospitalization and outpatient care. We selected 10 categories for hospitalization (consultation, home care, medication, injection, treatment, surgery, examination, imaging, hospitalization, and others) and 9 items for outpatient care (consultation, home care, medication, injection, treatment, surgery, examination, imaging, and others). The medical costs of medications including immunosuppressants after discharge were extrapolated on the basis of immunosuppressants prescribed at the time of discharge. All medical costs were prospectively measured. Medical costs were calculated in Japanese yen for the years 1999-2002 and converted to US dollars (US$) for the year 2009 using PPP and CPI.

The health utility scores of 19 participants were determined using a general instrument, the EQ-5D Japanese version [69,70]. EQ-5D was self-administered by participants before LDLT and at 3, 6, 12, and 24 months post-LDLT. Survival rates were determined in 79 patients with LDLT between September 1997 and April 2004 in the First Division of Surgery, Hokkaido University Hospital. Data yielded a 1-year survival rate of 79.5% and a 3-year survival rate of 76.2%. Interpolated values were substituted for missing health utility scores and survival rates.

Medical costs per QALY ratio (MCQR) was derived as a result of cost-utility analysis. An annual discount rate of 0% was adopted, as recommended by Drummond *et al.* [71], and a societal perspective was used for both analyses.

One-way sensitivity analysis was implemented to assess the robustness of MCQR at 24 months post-LDLT. The variables were total medical costs, the 3 most expensive categories of all 19 categories in cost analysis, health utility score, survival rate, and discounted rate. Totals medical costs, the 3 most expensive categories, and health utility score were calculated within the 25th to 75th percentiles. Survival rate was calculated as ±10% of baseline values, and discounted rates of cost and utility analyses were determined as 0-10%.

## 5.3. Results of Cost-Utility Analysis of LDLT

The median age of the 11 participants in the cost analysis was 42 yr (range, 27-58 yr). The median duration of hospitalization was 119 days (range, 73-306 days). The indications for LDLT were fulminant hepatic failure (n = 4), primary biliary cirrhosis (n = 3), liver cirrhosis type B (n = 1), liver cirrhosis type C (n = 1), alcoholic liver diseases (n = 1), and liver cirrhosis type B plus liver cancer (n = 1). The cumulative medical costs from pre-LDLT to 24 months post-LDLT are shown in Table 8. During follow-up, medical costs were highest (US$136,176) at 1-3 months post-LDLT, whereas the increment during the late follow-up period (13-24 months post-LDLT) was only US$16,189.

**Table 8. Medical costs for patients with LDLT**

| | | Percentiles | | |
|---|---|---|---|---|
| | Mean | 25th | 50th | 75th |
| Medical costs pre- and post-LDLT (number of cases) | | | | |
| Pre-LDLT (n=7) | 8,962 | 5,359 | 9,122 | 12,568 |
| 1-3 months post-LDLT (n=9) | 139,695 | 112,017 | 136,176 | 154,965 |
| 1-3 months post-LDLT (n=10) | 12,264 | 5,453 | 10,295 | 13,615 |
| 1-3 months post-LDLT (n=10) | 15,963 | 7,843 | 12,615 | 22,528 |
| 1-3 months post-LDLT (n=11) | 22,609 | 14,025 | 16,189 | 27,682 |
| Cumulative medical cost | | | | |
| Pre- to 12 months post-LDLT | 176,885 | 130,673 | 168,207 | 203,675 |
| Pre- to 24 months post-LDLT | 199,494 | 144,697 | 184,397 | 231,358 |

LDLT; living donor liver transplantation.
US$, 2009.

The median age of the 19 participants in the utility analysis was 46 yr (range, 27-58 yr). The indications for LDLT were fulminant hepatic failure (n = 6), primary biliary cirrhosis (n = 5), liver cirrhosis type B (n = 1), liver cirrhosis type C (n = 1), liver cirrhosis type B plus liver cancer (n = 2), alcoholic liver disease (n = 1), epithelioid hemangioendothelioma (n = 1), acute exacerbation of chronic hepatitis B (n = 1), and primary sclerosing cholangitis (n = 1). The median health utility score [25th-75th percentiles] was 0.66 at pre-LDLT (range, 0.64-0.75; n = 13), compared with 1.00 at 3 months (range, 0.67-1.00; n = 9), 1.00 at 6 months (range, 0.86-1.00; n = 11), 1.00 at 12 months (range, 0.92-1.00; n = 8), and 1.00 at 24 months post-LDLT (range, 1.00-1.00; n = 2). The median health utility scores were improved at post-LDLT compared with pre-LDLT values. However, after adjusting for survival, no significant difference was observed in health utility score between pre- and post-LDLT.

Cumulative QALYs were 0.85 at 12 months post-LDLT and 1.60 at 24 months post-LDLT (Table 9). MCQR thus decreased from US$721,640/QALY at 3 months post-LDLT to US$112,300/QALY at 24 months post-LDLT (Table 9)

**Table 9. QALYs for patients with LDLT, and medical costs per QALY**

| Months post-LDLT | QALY | Cumulative QALY | Medical cost per QALY |
|---|---|---|---|
| 3 | 0.20 | 0.20 | 721,640 |
| 6 | 0.23 | 0.43 | 360,063 |
| 12 | 0.42 | 0.85 | 196,676 |
| 24 | 0.75 | 1.60 | 112,300 |

US$, 2009.

MCQR was relatively stable for health utility scores and survival rate. However, considerable variation in MCQR was observed with changes in medical cost (Table 10).

**Table 10. One-way sensitivity analysis of MCQR at 24 months post-LDLT**

| Variables | Low value (US$) | High value (US$) | Range of analysis |
|---|---|---|---|
| Total medical cost | 79,581 | 124,042 | 25th to 75th percentile |
| Administration | 110,610 | 118,973 | 25th to 75th percentile |
| Operation | 103,818 | 117,200 | 25th to 75th percentile |
| Injection | 103,815 | 129,605 | 25th to 75th percentile |
| Health utility scores | 111,258 | 125,995 | 25th to 75th percentile |
| Survival rates | 92,200 | 142,291 | +10% to -10% |
| Discount rates | 107,013 | 112,300 | 10% to 0% |

US$, 2009.

## 5.4. Interpretation, Limitation and Conclusion

Ishida et al.[8] showed that cost-effectiveness for LDLT increased progressively for patients with ESLD. The medical costs were highest at 1-3 months post-LDLT, and the costs after 1-3 months post-LDLT came to less than 10% of the costs during those 1-3 months.

Health utility score as measured in terms of QALY was not markedly different between pre- and post-LDLT.

To the best of our knowledge, cost-utility analysis of LDLT has rarely been performed to measure both medical costs and health utility. In this study, MCQR for LDLT (US$112,300/QALY) was comparable to published MCQRs for organ transplantations such as DDLT versus the absence of DDLT in patients with alcoholic liver disease in England and Wales (US$89,348/QALY: 95% bootstrap confidence intervals, US$22325-US$154,499) [17]. Results were also consistent with MCQR for heart transplantation versus optional conventional treatment in patients needing heart transplants (US$91,314/QALY) [72], and for lung transplantation versus standard care in patients with end-stage pulmonary disease in the Netherlands (US$210,860/QALY) [73]. Furthermore, the present results are within the standard range suggested by Laupacis et al. [60] (US$20,000 – US$100,000/QALY), although the panel on cost-effectiveness in health technologies notes that no absolute standards exist for deciding whether an intervention is cost-effective [74].

Several limitations need to be considered when interpreting the present findings. First, cost analysis did not include donor-related medical costs. The national fee schedule did not list the donor-related fee at the beginning of this survey, although the schedule did list the fees for some ESLDs in 2000. The addition of these costs (e.g., national fee for surgery of US$3,536 since 2000) should increase MCQR. Furthermore, cost analysis did not include indirect costs. For example, costs involving factors such as travel and suspended economic activity were not taken into account, thus underestimating the results. Conversely, the resumption of economic activities may exert a different impact. The influence of relevant indirect costs on MCQR must therefore be considered. Second, the subjects were derived from patients in a single center. Nevertheless, Ishida et al. [8] believe that the subjects were an approximately representative LDLT population in Japan, as medical costs of hospitalization ranged widely for subjects (US$83,120-US$259,973) and resembled those in the populations of other Japanese representative centers (US$38,996-US$310,059) [75-77], whereas survival rates (79.5% at 1 year and 76.2% at 3 years) mirrored those in 49 centers in Japan (80.8% at 1 year and 78.5% at 3 years). Finally, they were unable to set alternative treatments, owing to the relatively small number of DDLTs performed in Japan and the difficulty in measuring health utility for patients with ESLD not receiving LDLT, owing to ethical consideration.

In conclusion, this study indicates that LDLT becomes progressively more cost-effective over time. The procedure also improves HRQOL of post-LDLT survivors. LDLT appears to represent a cost-effective medical technology.

# 6. Discussion

Advances in medical technologies have made the treatment of previously untreatable conditions possible. However, these same advances in technologies have also resulted in escalating medical expenditures, resulting in a dilemma in which it is economically unfeasible to have limitless utilization of these technologies. HEA represents a tool to support the scientific decision-making process involved in maximizing the healthcare outcomes of the public with limited resources. The use of QALY as an outcome measure that can be

## Cost Effectiveness Analysis of Liver Transplantation 213

potentially applied to all types of medical technologies allows evaluations for selecting the most cost-effective technology available. However, these evaluations require the following two factors: the costs are appropriately estimated using standardized estimation methods, and the cost effectiveness and specific thresholds for evaluations have been determined.

## 6.1. Subjects of Cost Estimation in HEA in Liver Transplantations

The liver transplantation process can be divided into 3 different stages: pretransplantation, transplantation admission, and post-transplantation. It is consequently necessary to conduct cost estimations for each of these 3 stages in HEA of liver transplantation. The various costing items for the cost estimations in each stage are discussed below.

The notable costing items that contribute to the costs incurred in the pretransplantation period include the evaluation of recipient, maintenance of the recipient while on the waiting list, and pretransplantation admission. A specific consideration for evaluations of the pre-transplant period is that costs incurred during this period are not limited to patients who have successfully undergone the transplantation procedure, but must also include the costs of candidate patients who were unable to have the procedure. This is due to the fact that the majority of hospitals that conduct transplantations admit and treat both transplantation patients as well as patients who ultimately do not undergo the transplantations owing to insufficient donor organs, organ rejection, or death. In addition to conducting transplantation therapy, such aforementioned patients are consistently increasing in number. Additionally, it is essential to obtain information on the patients' whereabouts during the waiting period, because whether these patients are in their own homes, hospitals, or ICUs has been shown to have a heavy influence on the costs incurred during the pretransplant period [39]. Furthermore, in the case of LDLT, costing items associated with testing to ensure donor safety, donor evaluation costs, and costs of failed donor evaluation should also be taken into consideration.

In the transplant admission period, costing items that should be included in cost evaluations should include organ acquisition costs, management of complications, hospital stay, and professional fees. However, many liver transplantation cost estimation studies have included general estimates of these costing items. Additionally, the costs of donor hepatectomies should be included for studies involving LDLT.

As there may be abrupt changes in recipient patient conditions approximately two years after the transplantation, post-transplantation follow-up care and patient visits should be conducted for as long as possible. The cost of immunosuppressive drugs administered during this period may be considered to be a costing item that has a major influence on overall costs. Although the dosage of immunosuppressive drugs may be reduced in liver transplant recipients after stabilization, the fact that these drugs are in principle administered for life results in heavy accumulated drug expenditures. Additionally, a portion of patients have to be administered with costly pharmaceuticals such as preventive drugs against the recurrence of hepatitis B or interferons against hepatitis C for lengthy durations.

Next, liver transplantation costs can be categorized on the basis of perspectives, namely, "costing items that directly involve the patient" and "costing items related to departments that have no specific or direct involvement with the patient". The costing items as presented above belong in the former category, but in reality there are also numerous costs that belong in the latter. As the costing items in the latter category involve activities that are essential for the liver transplantation process, they should be included in cost estimates.

As the indirect costs associated with loss in labor productivity for liver transplant recipients are not an essential costing item for estimating the costs of the transplantation process, these costs have essentially not been included in the cost estimation studies reviewed in this chapter.

In addition to utilizing the aforementioned costing items in cost estimation studies of liver transplantation, it is strongly desired for researchers to report the detailed breakdown of costs by each costing item. This would improve the transferability of cost estimates, and increase the value of the estimate as information to support the decision-making process in third parties.

## 6.2. What is the Value of One QALY?

Although it is extremely difficult to clearly establish the value of a single QALY, the evaluation of insurance listings for new health technologies utilizes a value of £20,000-£30,000 per QALY in the UK [78]. Published studies from the US frequently appear to use a standard value of US$50,000 per QALY. However, these thresholds have not been supported by any scientific basis.

The first study that proposed specific thresholds for evaluating whether a medical technology is cost-effective or not was conducted by Kaplan and Bush in 1982 [79]. The guidelines for the adoption of medical technologies as recommended by Kaplan and Bush are presented in Table 11, with "cost effective", "controversial", and "questionable" evaluated at ICER < US$20,000, ICER = US$20,000 – US$100,000, and ICER > US$100,000, respectively. However, the bases for these calculations are not transparent. Furthermore, a Canadian research team led by Laupacis *et al.* [60] produced the following grades of recommendation for the evaluation to support the adoption of new technologies in 1992: "strong evidence", "moderate evidence", and "weak evidence" were evaluated at ICER < CA$ 20,000/QALY, ICER = CA$20,000 – CA$100,000/QALY, and ICER > CA$100,000/QALY (Table 12). As the 1982 value of the US dollar was more than twice that of the 1992 value of the Canadian dollar, it is important to note the large differences in thresholds between both sets of guidelines.

**Table 11. Guidelines for adoption of medical technologies**

| Cost per well-year | Policy implication |
| --- | --- |
| Less than $20,000 per well-year | Cost-effective by current standards |
| $20,000 to $100,000 per well-year | Possibly controversial, but justifiable by many current examples |
| Greater than $100,000 per well-year | Questionable in comparison with other health care expenditure |

Source: Kaplan and Bush 1982 [79].

## Table 12. Grades of recommendation for adoption of appropriate utilization of new technologies

| Grade | Recommendation |
|---|---|
| A. | Compelling evidence for the adoption and appropriate utilization. The new technology is as effective as or more effective than the existing one and is less costly. |
| B. | Strong evidence for adoption and appropriate utilization The new technology is more effective than the existing one and costs less than $20,000 per quality adjusted life year (QALY) gained. The new technology is less effective than the existing one, but its introduction would save more than $100,000/QALY gained. |
| C. | Moderate evidence for adoption and appropriate utilization. The new technology is more effective than the existing one and cost $20,000 to $100,000/QALY gained. The new technology is less effective than the existing one, but its introduction would save $20,000 to $100,000/QALY gained. |
| D. | Weak evidence for adoption and appropriate utilization The new technology is more effective than the existing one and costs more that $100,000/QALY gained. The new technology is less effective than the existing one, but its introduction would save less than $20,000/QALY gained. |
| E. | Compelling evidence for rejection The new technology is less effective than or as effective as the existing one and is more costly. |

Source: Laupacis *et al.* [60]

In a study using samples from Japan, South Korea, Taiwan, Australia, the UK and the US, Shiroiwa *et al.* [80] have utilized a standardized method (double-bound dichotomous choice and analysis by nonparametric Turnbull method) to contemporaneously estimate the WTP value of one QALY. The WTP estimates for a single QALY by country were as follows: Japan, JPY 5 million; South Korea, KWN 68 million; Taiwan, NT$ 2.1 million; Australia, AU$ 64,000; UK, £23,000, and the US, US$62,000.

Although the differences in estimation methodologies and intrinsic differences among countries do not allow for precise comparisons, the fact that the estimates for the value of life as produced by Kaplan and Bush in 1982 [79], Laupacis *et al.* in 1992 [60], and Shiroiwa *et al.* in 2010 [80] are very similar is of great interest. However, owing to the large differences in monetary value, the more recently reported estimates show a lower value of life. The reasons for this remain unclear.

## 6.3. Ethical Issues Associated with Fairness of Resource Allocation in Liver Transplantation

Although liver transplantation is an effective treatment for ESLD, the short supply of organ donors and the protraction of the waiting period for ESLD patients are becoming a social problem. The issue of selecting liver transplantation recipients from a large body of ESLD patients, all of whom require the procedure for survival, is an extremely important issue from the ethical perspective of fairness in resource allocation.

The US and the UK implemented an organ allocation system based on the model for end-stage liver disease (MELD) score, which places an emphasis on the disease severity of each patient, in February, 2002 and December, 2006, respectively. MELD score is calculated from the following three parameters to objectively evaluate the disease severity of each patient: serum bilirubin level, serum creatinine level, and the international normalized ratio for prothrombin time (INR). However, does this use of MELD score to prioritize patients for receipt of a donor liver actually ensure fairness in resource allocation in liver transplantation?

In the evaluation of the actual operational situation in the US, there are problems that still prevent the actualization of safe and fair resource allocation. There are two aspects wherein factors of inequities remain. The first of these, as shown in the review conducted in this chapter, is that liver transplantation requires immense healthcare costs. In the US, where there is no national public insurance system, it is possible that doctors and hospitals may not place a patient in need of a liver transplant on the waiting list if they do not appear to have the means to pay for the procedure. This possibility arises owing to the fact that these actions are deemed legal under the current laws, and these issues were even highlighted in the 2002 motion picture "John Q", in which Denzel Washington played a father whose son needed a heart transplant but was not placed on a recipient list as it was not covered by HMO insurance. As such, there exists an inequity in which patients with poor economical strength are unable to receive the benefits of new medical technologies. (However, this problem is not limited to organ transplants, but is a widespread problem in all aspects of healthcare.)

The second inequity is that in the US, it is not illegal for a single patient to be simultaneously placed on waiting lists in numerous different regions. In general, the specifics of when and where an organ donor may emerge are unknown, and it may be impossible for patients in normal circumstances to reach the appropriate hospital within the short timeframe where the donor organ is still viable for transplantation. However, patients with a sufficient economical clout may possess private jets or other various modes of transportation that allows them fast access to hospitals located in distant locales for medical procedures. A notable example of someone who could actualize this situation is Steve Jobs, the CEO of Apple Inc. Only four months after he took a leave of absence from his work, he was the recipient of a new liver. However, this transplantation was not conducted in the state of California, where he resides, but in Methodist University Hospital, Tennessee. This inequity, in which wealthy patients have a higher chance of benefiting from new medical technologies, is therefore shown to exist.

# 7. Conclusions

In this chapter, using the theme of Cost-Effectiveness Analysis of Liver Transplantation, we have highlighted the issues presented in the existing literature as well as elucidated the problems that need to be addressed in the future in the aspects of cost, effectiveness and cost-effectiveness.

Presently, there are approximately 40 studies of cost estimates of liver transplantations in the scientific literature, and comparative analyses have progressed. However, we have shown that due to differences in research subjects, scope of costing items, and cost estimation methodologies, it is extremely dangerous to directly use the published cost estimates in the decision-making process. It is therefore required for researchers who conduct cost estimation research to ensure the transparency of the estimation results. Readers should also conduct detailed examinations of the possible applications and suitability of these published cost estimates before applying them to settings in their own institutions and countries.

Despite the first cost-effectiveness analysis of liver transplantation being conducted 20 years ago, it has become clear that there is a scarcity of such studies up to the present. Liver transplantations are an established treatment for ESLD patients. However, although the procedure can help achieve desirable health outcomes, the extremely high costs involved highlight the need for more cost-effectiveness analyses of liver transplantation. The scope of costing for cost-effectiveness analyses generally includes costing items from the pretransplantation period until the post-transplantation period. If there are insufficient costing items included in the cost estimation, the costs of liver transplantations may be severely underestimated, which may in turn distort decision-making concerning medical resource allocation. Therefore, efforts must be made to improve the quality of cost estimation studies. In the case of studies that have not reported the detailed breakdown of costing items, it becomes impossible to determine if similar results would be obtained when applied to other jurisdictions even if these costs have been utilized in cost-effectiveness analyses. Therefore, details in the scope of costing and costing methodologies should be reported in studies that estimate the costs of liver transplantations, as this would enhance the transferability of resulting estimates. In this way, the value of the determined cost-effectiveness can be expected to increase.

Although there are no standardized and absolute criteria with which the cost-effectiveness of a technology can be determined, the scientific literature up to the present has largely determined that liver transplantation is in fact a cost-effective treatment.

# References

[1] United Network for Organ Sharing. http://www.unos.org/ Access: August 31, 2010.

[2] European Liver Transplant Registry. http://www.eltr.org/ Access: August 31, 2010.

[3] Japanese Liver Transplantation Society. Liver transplantation in Japan: registry by the Japanese Liver Transplantation Society. *Japanese Journal of Transplantation* 2009;44(6):559-571.

[4] Buchanan P, Dzebisashvili N, Lentine KL, Axelrod DA, Schnitzler MA, Salvalaggio PR. Liver transplantation cost in the model for end-stage liver disease era: looking beyond the transplant admission. *Liver Transpl* 2009;15(10):1270-1277.

[5] Markley ET, Cooil B, Rubin JE, Chari RS. Cost prediction in liver transplantation using pretransplant donor and recipient characteristics. *Transplantation* 2008;86(2):238-244.

[6] Passarani S, De Carlis L, Maione G, Alberti AB, Bevilacqua L, Baraldi S. Cost analysis of living donor liver transplantation: the first Italian economical data. *Minerva Anestesiol* 2007;73(10):491-499.

[7] Englesbe MJ, Dimick J, Mathur A, *et al*. Who pays for biliary complications following liver transplant? A business case for quality improvement. *Am J Transplant* 2006;6 (12):2978-2982.

[8] Ishida K, Imai H, Ogasawara K, *et al*. Cost-utility of living donor liver transplantation in a single Japanese center. *Hepatogastroenterology* 2006;53(70):588-591.

[9] Kogure T, Ueno Y, Kawagishi N, *et al*. The model for end-stage liver disease score is useful for predicting economic outcomes in adult cases of living donor liver transplantation. *J Gastroenterol* 2006;41(10):1005-1010.

[10] Washburn WK, Pollock BH, Nichols L, Speeg KV, Halff G. Impact of recipient MELD score on resource utilization. *Am J Transplant* 2006;6(10):2449-2454.

[11] Kraus TW, Mieth M, Schneider T, *et al*. Cost distribution of orthotopic liver trans-plantation: single-center analysis under DRG-based reimbursement. *Trans-plantation* 2005;80(1 Suppl):S97-S100.

[12] Oostenbrink JB, Kok ET, Verheul RM. A comparative study of resource use and costs of renal, liver and heart transplantation. *Transpl Int* 2005;18(4):437-443.

[13] Reed A, Howard RJ, Fujita S, *et al*. Liver retransplantation: a single-center outcome and financial analysis. *Transplant Proc* 2005;37(2):1161-1163.

[14] Brand DA, Viola D, Rampersaud P, Patrick PA, Rosenthal WS, Wolf DC. Waiting for a liver: hidden costs of the organ shortage. *Liver Transpl* 2004;10(8):1001-1010.

[15] Cole CR, Bucuvalas JC, Hornung R, *et al*. Outcome after pediatric liver transplantation impact of living donor transplantation on cost. *J Pediatr* 2004;144(6):729-735.

[16] Filipponi F, Pisati R, Cavicchini G, Ulivieri MI, Ferrara R, Mosca F. Cost and outcome analysis and cost determinants of liver transplantation in a European National Health Service hospital. *Transplantation* 2003;75(10):1731-1736.

[17] Longworth L, Young T, Buxton MJ, *et al*. Midterm cost-effectiveness of the liver transplantation program of England and Wales for three disease groups. *Liver Transpl* 2003;9(12):1295-1307.

[18] Trotter JF, Mackenzie S, Wachs M, *et al*. Comprehensive cost comparison of adult-adult right hepatic lobe living-donor liver transplantation with cadaveric transplantation. *Transplantation* 2003;75(4):473-476.

[19] Azoulay D, Linhares MM, Huguet E, *et al*. Decision for retransplantation of the liver: an experience- and cost-based analysis. *Ann Surg* 2002;236(6):713-721.

[20] Sagmeister M, Mullhaupt B, Kadry Z, Kullak-Ublick GA, Clavien PA, Renner EL. Cost-effectiveness of cadaveric and living-donor liver transplantation. *Transplantation* 2002;73(4):616-622.

[21] Taylor MC, Greig PD, Detsky AS, McLeod RS, Abdoh A, Krahn MD. Factors associated with the high cost of liver transplantation in adults. *Can J Surg* 2002; 45(6):425-434.

[22] Skeie B, Mishra V, Vaaler S, Amlie E. A comparison of actual cost, DRG-based cost, and hospital reimbursement for liver transplant patients. *Transpl Int* 2002;15(9-10):439-445.

[23] Best JH, Veenstra DL, Geppert J. Trends in expenditures for Medicare liver transplant recipients. *Liver Transpl* 2001;7(10):858-862.

[24] Bucuvalas JC, Ryckman FC, Atherton H, Alonso MP, Balistreri WF, Kotagal U. Predictors of cost of liver transplantation in children: a single center study. *J Pediatr* 2001;139(1):66-74.

[25] Nair S, Cohen DB, Cohen MP, Tan H, Maley W, Thuluvath PJ. Postoperative morbidity, mortality, costs, and long-term survival in severely obese patients undergoing orthotopic liver transplantation. *Am J Gastroenterol* 2001;96(3):842-845.

[26] Schnitzler MA, Woodward RS, Brennan DC, Whiting JF, Tesi RJ, Lowell JA. The economic impact of preservation time in cadaveric liver transplantation. *Am J Transplant* 2001;1(4):360-365.

[27] van Agthoven M, Metselaar HJ, Tilanus HW, *et al*. A comparison of the costs and effects of liver transplantation for acute and for chronic liver failure. *Transpl Int* 2001;14(2):87-94.

[28] Freeman R, Tsunoda S, Supran S, *et al*. Direct costs for one year of liver transplant care are directly associated with disease severity at transplant. *Transplant Proc* 2001;33(1-2):1436-1437.

[29] Gilbert JR, Pascual M, Schoenfeld DA, Rubin RH, Delmonico FL, Cosimi AB. Evolving trends in liver transplantation: an outcome and charge analysis. *Transplantation* 1999;67(2):246-253.

[30] Rufat P, Fourquet F, Conti F, Le Gales C, Houssin D, Coste J. Costs and outcomes of liver transplantation in adults: a prospective, 1-year, follow-up study. GRETHECO study group. *Transplantation* 1999;68(1):76-83.

[31] Showstack J, Katz PP, Lake JR, *et al*. Resource utilization in liver transplantation: effects of patient characteristics and clinical practice. *JAMA* 1999;281(15):1381-1386.

[32] Brown RS Jr, Lake JR, Ascher NL, Emond JC, Roberts JP. Predictors of the cost of liver transplantation. *Liver Transpl Surg* 1998;4(2):170-176.

[33] Geevarghese SK, Bradley AE, Wright JK, *et al*. Outcomes analysis in 100 liver transplantation patients. *Am J Surg* 1998;175(5):348-353.

[34] Russo MW, Sandler RS, Mandelkehr L, Fair JH, Johnson MW, Brown RS Jr. Payer status, but not race, affects the cost of liver transplantation. *Liver Transpl Surg* 1998;4(5):370-377.

[35] Schulak JA, Ferguson RM, Hanto DW, Ryckman FC, Vogt DP, Bohnengel A. Liver transplantation in Ohio. *Surgery* 1997;122(4):842-848

[36] Brown RS Jr, Ascher NL, Lake JR, *et al*. The impact of surgical complications after liver transplantation on resource utilization. *Arch Surg* 1997;132(10):1098-1103.

[37] Smith DG, Henley KS, Remmert CS, Hass SL, Campbell DAJr, McLaren ID. A cost analysis of alprostadil in liver transplantation. *Pharmacoeconomics* 1996;9(6):517-524.

[38] Pageaux GP, Souche B, Perney P, *et al*. Results and cost of orthotopic liver transplantation for alcoholic cirrhosis. *Transplant Proc* 1993;25(1 Pt 2):1135-1136.

[39] Evans RW, Manninen DL, Dong FB. An economic analysis of liver transplantation: costs, insurance coverage, and reimbursement. *Gastroenterol Clin North Am* 1993;22(2):451-473.

[40] Burroughs AK, Blake J, Thorne S, Else M, Rolles K. Comparative hospital costs of liver transplantation and the treatment of complications of cirrhosis. A prospective study. *Eur J Gastroenterol Hepatol* 1992;4:123-128.

[41] Bonsel GJ, Essink-Bot ML, de Charro FT, van der Maas PJ, Habbema JD. Orthotopic liver transplantation in The Netherlands. The results and impact of a medical technology assessment. *Health Policy* 1990;16(2):147-161.

[42] Sculpher MJ, Pang FS, Manca A, *et al*. Generalisability in economic evaluation studies in healthcare: a review and case studies. *Health Technol Assess* 2004;8:1-192.

[43] O'Brien BJ. A tale of two (or more) cities: geographic transferability of pharmacoeconomic data. *Am J Manag Care* 1997;3:S33-S39.

[44] Goeree R, Burke N, O'Reilly D, Manca A, Blackhouse G, Tarride JE. Transferability of economic evaluations: approaches and factors to consider when using results from one geographic area for another. *Curr Med Res Opin* 2007;23(4):671-682.

[45] Cronbach LJ. Beyond the two disciplines of scientific psychology. *Am Psychol* 1975;30(2):116-127.

[46] Sherman KE, Sherman SN, Chenier T, Tsevat J. Health values of patients with chronic hepatitis C infection. *Arch Intern Med* 2004;164(21):2377-2382.

[47] Longworth L, Bryan S. An empirical comparison of EQ-5D and SF-6D in liver transplant patients. *Health Econ* 2003;12(12):1061-1067.

[48] Ratcliffe J, Longworth L, Young T, *et al.* Assessing health-related quality of life pre- and post-liver transplantation: a prospective multicenter study. *Liver Transpl* 2002;8(3):263-270.

[49] Ratcliffe J, Young T, Longworth L, Buxton M. An assessment of the impact of informative dropout and nonresponse in measuring health-related quality of life using the EuroQol (EQ-5D) descriptive system. *Value Health* 2005;8(1):53-58.

[50] Chong CA, Gulamhussein A, Heathcote EJ, *et al.* Health-state utilities and quality of life in hepatitis C patients. *Am J Gastroenterol* 2003;98(3):630-638.

[51] Siebert U, Sroczynski G, Rossol S, *et al.* Cost effectiveness of peginterferon alpha-2b plus ribavirin versus interferon alpha-2b plus ribavirin for initial treatment of chronic hepatitis C. *Gut* 2003;52(3):425-432.

[52] Bryan S, Ratcliffe J, Neuberger JM, Burroughs AK, Gunson BK, Buxton MJ. Health-related quality of life following liver transplantation. *Qual Life Res* 1998;7(2):115-120.

[53] Lewis MB, Howdle PD. Cognitive dysfunction and health-related quality of life in long-term liver transplant survivors. *Liver Transpl* 2003;9(11):1145-1148.

[54] Ishida K, Imai H, Ogasawara K, Tamashiro H. A review of health economic assessment for liver transplantation: toward social acceptance of liver transplantation in Japan. *Nippon Koshu Eisei Zasshi* 2004;51(4):233-239. (in Japanese)

[55] Kankaanpaa J. Cost-effectiveness of liver transplantations: how to apply the results in resource allocation. *Prev Med* 1990;19(6):700-704.

[56] Bonsel GJ, Klompmaker IJ, Essink-Bot ML, Habbema JD, Slooff MJ. Cost-effectiveness analysis of the Dutch liver transplantation programme. *Transplant Proc* 1990;22(4):1481-1484.

[57] Hisashige A, Katayama T, Mikasa H. Technology assessment of organ transplantation in Japan: economic evaluation of liver transplantation from a living donor. *Joint Conference on Medical Informatics* 1997; 400-401. (in Japanese)

[58] Northup PG, Abecassis MM, Englesbe MJ, *et al.* Addition of adult-to-adult living donation to liver transplant programs improves survival but at an increased cost. *Liver Transpl* 2009;15(2):148-162.

[59] Ouwens JP, van Enckevort PJ, TenVergert EM, *et al.* The cost effectiveness of lung transplantation compared with that of heart and liver transplantation in the Netherlands. *Transpl Int* 2003;16(2):123-127.

[60] Laupacis A, Feeny D, Detsky AS, Tugwell PX. How attractive does a new technology have to be to warrant adoption and utilization? Tentative guidelines for using clinical and economic evaluations. *CMAJ* 1992;146(4):473-481.

[61] Seek AL, Sullivan MA, Pomfret EA. Transplantation of the right hepatic lobe. *N Engl J Med* 2002;347(8):615-618.

[62] Fan ST, Lo CM, Liu CL, Yong BH, Chan JK, Ng IO. Safety of donors in live donor liver transplantation using right lobe grafts. *Arch Surg* 2000;135(3):336-340.

[63] Chisuwa H, Hashikura Y, Mita A, *et al.* Living liver donation: preoperative assessment, anatomic considerations, and long-term outcome. *Transplantation* 2003;75(10):1670-1676.

[64] Singer PA, Siegler M, Whitington PF, *et al.* Ethics of liver transplantation with living donors. *N Engl J Med* 1989;321(9):620-622.

[65] Malago M, Testa G, Marcos A, *et al.* Ethical considerations and rationale of adult-to-adult living donor liver transplantation. *Liver Transpl* 2001;7(10):921-927.

[66] Colardyn F. Organizational and ethical aspects of living donor liver transplantation. *Liver Transpl* 2003;9(9):S2-S5.

[67] de Villa VH, Lo CM, Chen CL. Ethics and rationale of living-donor liver transplantation in Asia. *Transplantation* 2003;75(3 Suppl): S2-S5.

[68] Finkler SA. The distinction between cost and charges. *Ann Intern Med* 1982;96(1):102-109.

[69] The Japanese EuroQol Translation Team. The development of the Japanese EuroQol instrument. *J Health Care Soc* 1998;8:109-117. (in Japanese)

[70] Ikeda S, Ikegami N. Health status in Japanese population. Results from Japanese EuroQol study. *J Health Care Soc* 1999;9:83-91. (in Japanese)

[71] Drummond MF, O'Brien B, Stoddart GL, Torrance GW. *Methods for the Economic Evaluation of Health Care Programmes.* 2nd Edition. Oxford: Oxford University Press, 1997.

[72] van Hout B, Bonsel G, Habbema D, van der Maas P, de Charro F. Heart transplantation in the Netherlands; costs, effects and scenarios. *J Health Econ* 1993;12(1):73-93.

[73] Ramsey SD, Patrick DL, Albert RK, Larson EB, Wood DE, Raghu G. The cost-effectiveness of lung transplantation. A pilot study. *Chest* 1995;108(6):1594-1601.

[74] Evans C, Tavakoli M, Crawford B. Use of quality adjusted life years and life years gained as benchmarks in economic evaluations: a critical appraisal. *Health Care Manag Sci* 2004;7(1):43-49.

[75] Matunami H, Kawasaki S, Hashikura Y, *et al.* Cost of living-related liver transplantation. *Kan Tan Sui* 1996;33:95-98. (in Japanese)

[76] Yagi T, Urushihara N, Oishi M, *et al.* Problems in living donor liver transplantation in adults: postoperative management, complications, and costs. *Transplant Proc* 2000;32(7):2156-2157.

[77] Nakata S, Umeshita K, Ueyama H, *et al.* Cost analysis of operative procedure for transplant patients. *Transplant Proc* 2001;33(1-2):1904-1906.

[78] NICE. *Guide to the Methods of Technology Appraisal.* 2008. (Available from: http://www.nice.org.uk/ [31 August 2010].)

[79] Kaplan RM, Bush JW. Health-related quality of life measurement for evaluation research and policy analysis. *Health Psychology* 1982;1:61–80.

[80] Shiroiwa T, Sung YK, Fukuda T, Lang HC, Bae SC, Tsutani K. International survey on willingness-to-pay (WTP) for one additional QALY gained: what is the threshold of cost effectiveness? *Health Econ* 2010;19(4):422-437.

In: Liver Cancer: Causes, Diagnosis and Treatment
Editor: Benjamin J. Valverde

ISBN: 978-1-61209-115-0
©2011 Nova Science Publishers, Inc.

*Chapter VIII*

# Imaging Hepatocellular Carcinoma Using Positron Emission Tomography

*Zhenghong Lee,*[*1,2] *Nicolas Salem,*[2] *Yu Kuang,*[2] *Haibin Tian,*[1] *and Pablo Ros*[1]

[1]Department of Radiology, Case Western Reserve University, Cleveland, Ohio, U.S.A.
[2]Department of Biomedical Engineering, Case Western Reserve University,
Cleveland, Ohio, U.S.A.

## Abstract

Hepatocellular carcinoma (HCC) is the fifth most common tumor and the third most common cause of cancer death worldwide with a dismal survival rate < 3 month. Positron emission tomography (PET) played a minor role in HCC imaging so far largely due to the fact that the commonly used radiotracer, 2-[$^{18}$F]-2-deoxy-D-glucose (FDG) has little uptake in a number of HCC cases leading to a high false positive rate. In addition, the cost associated with a PET scan prevented it from becoming surveillance or screening tool. Several existing small molecule PET tracers, which were initially developed for other studies, have shown uptake in HCC. These include [$^{11}$C]-acetate, [$^{11}$C]-methionine, [$^{11}$C]-choline as well as [$^{18}$F]-labeled fluorinated choline analogs. For each of these tracers, the uptake mechanisms were studied extensively with an animal model of hepatitis viral infection induced HCC for correlation with preliminary clinical PET scans of HCC using the same tracer if performed. However, the full clinical utility of each tracer needs to be further investigated through patient studies to determine if any of them is useful for early detection, staging, and/or treatment evaluation. The promising PET tracers such as 3'-deoxy-3'-fluorothymidine (FLT) or 2'-[$^{18}$F]fluoro-5-methyl-1-β-D-arabinofuranosyluracil (FMAU), both thymidine analogs designed for imaging tumor proliferation, may not be suitable for imaging HCC due to their degradation in the liver. Currently, an imaging biomarker for tumor proliferation in HCC is actively sought after. The combined PET/CT scanner offers advantage than the stand-alone PET by providing

---

\* Corresponding author: Zhenghong Lee, Ph.D.

anatomical reference for localizing tumor uptake as well as CT-based attenuation correction for PET tracer uptake quantification.

# Introduction

Ultrasound imaging and computed tomography (CT) in combination with routine measurements of serum alpha-fetoprotein levels are currently the routine clinical tests for early lesion detection in patients at risk [1-3]. Magnetic resonance imaging provides another method to enhance the sensitivity to neoplasm using new imaging sequences and contrast agents [4-6]. However, for smaller lesions of HCC, e.g., less than 1 cm in diameter, the percentage of failure in detecting HCC increased as size- or density-based (anatomic) imaging modalities often fail to convey information regarding the malignancy of these smaller nodules despite of the ever improving spatial resolution of modern scanners [7]. The presence of other liver conditions or diseases such as fibrosis and cirrhosis compounded the issue further. Early detection of HCC is of major clinical significance since many patients who present with advanced stage of HCC upon first diagnosis are usually too late for viable treatment options. If liver cancer such as HCC is detected at an early stage, treatment can be more successful and better prognosis can often be expected. Recent development with dynamic contrast-enhanced MRI (DCE-MRI), diffusion-weighted MRI (DWI), MR spectroscopy (MRS), and contrast-enhance ultrasound depart from the traditional morphological imaging and move toward physiology-based or even molecular imaging [8]. The utility of these approaches for early detection of HCC, treatment evaluation, recurrence detection, etc., has yet to be studied thoroughly, especially the correlation between what is actually measured (surrogate marker) and the biological characteristics of HCC.

PET imaging utilizes molecular probes, usually a small molecule radiotracer, to examine a specific metabolic pathway by design and to obtain information along that pathway by making use of tracer's uptake kinetics as well as cellular metabolism and retention, which can be quantitatively mapped out by way of mathematical modeling and parameter estimation based on dynamically acquired PET image data [9]. FDG-PET is widely used to detect cancer due to the generally upregulated glycolytic pathway in cancers. However, there are inconsistent results about the usefulness of FDG-PET for detecting HCC. While some studies have demonstrated its value in predicting the outcome for patients with liver cancer [10, 11], others have reported false-negative rates in detection, approaching 50% [12, 13]. Increased glycolysis may not be the preferred kinetic pathway in some HCCs, especially early-stage HCC. We have confirmed this performance of FDG on an animal model of HCC, and we therefore looked into other simple (small molecule) tracers for their potential in HCC imaging with PET.

# Imaging with Acetate

Acetate in the solution is often in the form of sodium acetate ($CH_3COONa$), a cell permeable simple molecule. Endogenous acetate and other short chain fatty acids (SCFA) are produced in several parts of the gastrointestinal tract of humans and animals (almost 10% of total daily energy requirements [14]) through the process of bacterial fermentation, mainly from the fermentation of plant materials such as cellulose, fibers, starch and sugars or mucus. [$^{11}$C]-Acetate was originally developed as a tracer for tricarboxylic acid (TCA) cycle influx, and thus the overall oxidation in myocardium [15], which was used to assess myocardial viability. The principle behind such application is that all major myocardium oxidative fuels such as fatty acid, glucose, lactate, pyruvate, ketone bodies and some amino acids are oxidized via conversion to acetyl-CoA and oxidation through the TCA cycle in mitochondria to produce large amount of adenosine triphosphate (ATP) for myocardium contractile work. Radio-synthesis of [$^{11}$C]-Acetate mostly followed procedure by Langstrom's group [16].

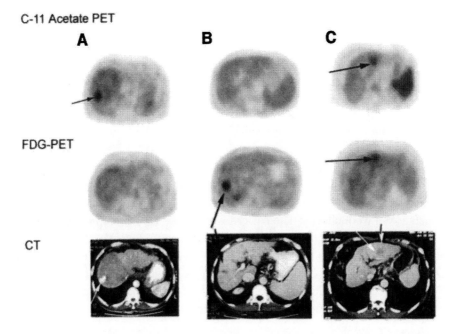

Figure 1. Dual-tracer PET imaging of HCC. Top row, PET imaging with [11C]-acetate depicts well-differentiated HCC (A), but not poorly-differentiated HCC (B). In contrast, FDG-PET in the middle row shows no uptake in well-differentiated HCC (A), but focal uptake in poorly-differentiated HCC (B). Column C is a patient with moderately-differentiated HCC, in which [11C]-acetate and FDG depict different portions of the same HCC. The bottom row shows the accompanying CT scans depicting the morphology of liver nodules. Reprint from Journal of Nuclear Medicine Vol. 44 No. 2 213-221, 2003, with permission from the Society of Nuclear Medicine.

## Human Studies

[$^{11}$C]-acetate has shown uptake for the well-differentiated HCC (an early stage of HCC) in our woodchuck models and holds promise for early detection of HCC. That echoed published clinical studies shown in *Figure 1*. In the figure, Columns *A, B* and *C* represent three patients with well-, poorly- and moderately-differentiated HCC, respectively. The three rows represent the imaging modalities: top is PET imaging with [$^{11}$C]-acetate, middle is PET imaging with [$^{18}$F]-FDG, and bottom is CT scan of the same abdominal region. It is convincing that acetate and FDG picked up different stages of HCC. In Patient **C**, however, different portions of the same tumor were lighted up by either acetate (well-differentiated) or

FDG (poorly-differentiated) due to the heterogeneity of this HCC. However, this type of two-tracer PET scanning protocol is not suitable for routine clinical use although it is well-designed to show-case what dual-tracer PET scans can reveal. Besides, [$^{11}$C]-acetate showed increased uptake in the benign lesions, such as adenoma, hemangioma and focal nodular hyperplasia etc, as compared to the surrounding hepatic tissues. Therefore, the specificity of acetate for HCC detection can be an issue. It is vital to have differential uptake between pre-cancerous and cancerous lesions. In brief, acetate or FDG alone cannot be an effective PET tracer for imaging HCC. Logistic hurdles and current health-economy prevented the implementation of the dual-tracer study as a clinical routine.

## Uptake Mechanisms of Acetate in Early-Stage HCC

The lipids are a heterogeneous group of compounds that are relatively insoluble in water and soluble in non-polar solvents such as chloroform. The relationship between lipids and cancer is a complex topic. Different from the situation in myocardium, the main pathway for *de novo* synthesis of fatty acids (lipogenesis) occurs in the cytosol of liver and adipose tissues. Acetyl-CoA is the immediate substrate, and free palmitate, the 16 carbon saturated fatty acid (with no double bond) is the end product. Acetyl-CoA, a common metabolite of nearly all products of digestion including carbohydrate, fat, and protein, is thus the major building block for long-chain fatty acid synthesis in nonruminants including the humans and animals such as the woodchucks. The eastern woodchuck (*Marmota monax*) was used in our study as the animal model. This woodchuck hepatitis virus (WHV) infection-induced HCC model is useful for studying human HCC. WHV is a member of Hepadnaviridae family, genus *Orthohepadnavirus*, of which human hepatitis B virus (HBV) is the prototype. Like HBV, WHV infects a woodchuck and can cause acute hepatitis that turns chronic. The chronic carriers usually develop HCC within 2–4 years of life [17].

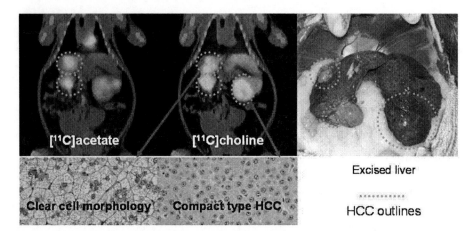

Figure 2. Tracer comparison study using the same animal. As choline showed in all three tumors, acetate clearly picked up two. While background in normal liver is high with choline, the TCA cycle can be seen in the heart with acetate.

Injected acetate is quickly converted into acetyl-CoA by enzyme acetyl-CoA synthetase (ACAS) [18-21], whose activity is up-regulated in HCC [22]. An uptake study using different tumor cell lines showed that labeled acetate was incorporated into the lipids, mostly of phosphatidylcholine (PC) and neutral lipids, in the tumor cells more prominently than into fibroblasts [23]. Our combined in vivo (imaging) and ex vivo (metabolites) studies in the woodchuck models of HCC concurred that. Tissues extracted from the regions of HCCs with the highest [11C]-Acetate uptake demonstrated a much greater amount of phosphatidylcholine (PC) and triacylglycerol (TG) accumulated within than in the surrounding hepatic tissues [24]. The first panel of *Figure 2* showed the performance of Acetate in HCC. Please notice the signals in myocardium as different metabolic pathways were involved as discussed above.

## Acetate Variants as Alternatives

There are several acetate related compounds. The first is fluoroacetate, which is a fluorinated analog of acetate. What we know is that it is converted to fluoroacetyl-CoA by the same ACAS and then enters the TCA cycle where it is transformed into fluorocitrate, which inhibits the enzyme aconitase (aconitate hydratase), leading to the buildup of citrate and limitation of cellular ATP production in various tissues with high metabolic rates. The toxicity and death associated with fluoroacetate are generally considered to be caused by severe impairment of energy production. Fluoroacetate is found to be rapidly metabolized and excreted with highest concentration in the blood, moderate level in the muscle and kidneys, and the lowest concentration in the liver [25]. This low background in normal liver may offer an opportunity for imaging. The bigger question, as asked in other studies [26], is whether [18F]-fluoroacetate mimics [11C]-acetate along the lipogenesis pathway in HCC. The second concern is its perceived toxicity. Although we believe that the tracer amount of labeled fluoroacetate is below the effective non-toxic level of fluoroacetate (determined by myocardium and CNS toxicity), safety study using tracer amount of fluoroacetate in the animal models will have to be performed before the imaging studies.

Another potential, but probably not dominant pathway for labeled acetate is ketogensis during fast state, during which ketone bodies are generated, transported outside liver as fuels in extrahepatic tissues. Although it seems unlikely that the amount of acetate going through this pathway contributes to PET imaging of HCC, it will be interesting to know if liver cancer produce more ketone bodies than the surrounding tissues, or vice versa. Based on the findings, we can estimate the level of ketogenesis in liver and HCC, and to determine if [11C]-acetoacetate can be an alternative for use in HCC imaging since acetoacetate can be a source for acetyl-CoA if ketogensis is negligible in HCC.

# Imaging with Choline Tracers

Choline is classified as a water-soluble essential nutrient and usually grouped into the Vitamin B complex. Choline and its metabolites are needed by the body for three main physiological purposes: structural integrity of cell membranes via its metabolite phosphatidyl-choline (PC); cholinergic neurotransmission via acetylcholine; and as a major source for methyl group via trimethylglycine (betaine). The major source of choline in the food is PC, which is abundant in egg, soy and cooked beef, chicken, veal and turkey livers. The digestive process converts PC back to choline. Many foods contain trace amounts of free choline such as iceberg lettuce. The commonly available choline dietary supplement lecithin is mostly PC, which is derived from soy or egg yolks.

## Human Studies with Choline and FCh

Using choline for HCC imaging, which has no uptake in pre-cancerous lesions, the quantitative issue in data analysis in terms of distinguishing different grades of HCC, well-, moderately-, and poorly-differentiated has not been satisfactorily addressed. Therefore, its clinical utility is not entirely clear at the moment. In a prove-of-concept study [27], [$^{18}$F]-fluorocholine (FCh) uptake by HCC was compared with that by FDG scanned one week apart in a small number of patients confirmed with HCC. FCh detected HCC for all patients while FDG missed some HCCs. Higher FCh uptake were obtained from well-differentiated HCC comparing with that from poorly-differentiated HCC [27]. A Phase III clinical trial for applying FCh in HCC imaging is on the way based on the positive results from this study. We also performed imaging studies using [$^{11}$C]/[$^{18}$F]-choline on the woodchuck models of HCC and compared the results with that from [$^{11}$C]-acetate PET scans on the same animal models [28]. As the middle panel of the PET/CT overlay showed in *Figure 2*, the woodchuck imaging results echoed that from the human FCh study. Choline picked up all HCCs, well-differentiated or poorly-differentiated. There is no cardiac uptake although a liver background exists with choline due to the betaine or phosphoethanolamine (PE)-methylation pathway discussed later.

## Mechanism of Choline Uptake in HCC

As summarized at the beginning of this section, among the three possible metabolic pathways of choline shown in *Figure 3*, only two will happen in the liver. The liver background is the result of betaine production along the slower (blue) PE-methylation pathway at least for early time points [29]. HCC, in contrast, quickly accumulated a higher uptake via the cytidine 5-diphosphocholine (CDP-Choline) pathway than did the surrounding hepatic tissues, and both choline transport and choline kinase activity in HCC are found to be up-regulated [30]. As HCC advances to a more malignant stage, the high HCC uptake would come down a bit (while still while still higher than the background uptake) at later time points due largely to a possibly shift from the CDP-choline pathway to the PE-methylation pathway, and CTP:phosphocholine cytidylyltransferase (CCT) seems to be the rate-limiting factor for PC synthesis via choline's CDP-choline pathway [30]. Further mechanistic studies are needed to confirm choline tracers' complex metabolite pathways in different stages of liver cancer. Nevertheless, it is possible that radio-choline can be used not only for detection, but also for staging HCC since it has the potential to be a one-stop tracer for HCC applications.

## Comparing Choline with Fluorinated Cholines

The general form of choline is shown in *Figure 4*. When $R_1$, $R_2$ and $R_3$ are all methyl groups and $R_4$ is the ehthyl alcohol group ($CH_2CH_2OH$), it has the basic form ($CH3$)$3N+CH2CH2OH$ $X^-$, where $X^-$ is a counterion such as chloride for choline chloride. The native choline with C-11 label limits its usage only to academic PET centers due to the very short half life of C-11 (20 minutes). Fluorinated cholines with F-18 label will practically make PET imaging clinically viable. The choices of $R_1$-$R_4$ enabled a great number of variations. However, almost all these analogs are not suitable as a candidate for radiolabeling for tracer production due to the requirement for transport efficiency and binding affinity for the key enzyme choline kinase that is involved with PET imaging. Devés and Krupka's [31] study limited the structure of choline analog. Small increases in the size of the quaternary ammonium head, as in triethylcholine ($R_1$, $R_2$ and $R_3$ all with an ethyl group), sharply lowered affinity for the transporter as large choline failed to penetrate the cells. In addition, Clary, Tsai and Guynn's [32] study found that none of the choline analogs they tested were better substrates than the simplest choline for choline kinase with the only exception of ethylcholine ($R_1$ is an ethyl group). Based on these results, besides the native choline, the choice of fluorinated choline analogs is limited to either fluorocholine (FCh) or fluoroethylcholine (FEC) first radiolabeled with F-18 by DeGrado [33] and Hara [34], respectively, for prostate cancer imaging. Application for HCC imaging is a new development. The obvious advantage of fluorocholine over other simple tracers such as FDG and acetate is that it offers a one-stop approach that will be sufficient for use in both early detection and grading/staging of HCC without combined use with other PET tracers. As discussed, only two small-scale clinical studies have been published [27, 35] so far although more are forth coming [36].

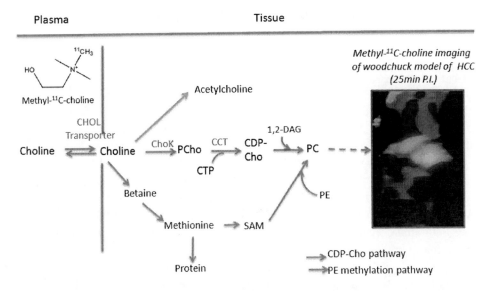

Figure 3. Metabolic fate of radiolabeled choline. 1, 2-DAG: 1,2-diacylglycerol; CCT: CTP:phosphocholine cytidylyltransferase; CDP-Cho: cytidine 5-diphosphocholine; ChoK; choline kinase; PCho: phosphocholine; PC: phosphatidylcholine; PE: phosphoethanolamine; SAM: S-adenosylmethionine; P.I.: post injection.

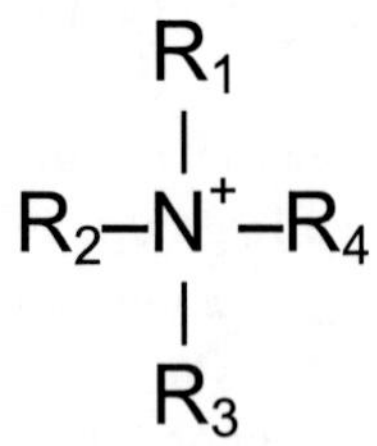

$$R_2-N^+-R_4$$

with $R_1$ above and $R_3$ below the central $N^+$.

Figure 4. Choline.

We used FEC in comparison with choline on the same animal model of woodchuck HCC. The contrast uptake with choline was shown to be higher than that with FEC for all animals studied, but the difference was found to be not statistically significant for the same-day studies. There might be a difference in the efficiency of choline transporter for choline and FEC; additionally, cellular enzymes such as choline kinase, CCT and others that influence the tracers' metabolism might differ in binding affinity or substrate selectivity for choline and FEC. However, our animal data demonstrate that both tracers can be used for HCC imaging with similar results [37].

In addition, overnight fasting is required for FDG-PET imaging to reduce endogenous glucose and competition with its radiotracer analog for transport and accumulation. Fasting can be an issue for some patients. Therefore, we compared choline and FEC when they were fed or fasted to evaluate the effect of fasting on the two tracers' contrast uptake in HCC comparing to the surrounding hepatic tissues. Fasting was not found to affect tumor contrast [37]. This is encouraging, but a range of diets (fatty foods vs. standard-care diet) needs be tested.

# Imaging with Methionine

Methionine may 1) be utilized for protein synthesis or 2) be converted to S-adenosylmethionine (SAM), which is the primary methyl donor in the body and a precursor in polyamine synthesis. During methylation, the methyl group of SAM is transferred to a large variety of methyl acceptors [38]. Although there are a large number of SAM-dependent methyltransferases [39, 40], the three reactions that quantitatively contribute most to the transmethylation flux are methylation of glycine by glycine N-methyltransferase (GNMT) to form sarcosine (N-methylglycine), methylation of guanidinoacetate by guanidinoacetate N-methyltransferase (GAMT) to form creatine, and methylation of PE by PEMT to form PC (specifically in the liver), which is of main interest to our imaging study.

As mentioned above, radiolabeled methionine (Met) was originally developed for imaging both amino acid transport and protein synthesis, which is believed to be generally increased during malignant transformation. In principle, local protein synthesis rates in tissue can be quantified via kinetic modeling by use of *in vivo* PET imaging data with positron-emitting amino acids, or amino acid analogues. After being transported into the cell, an *L*-amino acid is converted primarily into amino-acyl-tRNA by the enzyme amino-acyl RNA synthetase. This process is the first step in protein synthesis. The rate of incorporation of such *L*-amino acids into proteins reflects the protein synthesis rate (PSR) in tissue [41]. As a PET tracer, L-[methy-$^{11}$C]-Met has been applied for imaging brain, head and neck cancers, etc., for years. The uptake attained a constant radioactivity level after an initial rapid clearance with increase in the protein-bound frac*tion*. Significant accumulation was found in a variety of extracranial malignant tumors including lung cancer, head and neck cancers, breast cancer, sarcomas, and malignant lymphomas [42-48]. Most of PET imaging studies with L-[methyl-$^{11}$C]-Met were actually performed for brain tumors. The main reason for this was that its transport through normal BBB was well defined [49]. L-methionine's metabolic fate seems to be relatively simple in normal brain as most of the Met molecules will be incorporated in protein synthesis whereas the transmethylation pathway is negligible [50]. In the case of tumors, the parenchymal metabolic routes are far from being well identified. The transmethylation route can no longer be neglected, and incorporation in protein synthesis follows complex pathways [49].

Met was synthesized following a published procedure [51], and has been used by us as a biomarker for several clinical trials involving brain tumor therapeutics. In our preliminary study, several woodchucks with liver nodules seen on ultrasound were selected for PET imaging. Like all previous studies, the scans were conducted on the clinical PET/CT scanner, the GEMINI-TF (Philips Medical Systems, Cleveland, Ohio). PET/CT overlay nicely display HCC uptake in comparison to the surrounding hepatic background. Both regions of the tumor and the surrounding hepatic tissues were drawn to generate the time activity curves shown in **Figure 5**. The results showed that although there is a liver background, L-[mehtyl-$^{11}$C]-Met's uptake stabilized in the tumor quickly after injection, and maintained a ratio above 2:1 over the surrounding hepatic tissues throughout the dynamic scans.

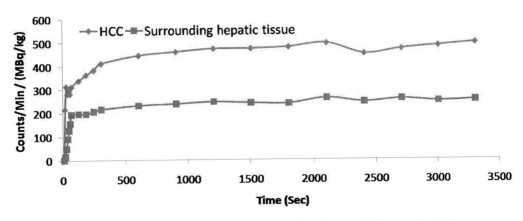

Figure 5. Time activity curve from dynamic PET imaging showing tumor/ liver ratio at 2.0.

## Imaging the Proliferative Aspect of HCC

During tumorigenesis of HCC, there are two highly proliferative periods [52]: one at very early stage with the development of well-differentiated small HCC (< 2.0 cm) within the precancerous dysplasia nodule; the other at a stage advancing towards high grade HCC when less-differentiated HCC was surrounded by well-differentiated HCC. In both cases, the highly proliferative cells in the core/center encircled by less-proliferative surrounding tissues always rendered a "nodule-in-nodule" appearance. [$^{11}$C]-thymidine (TdR, as *Figure 6a*) was first developed to image tumor proliferation through integration into DNA whose synthesis is usually up-regulated during the proliferation phase. However, it was quickly found to be of limited use due to severe catabolism even outside liver as TdR is rapidly metabolized and degraded. From labeled TdR to its analogs such as [$^{18}$F]-fluoro-3'-deoxy-3'-D-fluorothymidine ([$^{18}$F]-FLT as *Figure 6b*), 1-(2'-deoxy-2'-[$^{18}$F]fluoro-β-D-arabinofuranosyl) thymine (D-[$^{18}$F]-FMAU as *Figure 6c*), all D-isomers as the naturally occurring nucleosides, the main issue is their degradation in the liver. *Figure 7* demonstrated D-FMAU's performance in the liver where metastasized liver cancer appeared as a cold spot while the tracer was degradated in the liver parenchyma [53]. Similar performance can be found for FLT applied to human liver [54, 55]. That is the reason FLT or other D-isomers within the thymidine analogs cannot be effectively used to imaging proliferation of liver cancer [56].

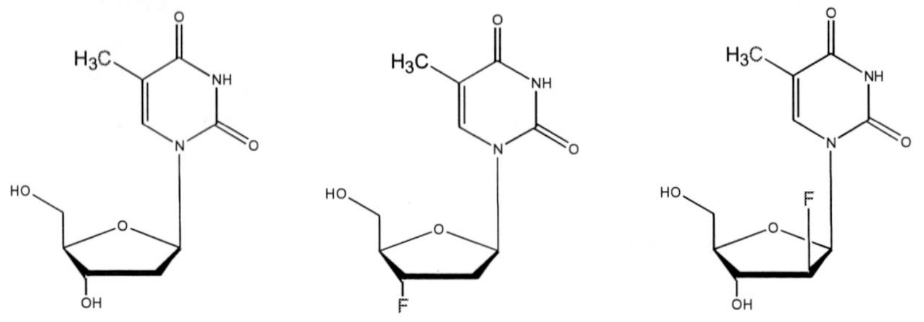

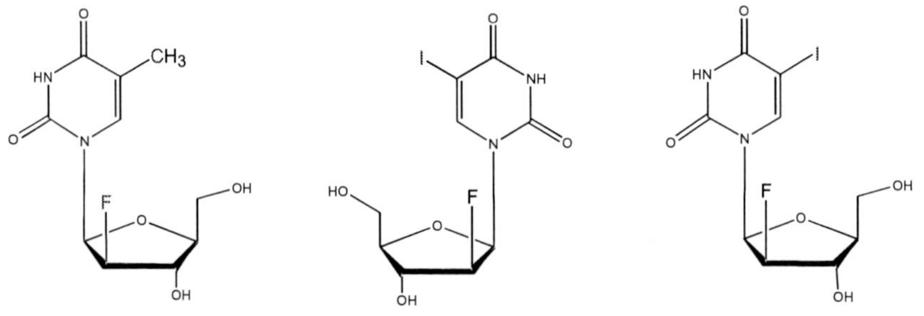

Figure 6. Thymidine (TdR) and its analogs. Red-colored atoms are the positions for radiolabels: C for C-11/C-14, F for F-18, I for radioiodide. FMAU can have F-18 or C-11.

On the other hand, there exists 1-(2'-deoxy-2'-[$^{18}$F]fluoro-β-L-arabinofuranosyl)thymine (also named 2'-[$^{18}$F]fluoro-5-methyl-1-β-L-arabinofuranosyluracil or L-[$^{18}$F]-FMAU as *Figure 6d*), a new PET tracer th great potential in imaging primary liver cancer such as HCC. L-FMAU, the enantiomer or mirrored stereoisomer to D-FMAU, is a non-natural nucleoside analog and a potent antiviral drug that has shown great promise for the treatment of hepatitis viral B infection. L-[$^{18}$F]-FMAU, being a non-natural nucleoside (L-isomer), is resistant to hepatic degradation and its contrast uptake in liver cancer can potentially be used for detecting the prolific aspect of HCC and for assessing the response to the treatment if the treatment impairs HCC proliferation. To ensure that L-FMAU is an effective PET tracer for imaging primary liver cancer, clinical study will eventually be needed to investigate the key issue relating to L-FMAU's metabolism, degradation (or lack of it) and clearance in liver cancer as well as the surrounding hepatic tissues.

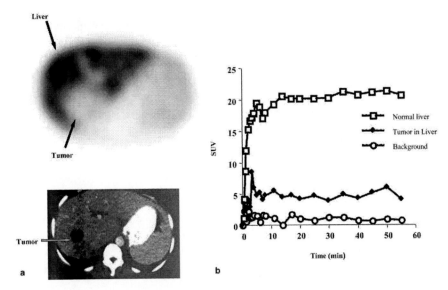

Figure 7. a D-[$^{18}$F]-FMAU PET (*above*) and CT (*below*) images of a liver metastasis in a patient with colorectal cancer. b D-[$^{18}$F]-FMAU retention time–activity curves. Reprint from Eur J Nucl Med Mol Imaging (2005) 32:15–22 with permission from Springer.

## Conclusion

Primary liver cancer such as hepatocellular carcinoma is a global health issue. An effective molecular imaging approach has been actively sought for clinical use in diagnosis, staging, and treatment assessment to completed existing medical imaging technology such as CT, MRI and ultrasound imaging. This chapter briefly reviewed several PET imaging approaches including work in progress. Admittedly, PET scans will probably not ne a screening tool for the general mass due to current issues with health economics. However, understanding the mechanism(s) regarding how each PET tracer works in hepatocellular carcinoma will be beneficial to evaluate their clinical utilities.

## References

[1] Kudo M, Zheng RQ, Kim SR, et al. Diagnostic accuracy of imaging for liver cirrhosis compared to histologically proven liver cirrhosis. A multicenter collaborative study. *Intervirology* 2008;51 Suppl 1:17-26.

[2] Teefey SA, Hildeboldt CC, Dehdashti F, et al. Detection of primary hepatic malignancy in liver transplant candidates: prospective comparison of CT, MR imaging, US, and PET. *Radiology* 2003;226:533-42.

[3] Tremolda F, Benevegnu L, Drago C, et al. Early detection of hepatocellular carcinoma in patients with cirrhosis by alphafetoprotein, ultrasound and fine-needle biopsy. *Hepatogastroenterology* 1989;36:519-21.

[4] Choi D, Kim SH, Lim JH, et al. Detection of hepatocellular carcinoma: combined T2-weighted and dynamic gadolinium-enhanced MRI versus combined CT during arterial portography and CT hepatic arteriography. *J Comput Assist Tomogr* 2001;25:777-85.

[5] Fujita T, Ito K, Honjo K, Okazaki H, Matsumoto T, Matsunaga N. Detection of hepatocellular carcinoma: comparison of T2-weighted breath-hold fast spin-echo sequences and high-resolution dynamic MR imaging with a phased-array body coil. *J Magn Reson Imaging* 1999;9:274-9.

[6] Tang Y, Yamashita Y, Arakawa A, et al. Detection of hepatocellular carcinoma arising in cirrhotic livers: comparison of gadolinium- and ferumoxides-enhanced MR imaging. *AJR Am J Roentgenol* 1999;172:1547-54.

[7] Sahani DV, Kalva SP. Imaging the liver. *Oncologist* 2004;9:385-97.

[8] Weber WA, Czernin J, Phelps ME, Herschman HR. Technology Insight: novel imaging of molecular targets is an emerging area crucial to the development of targeted drugs. *Nat Clin Pract Oncol* 2008;5:44-54.

[9] Phelps ME. Nuclear medicine, molecular imaging, and molecular medicine. *J Nucl Med* 2002;43:13N-4N.

[10] Kong YH, Han CJ, Lee SD, et al. [Positron emission tomography with fluorine-18-fluorodeoxyglucose is useful for predicting the prognosis of patients with hepatocellular carcinoma]. *Korean J Hepatol* 2004;10:279-87.

[11] Wudel LJ, Jr., Delbeke D, Morris D, et al. The role of [18F]fluorodeoxyglucose positron emission tomography imaging in the evaluation of hepatocellular carcinoma. *Am Surg* 2003;69:117-24; discussion 24-6.

[12] Jeng LB, Changlai SP, Shen YY, Lin CC, Tsai CH, Kao CH. Limited value of 18F-2-deoxyglucose positron emission tomography to detect hepatocellular carcinoma in hepatitis B virus carriers. *Hepatogastroenterology* 2003;50:2154-6.

[13] Khan MA, Combs CS, Brunt EM, et al. Positron emission tomography scanning in the evaluation of hepatocellular carcinoma. *J Hepatol* 2000;32:792-7.

[14] Bergman EN. Energy contributions of volatile fatty acids from the gastrointestinal tract in various species. *Physiol Rev* 1990;70:567-90.

[15] Ng CK, Huang SC, Schelbert HR, Buxton DB. Validation of a model for [1-11C]acetate as a tracer of cardiac oxidative metabolism. *Am J Physiol* 1994;266:H1304-15.

[16] Kihlberg T, Valind S, Langstrom B. Synthesis of [1-11C], [2-11C], [1-11C](2H3) and [2-11C](2H3)acetate for in vivo studies of myocardium using PET. *Nucl Med Biol* 1994;21:1067-72.

[17] Tennant BC, Toshkov IA, Peek SF, et al. Hepatocellular carcinoma in the woodchuck model of hepatitis B virus infection. *Gastroenterology* 2004;127:S283-93.

[18] Baranyai JM, Blum JJ. Quantitative analysis of intermediary metabolism in rat hepatocytes incubated in the presence and absence of ethanol with a substrate mixture including ketoleucine. *Biochem J* 1989;258:121-40.

[19] Barth C, Sladek M, Decker K. Dietary changes of cytoplasmic acetyl-CoA synthetase in different rat tissues. *Biochim Biophys Acta* 1972;260:1-9.

[20] Crabtree B, Gordon MJ, Christie SL. Measurement of the rates of acetyl-CoA hydrolysis and synthesis from acetate in rat hepatocytes and the role of these fluxes in substrate cycling. *Biochem J* 1990;270:219-25.

[21] Goldberg RP, Brunengraber H. Contributions of cytosolic and mitochondrial acetyl-CoA syntheses to the activation of lipogenic acetate in rat liver. *Adv Exp Med Biol* 1980;132:413-8.

[22] Kuang Y, Salem N, Wang F, Schomisch SJ, Chandramouli V, Lee Z. A colorimetric assay method to measure acetyl-CoA synthetase activity: application to woodchuck model of hepatitis virus-induced hepatocellular carcinoma. *J Biochem Biophys Methods* 2007;70:649-55.

[23] Yoshimoto M, Waki A, Yonekura Y, et al. Characterization of acetate metabolism in tumor cells in relation to cell proliferation: acetate metabolism in tumor cells. *Nucl Med Biol* 2001;28:117-22.

[24] Salem N, Kuang Y, Corn D, et al. [(Methyl)1-(11)C]-Acetate Metabolism in Hepatocellular Carcinoma. *Mol Imaging Biol* 2010.

[25] Eason C. Sodium monofluoroacetate (1080) risk assessment and risk communication. *Toxicology* 2002;181-182:523-30.

[26] Lindhe O, Sun A, Ulin J, Rahman O, Langstrom B, Sorensen J. [(18)F]Fluoroacetate is not a functional analogue of [(11)C]acetate in normal physiology. *Eur J Nucl Med Mol Imaging* 2009;36:1453-9.

[27] Talbot JN, Gutman F, Fartoux L, et al. PET/CT in patients with hepatocellular carcinoma using [(18)F]fluorocholine: preliminary comparison with [ (18)F]FDG PET/CT. *Eur J Nucl Med Mol Imaging* 2006;33:1285-9.

[28] Salem N, Brunengraber H, Tennant BC, Lee Z. Tracer kinetic modeling using [C-11]-acetate PET imaging on the woodchuck model of hepatocellular carcinoma. *J Nucl Med* 2006;47:426p.

[29] Kuang Y, Salem N, Tian H, et al. Imaging Lipid Synthesis in Hepatocellular Carcinoma with [Methyl-11C]Choline: Correlation with in vivo Metabolic Studies *Journal of Nuclear Medicine* (in press).

[30] Kuang Y, Salem N, Corn DJ, et al. Transport and Metabolism of Radiolabeled Choline in Hepatocellular Carcinoma. *Mol Pharm* 2010.

[31] Deves R, Krupka RM. The binding and translocation steps in transport as related to substrate structure. A study of the choline carrier of erythrocytes. *Biochim Biophys Acta* 1979;557:469-85.

[32] Clary GL, Tsai CF, Guynn RW. Substrate specificity of choline kinase. *Arch Biochem Biophys* 1987;254:214-21.

[33] DeGrado TR, Coleman RE, Wang S, et al. Synthesis and evaluation of 18F-labeled choline as an oncologic tracer for positron emission tomography: initial findings in prostate cancer. *Cancer Res* 2001;61:110-7.

[34] Hara T, Kosaka N, Kishi H. Development of (18)F-fluoroethylcholine for cancer imaging with PET: synthesis, biochemistry, and prostate cancer imaging. *J Nucl Med* 2002;43:187-99.

[35] Yamamoto Y, Nishiyama Y, Kameyama R, et al. Detection of hepatocellular carcinoma using 11C-choline PET: comparison with 18F-FDG PET. *J Nucl Med* 2008;49:1245-8.

[36] Balogova S, Bumsel F, Kerrou K, et al. La fluorocholine(18F) a une utilité clinique dans le cancer de la prostate et le carcinome hépatocellulaire. . . parfois chez le même malade. *Médecine Nucléaire* 2010;34:378-82.

[37] Kolthammer JA, Corn DJ, Tenley N, et al. PET Imaging of Hepatocellular Carcinoma with 18F-Fluoroethylcholine and 11C-Choline. *European Journal of Nuclear Medicine and Molecular Imaging* (under review).

[38] Poirier LA. The effects of diet, genetics and chemicals on toxicity and aberrant DNA methylation: an introduction. *J Nutr* 2002;132:2336S-9S.

[39] Mudd SH, Brosnan JT, Brosnan ME, et al. Methyl balance and transmethylation fluxes in humans. *Am J Clin Nutr* 2007;85:19-25.

[40] Mato JM, Martinez-Chantar ML, Lu SC. Methionine metabolism and liver disease. *Annu Rev Nutr* 2008;28:273-93.

[41] Vaalburg W, Coenen HH, Crouzel C, et al. Amino acids for the measurement of protein synthesis in vivo by PET. *Int J Rad Appl Instrum B* 1992;19:227-37.

[42] Leskinen-Kallio S, Lindholm P, Lapela M, Joensuu H, Nordman E. Imaging of head and neck tumors with positron emission tomography and [11C]methionine. *Int J Radiat Oncol Biol Phys* 1994;30:1195-9.

[43] Jager PL, Vaalburg W, Pruim J, de Vries EG, Langen KJ, Piers DA. Radiolabeled amino acids: basic aspects and clinical applications in oncology. *J Nucl Med* 2001;42:432-45.

[44] Leskinen-Kallio S, Ruotsalainen U, Nagren K, Teras M, Joensuu H. Uptake of carbon-11-methionine and fluorodeoxyglucose in non-Hodgkin's lymphoma: a PET study. *J Nucl Med* 1991;32:1211-8.

[45] Nettelbladt OS, Sundin AE, Valind SO, et al. Combined fluorine-18-FDG and carbon-11-methionine PET for diagnosis of tumors in lung and mediastinum. *J Nucl Med* 1998;39:640-7.

[46] Inoue T, Kim EE, Wong FC, et al. Comparison of fluorine-18-fluorodeoxyglucose and carbon-11-methionine PET in detection of malignant tumors. *J Nucl Med* 1996;37:1472-6.

[47] Deloar HM, Fujiwara T, Nakamura T, et al. Estimation of internal absorbed dose of L-[methyl-11C]methionine using whole-body positron emission tomography. *Eur J Nucl Med* 1998;25:629-33.

[48] Plathow C, Weber WA. Tumor cell metabolism imaging. *J Nucl Med* 2008;49 Suppl 2:43S-63S.

[49] Derlon JM, Bourdet C, Bustany P, et al. [11C]L-methionine uptake in gliomas. *Neurosurgery* 1989;25:720-8.

[50] Bustany P, Chatel M, Derlon JM, et al. Brain tumor protein synthesis and histological grades: a study by positron emission tomography (PET) with C11-L-Methionine. *J Neurooncol* 1986;3:397-404.

[51] Pascali C, Bogni A, Iwata R, Decise D, Crippa F, Bombardieri E. High efficiency preparation of L-[S-methyl-C-11]methionine by on-column [C-11]methylation on C18 Sep-Pak. *Journal of Labelled Compounds & Radiopharmaceuticals* 1999;42:715-24.

[52] Kojiro M. Histopathology of liver cancers. *Best Pract Res Clin Gastroenterol* 2005;19:39-62.

[53] Sun H, Mangner TJ, Collins JM, Muzik O, Douglas K, Shields AF. Imaging DNA synthesis in vivo with 18F-FMAU and PET. *J Nucl Med* 2005;46:292-6.

[54] Eckel F, Herrmann K, Schmidt S, et al. Imaging of proliferation in hepatocellular carcinoma with the in vivo marker 18F-fluorothymidine. *J Nucl Med* 2009;50:1441-7.

[55] Shields AF, Grierson JR, Dohmen BM, et al. Imaging proliferation in vivo with [F-18]FLT and positron emission tomography. *Nat Med* 1998;4:1334-6.

[56] Tehrani OS, Muzik O, Heilbrun LK, et al. Tumor imaging using 1-(2'-deoxy-2'-18F-fluoro-beta-D-arabinofuranosyl)thymine and PET. *J Nucl Med* 2007;48:1436-41.

# Index

## A

Abraham, 94
abuse, 68
access, 116, 216
accounting, 199, 201, 202, 203
acetaldehyde, 68, 71
acetylation, 42
acetylcholine, 227
acid, 3, 13, 14, 15, 20, 23, 25, 30, 32, 36, 37, 44, 46, 49, 50, 51, 57, 59, 113, 115, 127, 131, 225, 226, 230
active compound, 34
acute infection, 61
acute myeloid leukemia, 44
additives, 46
adenine, 110
adenocarcinoma, 9, 50, 145
adenoma, 54, 80, 226
adenomatous polyposis coli, 58
adenosine, 225
adenosine triphosphate, 225
adenovirus, 62
ADH, 54, 68
adhesion, 8, 20, 26, 47, 49, 64, 75, 79, 81, 83, 143, 144, 145, 147, 148, 154, 155, 156
adhesions, 147, 148
adipocyte, 59
adipose, 226
adipose tissue, 226
adjustment, 162
ADP, 63
adults, 7, 218, 219, 221
adverse effects, 120, 122, 123, 124
aetiology, 38
AFB1, 54, 69, 80, 82
aflatoxin, 1, 5, 38, 54, 71, 80, 83, 93, 100, 130

AFP glycoprotein, 1, 7
Africa, 2, 93, 105
age, 2, 4, 5, 56, 61, 210, 211
aggregation, 141
aggressiveness, 145, 146
agonist, 33, 74
AIDS, 36
alanine, 5, 30, 33, 38
alanine aminotransferase, 5, 38
albumin, 84, 165
alcohol abuse, 68
alcohol consumption, 5, 6, 38, 68, 71, 74, 105, 138
alcohol use, 1
alcoholic cirrhosis, 5, 219
alcoholic liver damage, 103
alcoholic liver disease, 5, 68, 206, 207, 210, 211, 212
alcoholics, 5
aldehydes, 68, 71
algorithm, 204
alimentary canal, 48
alkaloids, 20
alkylation, 82
allele, 76, 81
allelic loss, 99
alpha-fetoprotein, 30, 39, 40, 41, 42, 96, 173, 224
ALT, 33
alternative treatments, 212
alters, 68, 90
amino, 14, 32, 62, 80, 131, 144, 225, 230, 236
amino acid, 14, 32, 62, 80, 144, 225, 230, 236
amino acids, 14, 32, 62, 225, 230, 236
ampulla, 65
amyotrophic lateral sclerosis, 36
ancestors, 3
anchorage, 138, 141
androgen, 23, 45, 62, 90
aneuploid, 28

240 Index

angiogenesis, 20, 32, 34, 45, 62, 64, 75, 76, 82, 106, 117, 133, 139, 140, 146, 155
angiosarcoma, 54, 70
antibody, 4, 12, 73, 143
anti-cancer, 19, 25
anticancer drug, 111, 126
antigen, 4, 23, 30, 36, 54, 57, 116, 157
antioxidant, 2, 3, 4, 13, 18, 19, 27, 30, 33, 34, 35, 36, 37, 42, 46, 50, 68, 103, 106, 107, 108, 111, 119, 125, 126, 130, 131, 133, 134
antisense, 144
antitumor, 25, 47, 108, 111, 112, 126
APC, 58, 70, 76, 79, 87, 95
apigenin, 2, 19, 24, 25, 26, 46
apoptosis, 9, 19, 20, 23, 24, 26, 28, 29, 30, 31, 43, 44, 45, 46, 47, 48, 50, 51, 58, 59, 60, 62, 63, 64, 65, 66, 72, 73, 78, 81, 82, 85, 86, 87, 90, 91, 97, 99, 108, 109, 110, 111, 112, 114, 115, 116, 117, 127, 128, 131, 139, 141, 142, 143, 144, 147, 148, 150, 152, 159
appetite, 164, 166
apples, 14
arrest, 24, 26, 32, 44, 45, 62, 78, 81, 109, 111, 132, 143
arteries, 19
arteriography, 234
artery, 161, 166
aryl hydrocarbon receptor, 29, 48, 49, 129
ascites, 28, 108, 112
Asia, ix, 2, 56, 69, 104, 161, 173, 199, 221
Asian countries, 65
ASL, 54, 70, 71
aspartate, 30, 33
assessment, 161, 162, 163, 167, 169, 195, 203, 209, 219, 220, 221, 233
asthma, 25
atherosclerosis, 19, 27
atoms, 13, 232
ATP, 139, 151, 225, 227
attachment, 65, 157
Austria, 38
autoantibodies, 12
autoimmune diseases, 12
autosomal recessive, 70

**B**

B1 (AFB1), 5, 69, 80
background information, 86
bacteria, 32, 66, 68
bacterial fermentation, 225
bacterium, 67
base, 54, 78, 97, 141

BBB, 231
beef, 227
benchmarks, 221
beneficial effect, 28, 31, 126
benefits, 20, 25, 125, 166, 216
benign, 7, 41, 120, 123, 150, 157, 226
benzo(a)pyrene, 28, 34, 48, 51
beverages, 4, 14, 68, 111, 121, 123
Bible, 156
bile, 11, 53, 56, 65, 66, 70, 92, 163
bile acids, 66
bile duct, 11, 53, 56, 65, 66, 92, 163
biliary atresia, 207
biliary tract, 65
bilirubin, 30, 33, 165, 216
bioassay, 27, 28
bioavailability, 35, 43, 122, 123, 124, 125, 126, 134, 141
biochemistry, 37, 235
bioflavonoids, 46
bioinformatics, 111
biological activities, 107
biological fluids, 111, 133
biological processes, 138
biological responses, 45, 139
biologically active compounds, 19
biomarkers, 7, 40, 81, 122, 124, 134, 174
biomolecules, 3
biopsy, 234
birds, 3
black tea, 25, 27, 28, 46, 47, 48
bleeding, 105, 130
blood, 2, 6, 10, 56, 69, 121, 123, 133, 227
blood transfusion, 2
blood urea nitrogen, 123
blood vessels, 56
body image, 161, 163, 167
body weight, 26, 33, 116, 120
bone, 84, 152
bone marrow, 84
brain, 230, 231
brain tumor, 231
breakdown, 195, 200, 214, 217
breast cancer, 9, 27, 40, 45, 107, 131, 138, 231
breast carcinoma, 98
Bureau of Labor Statistics, 198

**C**

calcium, 57, 63, 64, 90, 91
Cambodia, 65
campaigns, 2
cancer cells, 24, 30, 34, 73, 104, 108, 114, 126, 128

## Index

cancer death, 53, 56, 71, 104, 223
cancer prevention, vii, 1, 21, 27, 35, 38, 46, 48, 106, 128, 130, 135
cancer progression, 31
candidates, 31, 105, 106, 117, 233
carbohydrate, 7, 226
carbon, 14, 50, 226, 236
carbon tetrachloride, 50
carcinoembryonic antigen, 1, 7, 30, 33, 40
carcinoembryonic antigen (CEA), 1, 7, 33
carcinogen, 2, 3, 5, 26, 29, 32, 59, 65, 66, 80, 88, 94, 106, 107, 113
carcinogenesis, 3, 4, 20, 25, 28, 31, 34, 37, 38, 45, 47, 48, 50, 51, 66, 70, 74, 78, 86, 92, 93, 97, 99, 100, 103, 106, 107, 116, 118, 125, 127, 129, 130, 131
carcinogenicity, 5, 68
carcinogens, 1, 3, 4, 20, 27, 65, 68, 100, 125
carcinoma, 29, 31, 32, 34, 38, 39, 40, 42, 49, 78, 86, 89, 93, 126, 129, 131, 133, 137, 159, 167, 169, 170, 174, 223, 233, 234
cardiovascular disease, 3, 13, 27, 43, 107
cardiovascular risk, 122
carotene, 127
carotenoids, 37, 43
cartilage, 152
case studies, 219
casein, 23
caspases, 20, 23, 26, 111
catabolism, 232
catalytic activity, 28, 33, 49
Caucasian population, 2
Caucasians, 6
causal relationship, 71
causation, 38, 92
CCA, 54, 65, 66
cDNA, 119, 151
cell culture, 26, 112, 130
cell cycle, 20, 24, 26, 28, 29, 32, 44, 45, 50, 59, 60, 64, 66, 78, 80, 81, 83, 88, 109, 110, 111, 112, 117, 132, 135, 149
cell death, 30, 90, 100, 111, 132
cell invasion, 27, 28, 33, 48, 81, 131, 132, 140
cell invasiveness, 29, 33
cell line, 20, 23, 24, 27, 29, 30, 31, 44, 60, 83, 88, 108, 129, 133, 138, 139, 141, 143, 149, 152, 153, 155, 156, 227
cell lines, 24, 27, 29, 30, 44, 60, 83, 108, 129, 139, 141, 143, 153, 155, 227
cell membranes, 227
cell metabolism, 64, 236
cell surface, 25, 139
cellular signaling pathway, 62, 67

cellulose, 225
central nervous system, 70
cervical cancer, 42
challenges, 104, 125
cheese, 4
chemical, 5, 12, 13, 27, 33, 59, 74, 94, 100, 106, 127, 128, 131
chemicals, 3, 32, 236
chemokines, 72
chemoprevention, 35, 47, 51, 103, 106, 116, 118, 125, 126, 127, 129, 130, 132
Chemoprevention, 1, 3, 37, 51, 103, 130, 133
chemopreventive agents, 2, 20, 31, 46, 119, 130
chemotherapeutic agent, 126, 132, 139
chemotherapy, 105, 138, 139, 155, 170
chicken, 227
childhood, 141, 156
children, 56, 162, 218
China, 3, 4, 65, 104, 173
chloroform, 226
cholangiocarcinoma, 41, 54, 61, 89, 91, 92, 101, 112, 133
cholangitis, 206, 207, 211
cholesterol, 23, 59, 112
choline, x, 73, 223, 226, 227, 228, 229, 230, 235
chromatography, 47, 133
chromosomal alterations, 57, 70
chromosomal instability, 94
chromosome, 64, 72, 79, 80, 81, 82, 88, 98, 99, 146, 150, 152, 158
chromosome 10, 98
chronic active hepatitis, 66, 156
chronic heavy alcohol use, 1
Chronic infection, 1
cigarette smoke, 20, 48, 70
cigarette smokers, 48
cigarette smoking, 6, 38
circulation, 8, 67
cirrhosis, 1, 4, 5, 6, 9, 37, 38, 39, 40, 41, 42, 61, 68, 69, 70, 72, 79, 81, 82, 86, 89, 99, 100, 106, 137, 138, 156, 157, 161, 170, 207, 210, 211, 219, 224, 233, 234
cirrhosis of the liver, 1
cities, 220
classes, 13, 19
classification, 14, 98, 150, 165, 166, 207
cleavage, 63, 142
climate, 69
clinical application, 236
clinical oncology, 168
clinical trials, 35, 107, 125, 127, 130, 162, 168, 169, 231
closure, 157

clothing, 94
clustering, 98
clusters, 169
CNS, 36, 70, 227
coding, 61
codon, 69, 80, 141
codon 249, 69, 80, 141
coffee, 32, 132
cognitive effort, 203
colitis, 74
collagen, 19, 68, 72
colon, 3, 8, 25, 27, 46, 50, 97, 107
colon cancer, 46, 107
colon carcinogenesis, 97
colonization, 67
color, iv, 19, 164
colorectal cancer, 10, 163, 233
communication, 235
community, 19, 128
competition, 230
complexity, 105, 137, 138
compliance, 124
complications, 69, 174, 213, 218, 219, 221
compounds, 2, 3, 4, 5, 12, 13, 19, 31, 33, 34, 35, 43, 46, 68, 111, 113, 125, 129, 132, 226, 227
computed tomography, ix, 173, 224
configuration, 19
conjugation, 70, 124
consent, 209
constipation, 164
constituents, 48
Constitution, 167
consumer price index, 198
consumption, 2, 27, 28, 48, 68, 71, 106, 107, 111, 122, 124, 135
contaminant, 69
contamination, 4
controversial, 209, 214
cooperation, 96, 156
copper, 70, 71
coronary heart disease, 13
correlation, 36, 58, 61, 84, 89, 107, 139, 223, 224
cost, 6, 7, 173, 195, 197, 199, 200, 201, 202, 203, 205, 206, 207, 208, 209, 210, 211, 212, 213, 214, 215, 216, 217, 218, 219, 220, 221, 223
cost effectiveness, 205, 213, 220, 221
coumarins, 14
CPI, 198, 210
creatine, 230
creatinine, 10, 123, 216
critical analysis, 39
cross-sectional study, 28
CT scan, 223, 225, 231

cultivation, 35
culture, 30, 67, 112, 139
culture medium, 30, 112
curative treatment, vii, 1
curcumin, 2, 20, 43
current limit, 104
cycling, 99, 235
cyclins, 20
cyclooxygenase, 23, 46, 54, 60, 64, 91, 104, 115, 130
Cydonia oblonga, 23
cysteine, 34
cytochrome, 23, 28, 31, 37, 48, 49, 51, 54, 68, 69, 92, 135
cytochrome p450, 23
cytokines, 1, 4, 11, 13, 20, 25, 67, 68, 72, 74, 86, 105, 132, 140
cytoplasm, 8, 20, 57, 58, 61, 76, 144, 145, 147, 148
cytoskeleton, 144, 147, 154
cytotoxicity, 30, 109, 111, 131, 135

## D

data analysis, 228
database, 197, 205
deacetylation, 34
deaths, 1, 2, 53, 104
deceased donor liver transplantation (DDLT), 195
decision-making process, 212, 214, 217
defects, 69, 88, 93
defence, 3
defense mechanisms, 11, 125
deficiency, 6, 8
deficit, 8
degradation, 58, 59, 60, 65, 66, 72, 76, 81, 83, 87, 118, 152, 223, 232
dementia, 150
deposition, 72
depression, 165, 166, 167
deregulation, 99
derivatives, 3, 5, 12, 111, 121
detectable, 121
detection, 7, 8, 9, 10, 11, 42, 117, 128, 133, 166, 173, 223, 224, 225, 228, 229, 234, 236
detoxification, 27
developed countries, 2, 4, 56, 203
developing countries, 2, 38, 104
diabetes, 6, 11, 38, 39
diacylglycerol, 229
diet, 12, 27, 31, 73, 113, 114, 115, 116, 121, 134, 170, 230, 236
dietary carcinogens, 103, 105
differential diagnosis, 41
diffusion, 224

digestion, 226
dimerization, 75
direct action, 85
direct cost, 208
direct costs, 208
disability, 203
disease progression, 143
diseases, 5, 11, 12, 25, 27, 31, 36, 47, 48, 53, 56, 93, 107, 174, 224
disintegrin, 142
disorder, 70, 165
dissociation, 144, 145, 147
distribution, 40, 123, 218
diversity, 144, 145
DNA, 3, 4, 5, 19, 20, 23, 24, 26, 31, 32, 34, 36, 43, 51, 54, 55, 57, 58, 59, 60, 61, 62, 63, 64, 66, 67, 68, 69, 70, 71, 73, 75, 78, 81, 82, 85, 86, 87, 88, 89, 92, 93, 96, 97, 99, 100, 109, 111, 127, 130, 134, 146, 231, 236
DNA damage, 3, 4, 19, 26, 34, 36, 51, 54, 60, 61, 64, 66, 70, 71, 78, 92, 97, 130
DNA lesions, 68, 127
DNA repair, 4, 54, 59, 66, 68, 69, 75, 78, 81, 82, 85, 86, 100
DNA strand breaks, 34, 70
doctors, 216
donors, 19, 196, 209, 215, 221
dosage, 213
dose-response relationship, 71
dosing, 123
down-regulation, 24, 26, 32, 33, 89, 159
drinking water, 4, 32, 116, 121, 123
drug abuse, 2
drug metabolism, 47
drug resistance, 113
drug therapy, 132
drugs, 3, 26, 213, 234
duodenum, 65
DWI, 224
dysplasia, 67, 231

## E

E-cadherin, 81, 99, 140, 141
economic activity, 212
economic evaluation, 219, 220, 221
economics, 195, 205, 209, 233
education, 165
egg, 227
electron, 31, 91
electron microscopy, 31
electrons, 18
ELISA, 10

e-mail, 53
emboli, 82, 165, 170
embolization, 165, 170
embryogenesis, 138, 152
emission, 223, 234
emotional well-being, 165
employees, 70
encoding, 58, 81, 99
encouragement, 126
endonuclease, 135
endothelial cells, 11, 76, 140
endothelium, 27
endotoxins, 20
end-stage liver disease (ESLD), 195
energy, 164, 225, 227
England, 207, 212, 218
enlargement, 158
environment, 35, 37, 162
environmental control, 70
environmental stress, 3, 23
environmental stresses, 23
enzymatic activity, 33
enzyme, 11, 27, 29, 31, 33, 68, 71, 81, 105, 120, 123, 130, 131, 226, 227, 229, 230
enzyme induction, 120, 131
enzymes, 3, 4, 5, 7, 13, 25, 27, 28, 29, 31, 33, 48, 49, 68, 92, 106, 107, 109, 111, 119, 121, 123, 124, 127, 128, 129, 130, 131, 133, 134, 230
epidemiology, 38, 56, 86, 93, 129
epidermis, 129
epigenetic alterations, 53, 56, 79, 83, 158
epigenetic modification, 60
epigenetic silencing, 81, 146
epithelial cells, 44, 46, 65, 81, 112
epithelium, 65, 66, 157
Epstein-Barr virus, 36, 62
erythrocytes, 120, 235
erythropoietin, 25
esophagus, 3, 25, 27, 132
ester, 26, 32, 37, 46, 51
estrogen, 25, 27, 74
ethanol, 68, 105, 234
ethers, 12
ethical issues, 196
ethics, 209
ethyl acetate, 34
etiology, 38, 103, 105
eukaryotic, 106, 144, 157
Europe, 2, 4, 105, 196, 197, 199, 200, 208
evidence, 4, 5, 10, 12, 20, 49, 51, 57, 67, 84, 101, 105, 107, 111, 113, 117, 118, 123, 126, 127, 137, 141, 155, 214, 215
exaggeration, 202

# Index

examinations, 209, 217
excision, 54, 55, 59, 78, 87, 97
excretion, 121, 122
exercise, 19
expenditures, 212, 213, 218
exposure, 1, 2, 5, 59, 69, 70, 71, 80, 83, 86, 94
external validity, 202
extracellular matrix, 72, 86
extracts, 42, 96, 131

## F

factories, 70
fairness, 216
false positive, x, 223
families, 209
family history, 6
family members, 26, 144, 145, 147
fasting, 124, 230
fat, 92, 226
fatty acids, 224, 226, 234
FDA, 7, 8
FDA approval, 7
feelings, 162, 166
female rat, 104, 120, 121, 123
fermentation, 27, 225
fetus, 7
fiber, 20, 144
fibers, 147, 225
fibroblast growth factor, 25
fibroblasts, 66, 227
fibrogenesis, 65, 94
fibrosarcoma, 29, 49
fibrosis, 61, 65, 66, 68, 71, 72, 78, 82, 86, 94, 100,
  106, 128, 129, 224
financial, 218
Finland, 3
fish, 5, 65
flavonoids, 3, 12, 14, 18, 19, 20, 26, 27, 34, 37, 43,
  46, 49
flowers, 19, 30, 50
fluorescence, 129
fluorine, 234, 236
food, 1, 44, 47, 69, 92, 103, 107, 112, 116, 122, 124,
  130, 134, 164, 227
food additives, 1
force, 106, 148
formation, 4, 26, 30, 33, 48, 58, 62, 64, 66, 68, 69,
  70, 71, 74, 78, 84, 94, 101, 107, 113, 115, 116,
  117, 131, 134, 140, 144, 145, 146, 148, 149, 155
foundations, 168
fragile site, 57
frameshift mutation, 80

France, 4, 198, 199, 200
free radicals, 3, 12, 18, 19, 20, 30, 78, 85
fruits, 14, 19, 20, 23, 25, 32, 35, 103, 107
fucosylated variant, 1, 7
fungal metabolite, 5
fungal toxins (aflatoxins), vii, 1
fungus, 69
fusion, 57

## G

gadolinium, 234
gallbladder, 65, 66, 163
gastrointestinal tract, 68, 224, 234
GDP, 144, 145, 146, 147, 198
gene expression, 4, 44, 46, 58, 61, 64, 83, 88, 90, 92,
  111, 113, 119, 128, 132, 150, 151, 159
gene promoter, 99
gene silencing, 96
generalizability, 200
genes, 19, 20, 23, 24, 25, 46, 57, 58, 60, 64, 66, 69,
  70, 75, 76, 79, 80, 81, 82, 83, 84, 95, 99, 106,
  120, 123, 130, 133, 138, 142, 153, 159
genetic alteration, 7, 79
genetic factors, 69
genetic information, 81
genetic mutations, 69, 79, 83
genetics, 236
genistein, 2, 13, 20, 24, 25, 45
genome, 57, 60, 61
genomic instability, 57, 59, 60, 61, 67, 70, 73
genomic stability, 24, 57, 67, 73
genomics, 131
genotype, 5, 60, 87, 89, 153
genus, 226
Georgia, 1
Germany, 199
ginseng, 34, 51
glioma, 130, 132
glucose, 223, 225, 230
glutamine, 41
glutathione, 23, 28, 30, 33, 54, 64, 70, 92, 100, 104,
  113, 115, 156
glycans, x, 174
glycine, 230
glycogen, 54, 58
glycolysis, 224
glycoproteins, 11, 41, 61
glycoside, 124
glycosylation, 174
grades, 214, 228, 236
grading, 229
grants, 86

# Index 245

green tea polyphenols, 2, 25, 44

gross domestic product, 197

growth, 1, 4, 9, 10, 11, 20, 23, 24, 25, 26, 28, 33, 34, 41, 42, 44, 47, 48, 49, 51, 54, 55, 57, 59, 60, 62, 63, 64, 66, 69, 72, 75, 76, 77, 78, 87, 88, 89, 92, 95, 96, 99, 107, 108, 110, 111, 112, 114, 129, 130, 132, 133, 137, 138, 139, 141, 142, 143, 147, 148, 149, 150, 151, 152, 153, 154, 155, 156, 157, 158, 159

growth arrest, 62, 63

growth factor, 1, 11, 20, 23, 25, 28, 34, 41, 42, 48, 49, 54, 55, 57, 59, 60, 63, 66, 72, 75, 76, 77, 78, 87, 88, 89, 92, 95, 96, 99, 108, 110, 111, 129, 130, 132, 137, 138, 139, 143, 149, 150, 151, 152, 153, 154, 155, 156, 157, 158

GTPases, 144, 145, 146, 147, 148, 152, 153

guanine, 58, 70, 82, 110, 112, 144, 145

guidelines, 40, 214, 220

## H

half-life, 121, 124

happiness, 162

HBV, 2, 4, 5, 6, 50, 54, 56, 57, 58, 59, 60, 61, 63, 67, 69, 75, 79, 82, 85, 86, 87, 88, 100, 145, 146, 147, 150, 226

HBV infection, 4, 5, 56, 59, 61, 69, 79

HCC, 1, 2, 4, 5, 6, 7, 8, 9, 10, 11, 12, 26, 30, 33, 34, 39, 54, 56, 57, 58, 59, 60, 61, 63, 64, 65, 66, 67, 69, 70, 71, 72, 73, 74, 75, 77, 78, 79, 80, 81, 82, 83, 84, 88, 95, 98, 103, 104, 105, 106, 111, 113, 116, 117, 125, 133, 137, 138, 139, 140, 141, 142, 143, 144, 145, 146, 147, 148, 149, 150, 154, 155, 163, 164, 167, 223, 224, 225, 226, 227, 228, 229, 230, 231, 232

HDAC, 34

head and neck cancer, 230

healing, 34, 72, 105

health, 20, 38, 93, 161, 162, 165, 166, 167, 168, 169, 170, 195, 203, 207, 209, 210, 211, 212, 214, 217, 220, 226, 233

health care, 161, 162, 168, 214

health insurance, 195

health locus of control, 165, 166

health status, 162, 167, 203

Health-related quality of life (HRQOL), ix, 161

heart attack, 19

heart disease, 47, 162

heart transplantation, 212, 218

heat shock protein, 115, 117

Helicobacter, 53, 56, 66, 67, 92

hemangioma, 226

heme, 23

heme oxygenase, 23

hemochromatosis, 6, 39, 54, 69, 71, 80, 93, 98

hemodialysis, 37

hepatic encephalopathy, 170

hepatic failure, 210, 211

hepatic fibrosis, 86

hepatic injury, 72

hepatic stellate cells, 68, 72, 76, 86

hepatitis, 1, 2, 4, 5, 6, 7, 9, 37, 38, 39, 42, 53, 54, 56, 57, 71, 72, 73, 75, 78, 81, 82, 84, 87, 88, 89, 90, 91, 92, 93, 94, 95, 97, 99, 100, 101, 103, 105, 125, 133, 137, 138, 145, 150, 151, 153, 154, 157, 161, 204, 211, 213, 220, 223, 226, 232, 234, 235

hepatitis a, 38, 72, 75, 81, 82, 99, 151

hepatocarcinogen, 113

hepatocarcinogenesis, 3, 4, 26, 28, 30, 31, 32, 33, 35, 36, 37, 48, 53, 56, 57, 59, 60, 61, 63, 64, 65, 66, 67, 69, 70, 71, 73, 74, 75, 76, 77, 78, 79, 80, 83, 84, 85, 86, 87, 88, 89, 91, 93, 94, 95, 97, 98, 101, 103, 113, 114, 115, 116, 117, 118, 119, 127, 128, 131, 132, 141, 143, 146, 150, 152, 154, 155, 156

hepatocellular cancer, 82, 97, 101, 126, 128, 133, 151

hepatocellular carcinoma, 1, 2, 26, 31, 32, 33, 35, 37, 38, 39, 40, 41, 42, 47, 48, 50, 51, 54, 56, 87, 89, 90, 93, 94, 95, 96, 97, 98, 99, 100, 101, 103, 104, 127, 128, 129, 130, 131, 132, 133, 134, 135, 150, 151, 152, 153, 154, 155, 156, 157, 158, 159, 163, 167, 168, 169, 170, 171, 173, 174, 233, 234, 235, 237

hepatocytes, 26, 30, 47, 50, 56, 58, 59, 60, 61, 63, 64, 67, 68, 71, 72, 73, 74, 75, 76, 77, 84, 85, 89, 118, 119, 133, 139, 140, 142, 143, 154, 156, 157, 234, 235

hepatoma, 11, 28, 42, 43, 48, 49, 51, 90, 94, 108, 111, 112, 114, 131, 132, 133, 135, 138, 144, 148, 152, 154, 155, 156

hepatomegaly, 146

hepatotoxicity, 3, 31, 123

heterogeneity, ix, 66, 137, 226

high-risk populations, vii, 2, 107, 125

Hispanic population, 2

histology, 120

histone, 34

histone deacetylase, 34

history, 39, 93, 106

HIV, 5, 36, 61, 134

HO-1, 23

homes, 213

Hong Kong, 137, 149

hormone, 13

hormones, 7

hospitalization, 6, 208, 209, 210, 212

host, 11, 61, 65, 113
hTERT, 42, 54, 57, 60
HTLV, 62
hub, 86
human genome, 57
human health, 3, 4, 13
human papilloma virus, 62
human subjects, 122, 123, 125
hybrid, 60, 120, 134
hydrogen, 19, 50
hydrogen peroxide, 50
hydrolysis, 144, 145, 146, 147, 235
hydroxyl, 12, 14, 19, 26
hydroxyl groups, 19
hyperlipidemia, 31, 50
hypermethylation, 75, 81, 82, 99, 100
hyperplasia, 3, 66, 71, 72, 86, 226
hypertension, 14
hypertrophy, 72
hypothyroidism, 11
hypoxia, 34, 76, 110, 111, 135, 146
hypoxia-inducible factor, 110, 111, 135, 146

# I

ICC, 61
ideal, 7, 10, 18, 117, 125
identification, vii, ix, 3, 5, 20, 37, 128, 134, 137
IFN, 23
IL-8, 23, 29, 49
image, 224, 231
images, 233
imaging modalities, ix, 173, 224, 225
immune response, 11, 66
immune system, 62, 63
immunity, 94, 130
immunoglobulin, 8
immunohistochemistry, 31, 116, 118
immunomodulation, 29
immunomodulatory, 7, 113, 114, 131
immunoreactivity, 119
immunosuppressive drugs, 213
immunosuppressive therapies, 209
immunotherapy, 12
impairments, 162
in vitro, 18, 29, 35, 45, 46, 47, 48, 49, 50, 104, 107, 108, 112, 129, 131, 133, 143, 144, 145, 147, 149, 151
in vivo, 26, 28, 29, 31, 33, 100, 104, 107, 112, 116, 119, 127, 131, 138, 141, 143, 144, 145, 146, 147, 149, 153, 227, 230, 234, 235, 236, 237

incidence, 1, 2, 5, 6, 32, 34, 35, 38, 39, 56, 60, 67, 73, 74, 83, 86, 103, 104, 107, 112, 115, 116, 128, 137, 138, 167
independence, 162
India, 1, 3
indirect measure, 203
individuals, 1, 5, 8, 56, 61, 63, 65, 66, 69, 70, 162, 174
inducer, 30, 147
induction, 3, 13, 24, 25, 26, 28, 44, 64, 68, 69, 71, 100, 108, 111, 116, 117, 119, 127, 129, 130, 131, 132, 133, 134, 144
industrial chemicals, 1
industrial emissions, 20
industry, 70
inequity, 216
infection, 1, 3, 4, 5, 37, 56, 61, 63, 64, 65, 66, 67, 69, 72, 85, 92, 138, 173, 220, 226, 232
inflammation, 3, 13, 20, 25, 32, 53, 54, 56, 61, 64, 65, 66, 67, 70, 71, 73, 74, 75, 76, 78, 84, 85, 86, 92, 93, 94, 97, 101, 103, 105, 106, 107, 117, 125, 126, 127, 129, 130, 132, 133, 138, 142
inflammatory cells, 66, 72, 74
inflammatory disease, 25, 130
inflammatory mediators, 73, 78, 105
inflammatory responses, 106, 118, 129
inflation, 206, 207
informed consent, 209
ingestion, viii, 34, 103, 132
ingredients, 3
inhibition, 2, 23, 26, 28, 31, 33, 34, 44, 46, 47, 49, 59, 62, 64, 65, 73, 75, 76, 101, 107, 111, 116, 117, 118, 127, 142, 143, 151, 154, 155, 156
inhibitor, 23, 26, 29, 32, 33, 34, 55, 60, 62, 72, 77, 80, 81, 83, 96, 100, 104, 110, 112, 117, 118, 143, 145, 148, 155
initiation, 20, 25, 33, 37, 73, 94, 105, 107, 116, 128, 134, 137, 144, 152, 157
injury, iv, 30, 33, 50, 65, 70, 71, 72, 84, 92, 107, 125, 142, 157, 158
insects, 3
institutions, 201, 217
insulin, 1, 25, 41, 54, 55, 65, 72, 76, 95, 99, 141, 150, 151, 153, 154, 155, 156, 157
insulin resistance, 55, 65
integration, 55, 57, 58, 67, 231
integrin, 27
integrins, 27
integrity, 227
interference, 111
interferon, 25, 38, 220
interferons, 213
interferon-$\gamma$, 25

## Index

internal validity, 202
intervention, 34, 117, 126, 166, 170, 202, 205, 207, 212
ionizing radiation, 126
iron, 6, 39, 46, 69, 70, 71, 93, 105
irradiation, 27
islands, 99
isoflavone, 44
isoflavonoids, 3, 13
isolation, 34
isomers, 232
isozymes, 25
Israel, 3, 88, 97
issues, 161, 163, 209, 216, 233
Italy, 3, 4, 6, 39, 198, 199, 200

### J

Japan, 2, 4, 6, 8, 37, 38, 40, 65, 95, 98, 196, 197, 198, 199, 200, 205, 206, 208, 209, 212, 215, 217, 220
jaundice, 161, 163, 164, 167
Jordan, 53

### K

kaempferol, 2, 19, 25, 46
karyotype, 80
keratinocyte, 23, 44
keratinocytes, 24, 44
kidney, 120, 130, 152, 156
kidneys, 70, 227
kinase activity, 228
kinetic model, 230, 235
kinetic parameters, 127
kinetics, 96, 224
Korea, 34, 65, 215

### L

labeling, 116
lactate dehydrogenase, 30, 110, 112
Laos, 65
Latin America, 2
laws, 216
LDL, 4, 13, 19, 114, 115, 121, 122
lead, 19, 20, 25, 58, 61, 66, 68, 69, 70, 71, 73, 76, 78, 79, 106, 127, 166
leakage, 30
lecithin, 228
legs, 164
lens, 1

lesions, 5, 28, 34, 36, 66, 73, 78, 93, 120, 150, 173, 224, 226, 228
leucine, 106
leukemia, 26, 49, 57, 66, 130
leukotrienes, 25
life cycle, 61
life expectancy, 104
life satisfaction, 162
lifetime, 106, 207
ligand, 29, 55, 76, 95, 141, 142
light, 3, 20, 27, 126, 148, 164
lignans, 12
lipid metabolism, 59, 62, 65
lipid peroxidation, 31, 43, 64, 68, 70, 71, 78, 93, 113, 114, 117, 127
lipids, 59, 226, 227
liquid chromatography, 124, 128, 134
liver cancer biomarker, 173
liver cells, 7, 29, 88, 90, 91, 93, 107, 139, 152
liver cirrhosis, 7, 8, 9, 10, 37, 38, 81, 105, 150, 156, 210, 211, 233
liver damage, 5, 78, 103
liver disease, 6, 8, 9, 12, 39, 40, 41, 48, 59, 61, 72, 84, 91, 92, 101, 103, 128, 129, 132, 158, 166, 169, 170, 195, 216, 217, 218, 236
liver enzymes, 120
liver failure, 71, 219
liver transplant, 103, 105, 149, 155, 195, 196, 197, 198, 199, 200, 203, 204, 205, 206, 207, 208, 210, 213, 214, 215, 216, 217, 218, 219, 220, 221, 233
liver transplantation, 103, 105, 149, 155, 195, 196, 197, 198, 199, 200, 203, 204, 205, 206, 207, 208, 210, 213, 214, 215, 216, 217, 218, 219, 220, 221
lobectomy, 207
localization, 32, 60, 87, 118, 126, 145, 147, 148, 154, 159
loci, 60, 83
locus, 76, 80, 81, 82, 167
longitudinal study, 169
loss of appetite, 166
low-density lipoprotein, 115, 134
lung cancer, 47, 50, 153, 169, 231
lung metastases, 146
Luo, 94, 131, 156, 170
lutein, 20
luteolin, 2, 25, 26, 47, 49
lycopene, 20
lymphocytes, 43
lymphoma, 236

### M

machinery, 20, 57, 81

248 Index

macrophages, 24, 46, 68, 74, 78
magnetic resonance, ix, 173, 174
magnetic resonance imaging, ix, 173, 174
magnetic resonance spectroscopy, 174
magnitude, 5
major issues, 196
majority, 41, 68, 69, 103, 105, 198, 199, 213
malignancy, 3, 56, 71, 73, 83, 84, 85, 104, 105, 112, 137, 138, 224, 233
malignant cells, 8, 84
malignant growth, 156
malignant tumors, 231, 236
management, 105, 133, 137, 138, 170, 213, 221
MAPK/ERK, 63, 90
mass, 71, 74, 124, 133, 134, 174, 233
mass spectrometry, 124, 134, 174
Mass spectrometry (MS), x, 174
mast cells, 31
materials, 3, 71, 225
matrix, 20, 23, 27, 29, 32, 34, 35, 47, 49, 50, 51, 55, 72, 76, 91, 104, 110, 111, 135, 139, 152, 158
matrix metalloproteinase, 29, 32, 34, 49, 50, 51, 55, 76, 91, 104, 110, 111, 135, 139, 158
matter, iv
measurement, 7, 40, 161, 163, 168, 203, 221, 236
measurements, 40, 163, 168, 224
median, 199, 204, 206, 210, 211
mediastinum, 236
medical, 6, 7, 162, 165, 166, 195, 197, 200, 203, 205, 206, 207, 209, 210, 211, 212, 214, 216, 217, 219, 233
Medicare, 201, 202, 203, 218
medication, 209
medicine, 3, 108, 234
MEK, 23, 24, 47, 58, 60, 111
melanoma, 26, 135
membranes, 147
mental health, 168
meta-analysis, 66
Metabolic, 229, 235
metabolic disorder, 72
metabolic disorders, 72
metabolic pathways, 59, 227, 228
metabolism, 3, 25, 26, 29, 36, 46, 65, 68, 69, 70, 120, 123, 125, 134, 224, 230, 233, 234, 235, 236
metabolites, 68, 85, 121, 122, 124, 126, 128, 134, 135, 227
metabolized, 68, 69, 70, 71, 227, 232
metabolizing, 3, 27, 28, 48, 71, 106, 121, 124, 128, 130
metalloproteinase, 34, 55, 72, 91, 104, 110, 112
metals, 37, 71

metastasis, 20, 25, 26, 33, 49, 51, 62, 81, 106, 112, 114, 117, 137, 138, 140, 142, 143, 144, 145, 146, 149, 150, 151, 152, 154, 155, 158, 159, 233
methodology, 200
methyl group, 227, 229, 230
methyl groups, 227, 229
methylation, 69, 75, 81, 82, 83, 96, 99, 100, 228, 230, 236
mice, 25, 27, 29, 30, 33, 34, 36, 38, 48, 49, 50, 51, 66, 67, 73, 74, 88, 91, 92, 94, 97, 101, 113, 114, 120, 123, 128, 130, 131, 132, 133, 134, 139, 141, 143, 146, 150, 151, 156, 157, 158, 159
micronucleus, 70
micronutrients, 20
microRNA, 55, 79, 101, 145
microsomes, 29
microspheres, 105, 165, 169
migration, 33, 75, 76, 82, 83, 95, 143, 145, 146, 152, 153, 155
mitochondria, 63, 64, 68, 225
mitogen, 23, 26, 44, 55, 58, 104, 110, 112, 139, 154
mitogens, 25, 66, 67, 72, 74, 77
mitosis, 29, 59, 64, 108, 113
MMP, 20, 23, 29, 31, 32, 34, 55, 83, 104, 109, 110, 112, 139, 140, 141, 145, 155, 156
MMP-2, 29, 31, 32, 33, 34, 83, 110, 112, 145, 155
MMP-9, 23, 29, 31, 32, 34, 109, 112, 145
MMPs, 76
model system, 114
models, 2, 3, 27, 30, 34, 57, 78, 104, 107, 112, 113, 125, 126, 131, 142, 145, 225, 227, 228
modifications, 4, 37, 51, 174
molecular medicine, 234
molecular oxygen, 68
molecular structure, 155
molecules, 20, 23, 60, 72, 74, 137, 143, 151, 231
monoclonal antibody, 139
Moon, 51, 88, 143, 154, 155
morbidity, ix, 105, 173, 219
morphogenesis, 76, 140
morphology, 71, 77, 153, 225
mortality, 2, 6, 71, 86, 93, 105, 138, 219
mosaic, 146
motif, 20, 55, 58, 87, 145
MRI, 173, 224, 233, 234
mRNA, 10, 29, 49, 61, 67, 82, 83, 96, 117, 138, 144, 150, 151, 152
mucosa, 46
mucus, 225
multiplication, 90
mutagenesis, 2, 68, 69, 79
mutant, 61, 96, 141, 143, 154
mutation, 61, 68, 69, 70, 79, 93, 98, 99, 100, 138

Index 249

mutations, 32, 59, 60, 64, 69, 70, 71, 76, 77, 78, 79, 80, 81, 83, 85, 93, 96, 97, 98, 99, 138, 141, 147, 156
mycotoxins, 38
myeloid cells, 26
myocardium, 225, 226, 227, 234
myofibroblasts, 29, 49, 140, 152, 155
myosin, 148

## N

nasopharyngeal carcinoma, 170
National Health Service, 207, 218
natural compound, 3, 13
natural killer cell, 90
nausea, 161, 163, 165, 167
neck cancer, 231
necrosis, 45, 74, 94, 132, 133
neolignans, 13
neoplasm, 120, 123, 224
neoplastic tissue, 69
nephropathy, 120, 123
Netherlands, 198, 199, 200, 205, 206, 212, 219, 220, 221
neurodegenerative diseases, 3, 107, 127, 138
neurological disease, 27
neurotransmission, 227
neutral, 227
neutral lipids, 227
neutrophils, 72, 78
New England, 40
New Zealand, 2, 120
NH2, 33, 41, 55, 58, 149, 151
nicotinamide, 110
nitric oxide, 23, 46, 54, 55, 64, 75, 91, 92, 104, 106, 110, 111, 115, 126, 130, 133, 135
nitric oxide synthase, 23, 46, 54, 64, 91, 92, 104, 106, 110, 111, 115, 126, 130, 133, 135
nitrogen, 55, 66, 71
nitrosamines, viii, 51, 68, 92, 103, 105, 106, 127
nitroso compounds, 66
N-N, 4, 128
nodules, 9, 31, 41, 70, 72, 77, 78, 86, 96, 99, 116, 137, 224, 225, 231
non-polar, 226
non-steroidal anti-inflammatory drugs, 36
North America, 2, 40, 105, 199
Norway, 198, 199
Nrf2, 23, 104, 106, 115, 117, 118, 119, 129, 130, 131, 132, 133
nuclei, 71
nucleus, 14, 16, 19, 20, 57, 58, 75, 76, 117, 118, 140, 147, 148

null, 82
nutraceutical, 19
nutrient, 227
nutrients, 3
nutrition, 3, 13, 20, 36, 164
nutritional status, 10

## O

obesity, 61, 105
oil, 20, 43
omission, 86, 202
oncogenes, 79, 80, 97
oncogenesis, 87, 154
oncoproteins, 23
operations, 200
oral cavity, 3, 27
organ, 2, 3, 68, 72, 74, 76, 85, 105, 121, 123, 209, 212, 213, 215, 216, 218, 220
organs, x, 34, 51, 69, 106, 107, 147, 195, 213
ovarian cancer, 9, 51, 139
overhead costs, 202
overlay, 228, 231
oxidation, 3, 4, 13, 19, 68, 225
oxidation products, 4
oxidative damage, 27, 69
oxidative stress, 4, 13, 19, 25, 26, 28, 37, 43, 47, 48, 50, 60, 61, 63, 64, 65, 67, 68, 69, 70, 71, 73, 88, 90, 94, 95, 103, 107, 109, 117, 119, 123, 127, 131, 132, 133, 134
oxygen, 4, 19, 47

## P

pain, 161, 162, 163, 164, 165, 166, 167
pancreas, 3, 25, 27
pancreatic cancer, 163
pancreatitis, 11
parallel, 94, 152
parameter estimation, 224
parasite, 65
parasitic infection, 71
parenchyma, 232
parenchymal cell, 69, 72, 73, 94, 95
participants, 71, 207, 209, 210, 211
pathogenesis, 31, 38, 88, 93, 137
pathology, 50, 137
pathophysiology, 93
pathways, 14, 19, 23, 26, 44, 45, 64, 66, 67, 72, 75, 76, 77, 78, 81, 84, 87, 91, 95, 98, 106, 112, 117, 125, 126, 132, 137, 139, 140, 141, 142, 149, 228, 231

PCR, 32
peptide, 33
peptides, 33
percentile, 211
peritonitis, 39
permeability, 68
permission, 116, 118, 119, 225, 233
peroxidation, 4, 46, 93
peroxide, 113
peroxynitrite, 66
PET, 173, 223, 224, 225, 227, 228, 229, 230, 231, 232, 233, 234, 235, 236, 237
PET scan, 223, 226, 228, 233
PGE, 23
pharmaceuticals, 213
pharmacokinetics, 124, 125
phenol, 13
phenolic compounds, 43
phenotype, 72, 79, 84, 96, 97, 111, 128, 139, 141, 150, 151, 153
phenotypes, 151
phenylalanine, 14
phosphate, 95, 99, 110
phosphatidylcholine, 227, 229
phospholipids, 25
phosphorylation, 24, 26, 33, 44, 45, 49, 58, 59, 64, 75, 76, 79, 82, 83, 140, 143, 147, 149, 151
physical fitness, 162
physical health, 162, 166
physical well-being, 162, 164, 165
physiology, 224, 235
pilot study, 221
plant polyphenols, 2, 4, 21, 22
plants, 2, 3, 12, 13, 14, 19, 35, 36
plaque, 19
plasma levels, 122, 123, 124, 132
plasma membrane, 9, 144, 145
plasma proteins, 122
plasminogen, 76
plastics, 70
platelet aggregation, 4, 13, 14
platelet count, 38
playing, 144
point mutation, 80
polarity, 144, 146
policy, 197, 221
policy makers, 197
pollination, 3
polyamine, 230
polychlorinated biphenyl, 113, 115
polymerase, 32, 57, 63, 83
polymerase chain reaction, 32
polymerization, 27

polymorphism, 75, 95, 124
polymorphisms, 95
polypeptide, 10
polyphenols, 2, 3, 12, 14, 18, 20, 21, 22, 23, 24, 25, 27, 28, 30, 31, 34, 43, 44, 45, 46, 47, 48, 50, 51, 129, 133
polyvinyl chloride, 70, 93
population, 2, 6, 28, 31, 39, 57, 70, 72, 83, 106, 112, 119, 140, 161, 162, 163, 164, 165, 169, 173, 204, 212, 221
population growth, 31
portal vein, 82
positive correlation, 165
positron, ix, 173, 230, 234, 235, 236, 237
positron emission tomography, 173, 234, 235, 236, 237
post-transplant, 198, 199, 204, 205, 206, 207, 208, 213, 217
potential benefits, 13
premature death, 69
preparation, 236
preservation, 209, 219
prevention, 1, 2, 3, 20, 21, 22, 23, 27, 30, 32, 34, 35, 36, 38, 39, 43, 46, 48, 53, 56, 93, 103, 106, 107, 119, 123, 125, 126, 127, 128, 130, 134, 135
primary biliary cirrhosis, 6, 39, 206, 207, 210, 211
primary cells, 57
Primary liver cancer, 1, 2, 56, 103, 128, 233
primary tumor, 152
progenitor cells, 84, 101
prognosis, 6, 7, 8, 80, 84, 97, 100, 103, 104, 125, 137, 138, 143, 144, 145, 151, 153, 154, 157, 161, 224, 234
pro-inflammatory, 67, 68, 72
proliferation, 3, 9, 10, 19, 20, 23, 24, 25, 26, 29, 30, 31, 44, 45, 47, 48, 57, 58, 59, 60, 61, 62, 66, 67, 73, 74, 75, 76, 77, 79, 81, 82, 83, 84, 85, 86, 88, 90, 91, 94, 97, 106, 108, 109, 110, 111, 114, 115, 116, 117, 127, 129, 131, 135, 138, 140, 141, 143, 144, 153, 155, 156, 158, 223, 231, 232, 235, 237
proline, 55, 58, 87
promoter, 4, 29, 46, 54, 60, 62, 63, 64, 74, 81, 82, 83, 89, 91, 92, 94, 99, 100, 140, 141, 152
propagation, 106
prostaglandins, 25, 105
prostate cancer, 24, 45, 229, 235
prostate carcinoma, 29, 44, 45, 46, 49
protease inhibitors, 59
protection, 4, 13, 26, 27, 132, 134, 135
protective role, 12, 28
protein family, 62
protein kinase C, 23, 55, 58, 142
protein kinases, 20, 144

protein oxidation, 4, 117, 120
protein synthesis, 19, 92, 170, 230, 236
proteinase, 33
proteins, 5, 20, 24, 25, 31, 32, 57, 58, 60, 61, 63, 64, 66, 67, 68, 72, 76, 77, 85, 89, 91, 95, 113, 131, 135, 139, 144, 147, 150, 158, 174, 230
prothrombin, vii, 1, 7, 8, 40, 216
proto-oncogene, 43, 80, 139, 150, 157
prototype, 226
psychological variables, 163, 166
psychological well-being, 166
psychology, 220
psychometric properties, 168
psychosocial factors, 166
psychosocial functioning, ix, 161, 162
psychosocial interventions, 166
PTEN, 32, 80, 83, 99, 101
public health, 137, 138
purchasing power, 197
purchasing power parity, 197
purification, 155
purines, 34, 51
purity, 134
PVC, 70

## Q

quality improvement, 218
quality of life, 161, 162, 167, 168, 169, 170, 203, 209, 220, 221
quantification, 134, 224
quaternary ammonium, 229
quercetin, 2, 3, 19, 20, 23, 25, 26, 29, 33, 34, 36, 37, 44, 47, 49, 132, 133
questionnaire, 163, 169, 204, 207

## R

Rab, 110
race, 7, 219
radiation, 20, 45, 166, 170
radiation therapy, 166, 170
radical formation, 4, 13, 78
radicals, 18, 33, 37, 85
radio, 20, 228
RANTES, 55, 72
RB1, 55, 80, 81
reactions, 230
reactive oxygen, 4, 5, 28, 30, 36, 43, 47, 55, 60, 66, 71, 91, 104, 106, 110, 132, 133, 156
reading, 55, 57, 126, 195
reality, 214

receptors, 25, 61, 63, 77, 90, 95, 96, 151, 155
recognition, 6, 40
recombination, 60
recommendations, iv, 196
recovery, 124, 166
recruiting, 60, 72
recurrence, 6, 105, 125, 137, 138, 143, 149, 155, 165, 166, 213, 224
red wine, 14, 49, 103, 107, 123, 124, 131, 132, 134
regenerate, 72
regeneration, 68, 72, 73, 75, 76, 77, 78, 79, 84, 86, 94, 96, 97, 142, 150, 153, 155, 158
regions of the world, 86, 124
registries, 2
Registry, 217
regression, 51, 113
regulations, 154
rehabilitation, 208
rejection, 213, 215
relatives, 14, 39
relaxation, 166
relevance, 101, 104, 138
reliability, 7
repair, 54, 55, 59, 72, 78, 82, 83, 87, 92, 97
replication, 4, 57, 58, 61, 82
repression, 87, 89, 90
repressor, 138
requirements, 225
researchers, 60, 111, 124, 201, 203, 214, 217
resection, 105, 138, 165, 166, 169
residues, 139, 147, 148
resistance, 20, 77, 96, 139, 143, 150, 151, 157
resolution, 99, 224, 234
resource allocation, 196, 205, 216, 217, 220
resource utilization, 218, 219
resources, 205, 209, 212
respiration, 68
response, 24, 35, 58, 59, 66, 72, 73, 75, 78, 79, 83, 85, 105, 106, 112, 127, 130, 131, 132, 139, 152, 155, 232
resveratrol, 20, 23, 24, 25, 27, 28, 29, 46, 47, 48, 49, 103, 107, 108, 109, 111, 112, 113, 114, 116, 117, 118, 119, 120, 121, 122, 123, 124, 125, 126, 127, 128, 129, 130, 131, 132, 133, 134, 135
reticulum, 54, 60, 88
retinoblastoma, 55, 60, 81, 98
reverse transcriptase, 42, 54, 57, 88, 119
ribonucleotide reductase, 49
ribose, 63
risk, 2, 3, 4, 5, 6, 7, 13, 14, 27, 34, 37, 38, 39, 48, 53, 56, 57, 60, 61, 65, 67, 69, 70, 71, 73, 75, 78, 79, 82, 85, 87, 91, 92, 93, 105, 107, 117, 125, 131, 133, 134, 138, 173, 224, 235

## 252 Index

risk assessment, 134, 235
risk factors, 4, 5, 6, 53, 56, 57, 67, 82, 85, 91, 92, 93, 105, 133, 138
risks, 161
RNA, 49, 57, 61, 64, 83, 119, 230
RNAi, 143, 146
rodents, 5, 112, 113, 119, 123
routes, 231
rural population, 5

## S

safety, 121, 123, 124, 125, 126, 127, 196, 209, 213, 227
saturated fat, 226
Saudi Arabia, 1
Scandinavia, 3
scar tissue, 72
scarcity, 217
scatter, 152, 156
scattering, 28, 108, 140, 141, 156
scope, 125, 198, 200, 201, 202, 203, 217
secrete, 65, 67, 70, 72, 76, 86
secretion, 29, 65, 72, 77, 140, 143, 146, 152
seed, 3, 35
segregation, 88
selectivity, 230
self-assessment, 168
senescence, 30, 50
sensing, 36, 42
sensitivity, 7, 8, 9, 10, 11, 113, 152, 210, 211, 224
serine, 24, 45, 58, 59, 87, 147, 148, 149
serum, 5, 7, 8, 9, 10, 11, 23, 28, 35, 38, 40, 41, 42, 57, 82, 100, 108, 113, 114, 121, 122, 123, 139, 140, 155, 156, 157, 165, 173, 216, 224
serum cholinesterase, 165
services, 165, 166
sex, 2, 4, 5, 13, 61, 94, 132, 133, 138
sex differences, 94, 132
sex ratio, 2
sheep, 94
short supply, 215
shortage, 105, 218
showing, 9, 74, 231
side effects, 105, 166
signal transduction, 19, 24, 29, 44, 62, 87, 91, 139, 140, 149
signaling pathway, 4, 20, 24, 25, 27, 35, 44, 45, 58, 60, 62, 63, 64, 66, 72, 76, 77, 82, 85, 90, 91, 105, 111, 117, 125, 130, 137, 140, 141, 142, 143, 144, 145, 149, 151, 154
signalling, 13, 150, 153
signals, 20, 26, 227

signs, 146
silver, 30
Singapore, 99
sister chromatid exchange, 70
skeleton, 13
skin, 3, 25, 27, 45, 65, 164
Slovakia, 173
small intestine, 3, 27
smoking, 38
social acceptance, 209, 220
social life, 162
social relations, 162
social relationships, 162
sodium, 224
solution, 138, 224
solvents, 226
somatic alterations, 97
South Korea, 215
Southeast Asia, 4
soybeans, 19
Spain, 3, 37
species, 4, 5, 28, 30, 36, 47, 55, 60, 65, 66, 71, 91, 92, 104, 106, 107, 110, 113, 122, 132, 133, 156, 234
spectroscopy, 174, 224
spin, 234
spindle, 64, 91
spleen, 8
Sprague-Dawley rats, 114, 116, 118
squamous cell, 135
squamous cell carcinoma, 135
stability, 2, 58, 79
stabilization, 64, 90, 213
starch, 225
starvation, 60, 88
state, 35, 72, 98, 106, 146, 162, 203, 216, 220, 227
states, 83, 144, 145, 207
statistics, 167
stem cells, 53, 56, 83, 84, 101, 139, 155
stigma, 166
stimulus, 72
stomach, 3, 13, 25, 27, 164, 166
storage, 69, 72, 93
stress, 4, 24, 28, 55, 58, 60, 61, 64, 70, 71, 83, 88, 91, 93, 103, 106, 117, 119, 127, 129, 130, 144, 147, 170
stroke, 19
structural protein, 67, 90
structure, 2, 12, 14, 18, 36, 46, 108, 155, 229, 235
subgroups, 163
sub-Saharan Africa, 56, 69, 105, 161
substitution, 60, 80
substrate, 63, 64, 141, 226, 230, 234, 235

# Index

substrates, 26, 76, 229

sulfate, 9, 41, 121, 122, 123, 124, 125

sulfuric acid, 26

Sun, 28, 42, 43, 48, 88, 91, 98, 100, 109, 111, 133, 135, 154, 169, 235, 236

supplementation, 31, 32, 123, 125, 163

suppression, 32, 33, 45, 78, 87, 89, 106, 107, 116, 138, 143, 154, 158

surgical resection, 103, 105

surgical technique, 209

surveillance, 7, 8, 9, 223

Surveillance, Epidemiology, and End Results (SEER), 53

survival, 1, 2, 7, 24, 45, 53, 56, 57, 60, 63, 72, 73, 75, 76, 77, 81, 82, 88, 90, 98, 106, 112, 139, 140, 141, 142, 155, 157, 158, 161, 162, 167, 168, 169, 171, 174, 195, 197, 203, 205, 208, 210, 211, 212, 216, 219, 220, 223

survival rate, 2, 53, 56, 161, 162, 167, 174, 197, 203, 205, 210, 211, 212, 223

survivors, 212, 220

susceptibility, 68, 71, 74, 106, 131, 155

swelling, 164, 166

Switzerland, 198, 199, 205, 206

symptoms, 162, 164, 165, 166, 167

syndrome, 69

synergistic effect, 5, 69, 111, 143

synthesis, 2, 4, 13, 28, 65, 68, 111, 134, 225, 226, 228, 230, 231, 235, 236

Syria, 37

## T

T cell, 72

Taiwan, 71, 93, 215

tannins, 13, 15

target, 2, 12, 20, 23, 32, 34, 46, 55, 60, 62, 75, 76, 82, 83, 101, 107, 111, 117, 118, 125, 132, 138, 148, 153, 154, 158

target organs, 107

tau, 150

TBP, 58

techniques, 7, 69

technologies, 212, 214

technology, 203, 212, 213, 214, 215, 217, 219, 220, 233

telephone, 53

telomere, 72, 78, 94

telomere shortening, 72, 94

terpenes, 20

testing, 10, 213

tetrachlorodibenzo-p-dioxin, 29

TGF, 10, 25, 26, 41, 55, 59, 62, 64, 67, 72, 84, 87, 89, 96, 101, 128, 142, 143, 154

Thailand, 65, 92

therapeutic agents, 111, 125, 128

therapeutic approaches, 103

therapeutic effects, 36, 117

therapeutic targets, 12, 98, 150

therapeutics, 231

therapy, 3, 7, 20, 22, 23, 35, 36, 38, 42, 79, 103, 105, 113, 123, 125, 126, 133, 138, 161, 165, 170, 195, 196, 197, 213

threonine, 24, 45, 148, 149

thrombin, 33

thymine, 232, 237

thymoma, 54, 60

time periods, 206

TIMP, 34, 55, 72, 100, 104, 110, 112

TIMP-1, 72, 110, 112

tissue, 6, 9, 10, 11, 34, 55, 58, 59, 66, 69, 70, 72, 73, 76, 81, 82, 89, 100, 104, 110, 112, 113, 116, 138, 156, 230

TLR, 55, 74

TNF, 20, 23, 24, 25, 43, 45, 90, 104, 111, 117

TNF-alpha, 90

TNF-$\alpha$, 104, 111, 117

tobacco, 4, 68, 92

tobacco smoke, 4, 68

tocopherols, 18

total costs, 199, 207

toxic industrial chemicals, 1

toxicity, 5, 31, 47, 49, 104, 113, 119, 120, 121, 123, 129, 227, 236

toxin, 67, 69

Toyota, 40, 99

TP53, 80

TPA, 23

trade, 203, 207

trade-off, 203, 207

trafficking, 144

trajectory, 166

transcatheter, 105, 161, 165, 166, 169, 170

transcription, 19, 20, 24, 29, 32, 43, 44, 45, 46, 49, 54, 55, 57, 58, 59, 62, 63, 64, 67, 73, 74, 75, 76, 81, 87, 90, 92, 106, 119, 129, 131, 133, 138, 139, 140, 152, 153, 156, 158

transcription factors, 19, 20, 24, 43, 58, 63, 64, 67, 74, 76, 106, 138, 158

transcripts, 83

transducer, 55, 58, 139

transfection, 88

transformation, 12, 20, 23, 29, 30, 44, 45, 57, 60, 61, 62, 63, 64, 66, 70, 71, 73, 75, 77, 78, 80, 84, 113, 146, 154, 230

# Index

transforming growth factor, 25, 47, 55, 87, 88, 91, 96, 142, 151, 154, 156, 158

transition metal, 70, 71, 85

translation, 57, 61, 83

translocation, 20, 63, 88, 117, 118, 159, 235

transmission, 32

transmission electron microscopy, 32

transparency, 201, 217

transplant, 213, 216, 217, 219, 221

transplantation, 105, 149, 195, 196, 197, 198, 199, 200, 203, 204, 205, 206, 207, 208, 209, 212, 213, 214, 216, 217, 218, 219, 220, 221

transport, 70, 91, 92, 112, 135, 228, 229, 230, 231, 235

transportation, 216

transthoracic echocardiography, 117

treatment, 1, 7, 26, 27, 30, 31, 33, 35, 36, 40, 46, 53, 56, 73, 74, 93, 103, 105, 106, 107, 111, 112, 113, 114, 116, 125, 126, 127, 128, 138, 139, 140, 143, 149, 156, 161, 163, 165, 166, 167, 173, 197, 200, 206, 207, 208, 209, 212, 215, 217, 219, 왬220, 223, 224, 232, 233

trial, 34, 39, 165, 209, 228

tricarboxylic acid, 225

triggers, 74, 91, 97

triglycerides, 114

tuberculosis, 2

tumor, 1, 3, 6, 7, 8, 9, 10, 11, 12, 19, 20, 23, 24, 25, 27, 28, 29, 30, 32, 33, 40, 41, 42, 43, 44, 45, 46, 49, 50, 55, 59, 60, 62, 63, 66, 67, 69, 71, 73, 76, 77, 78, 79, 80, 81, 82, 83, 84, 87, 88, 89, 90, 94, 97, 98, 100, 101, 104, 106, 107, 111, 112, 114, 125, 131, 132, 134, 135, 138, 140, 141, 143, 144, 146, 148, 150, 151, 152, 153, 154, 155, 156, 157, 158, 159, 174, 223, 225, 227, 230, 231, 235, 236

tumor cells, 8, 76, 84, 107, 113, 141, 152, 153, 155, 158, 227, 235

tumor development, 139

tumor growth, 19, 76, 88, 100, 113, 114, 125, 142, 154

tumor invasion, 148, 158

tumor metastasis, 157

tumor necrosis factor, 20, 23, 25, 43, 44, 45, 46, 55, 62, 63, 90, 94, 104, 111, 135

tumor progression, 62, 73, 78, 81, 156

tumorigenesis, 2, 3, 10, 24, 36, 43, 57, 58, 60, 67, 69, 71, 72, 75, 78, 83, 94, 116, 138, 144, 155, 157, 231

tumors, 4, 14, 30, 34, 74, 79, 81, 82, 83, 84, 97, 100, 105, 106, 107, 113, 126, 139, 140, 150, 167, 226, 231, 236

tumour growth, 48, 128

tumours, 98, 150

turnover, 72, 87, 92

tyrosine, 14, 26, 49, 55, 58, 75, 76, 77, 84, 130, 139, 142, 152, 153

## U

UK, 36, 43, 134, 161, 198, 199, 200, 206, 214, 215, 216

ultrasonography, 7, 173

ultrasound, 224, 231, 233, 234

UN, 202

underlying mechanisms, 109, 147

unit cost, 201, 202, 203

United, 4, 6, 35, 38, 39, 53, 56, 67, 105, 129, 217

United States, 4, 6, 35, 38, 39, 53, 56, 67, 105, 129

urban, 5

urine, 6, 10, 121, 122, 123, 124, 128, 130, 133, 135

urokinase, 28, 76

USA, 1, 3, 35, 36, 41, 43, 53, 103, 126, 198, 200, 206

UV, 3, 20, 23, 54, 59

UV irradiation, 3

UV radiation, 23

## V

validation, 11, 168

valuation, 39

vanadium, 127, 128

variables, 163, 166, 167, 210

variations, 138, 199, 202, 229

varieties, 42

vascular endothelial growth factor (VEGF), 20, 139

VCAM, 26

vector, 29

vegetables, 14, 19, 20, 25, 35, 103, 107

VEGF expression, 62, 135, 140

very low density lipoprotein, 65

Vietnam, 65

vinyl chloride, 55, 71, 80, 94

viral infection, 38, 58, 61, 74, 85, 87, 94, 100, 103, 107, 125, 223

virology, 56, 57, 61

virus infection, 37, 38, 56, 91, 95, 100, 234

virus replication, 157

viruses, 1, 20, 38, 53, 56, 62, 67, 71, 89

vitamin A, 72

vitamin C, 14, 19, 43

Vitamin C, 20

vitamin E, 43

vitamin K, 8, 40, 42

vitamins, 20

VLDL, 65, 114, 115

## W

Wales, 207, 212, 218
Washington, 37, 53, 95, 98, 134, 216
water, 1, 4, 27, 65, 226, 227
WD, 55, 70
wealth, 125
weight loss, 161, 163, 167
well-being, 162, 164, 165, 166, 167
West Africa, 38
western blot, 31
Western countries, 196
white blood corpuscle, 121
WHO, 5, 93, 167, 168, 173
wild type, 61
Wnt signaling, 77

workers, 70, 93, 124
World Health Organization, 53, 163, 167, 168
World Health Organization (WHO), 53
World War I, 2
worldwide, 1, 2, 5, 27, 53, 56, 104, 128, 137, 161, 223
worms, 65
wound healing, 140

## X

xenografts, 33, 113

## Y

yield, 125